Heart Disease and Diabetes

Edited by

Miles Fisher

Consultant Physician
Glasgow Royal Infirmary
Glasgow
UK

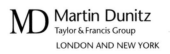

Martin Dunitz
Taylor & Francis Group

LONDON AND NEW YORK

First published in the United Kingdom in 2003
by Martin Dunitz, the Taylor & Francis Group plc, 11 New Fetter Lane,
London EC4P 4EE

Tel.: +44 (0) 20 7583 9855
Fax.: +44 (0) 20 7842 2298
E-mail: info@dunitz.co.uk
Website: http://www.dunitz.co.uk

A CIP record for this book is available from the British Library.

ISBN 1 84184 220 6

Although every effort has been made to ensure that all owners of copyright material
have been acknowledged in this publication, we would be glad to acknowledge in
subsequent reprints or editions any omissions brought to our attention.

Distributed in the USA by
Fulfilment Center
Taylor & Francis
10650 Tobben Drive
Independence, KY 41051, USA
Toll Free Tel.: +1 800 634 7064
E-mail: taylorandfrancis@thomsonlearning.com

Distributed in Canada by
Taylor & Francis
74 Rolark Drive
Scarborough, Ontario M1R 4G2, Canada
Toll Free Tel.: +1 877 226 2237
E-mail: tal_fran@istar.ca

Distributed in the rest of the world by
Thomson Publishing Services
Cheriton House
North Way
Andover, Hampshire SP10 5BE, UK
Tel.: +44 (0)1264 332424
E-mail: salesorder.tandf@thomsonpublishingservices.co.uk

Composition by Scribe Design, Gillingham, Kent
Printed in Great Britain by Biddles Ltd, Guildford and Kings Lynn

Contents

Contents

Contributors

Geraldine M Brennan
Ninewells Hospital
Dundee
Scotland
UK

Stephen J Cleland
Department of Medicine and
Therapeutics
Western Infirmary
Glasgow
Scotland
UK

John MC Connell
Western Infirmary
Glasgow
Scotland
UK

Jon Dowell
Tayside Centre for General
Practice
Dundee
Scotland
UK

Alastair Emslie-Smith
Tayside Centre for General
Practice
Dundee
Scotland
UK

Henrik Enhörning
Karolinska Hospital
Stockholm
Sweden

Iain Findlay
General Medicine, Diabetes and
Endocrinology
Royal Alexandra Hospital
Paisley
UK

John Hinnie
General Medicine, Diabetes and
Endocrinology
Royal Alexandra Hospital
Paisley
UK

Alison F Kirk
Cardiology Department
Royal Alexandra Hospital
Paisley
UK

Ian G Lawrence
Department of Diabetes and
Endocrinology
Leicester Royal Infirmary
Leicester
UK

Klas Malmberg
Department of Cardiology and
Thoracic Radiology
Karolinska Hospital
Stockholm
Sweden

Paul D MacIntyre
General Medicine, Diabetes and
Endocrinology
Royal Alexandra Hospital
Paisley
UK

Paul G McNally
Department of Diabetes and
Endocrinology
Leicester Royal Infirmary
Leicester
UK

Andrew D Morris
University Department of
Medicine
DARTS, Medicines Monitoring
Unit
University of Dundee
Ninewells Hospital & Medical
School
Dundee
UK

John R Petrie
University of Glasgow
Glasgow
Scotland
UK

Lars Rydén
Karolinska Hospital
Stockholm
Sweden

Frank Sullivan
Tayside Centre for General
Practice
Dundee
UK

Peter H Winocour
East and North Hertfordshire
NHS Trust
Queen Elizabeth II Hospital
Welwyn Garden City
UK

Series preface

Advances in Diabetes is a new series of monographs, each concerned with a hot or rapidly-evolving topic in diabetes. Our understanding of the processes involved in diabetes advances at the same time as new treatments emerge. There is a space for an up-to-date series of concise texts which outline these advances and this series is aimed at specialist medical and nursing practitioners in diabetes, together with their trainees. I hope that you find this series useful and stimulating as it brings together the latest information on each topic under review.

H Jonathan Bodansky
The General Infirmary at Leeds, Leeds, UK

Preface

The excessive cardiovascular morbidity and mortality that is associated with diabetes has been recognised for many years. To try and focus attention on the burden of cardiovascular disease in people with diabetes I suggested that diabetes should be defined as 'a state of premature cardiovascular death which is associated with chronic hyperglycaemia, and may also be associated with blindness and renal failure'.

My intention was two-fold; firstly to encourage diabetes specialists to take an interest in managing the large-vessel complications of diabetes and not just the small-vessel complications that are specific to diabetes, and secondly, to look beyond the control of blood glucose to other modifiable cardiovascular risk factors, and to other considerations that should be made when treating existing cardiovascular disease in people with diabetes.

It is clear that the pathophysiology of cardiac disease in diabetes is more complex than originally envisaged, and a large amount of vascular damage may accrue in the pre-diabetic period in association with insulin resistance (Chapter 1). People with diabetes may have additional problems with the diabetic cardiomyopathy, and the presence of diabetic autonomic neuropathy (Chapter 2) may mask some of the symptoms of coronary heart disease (Chapter 3), and may itself affect the functioning of the heart. Even in patients without autonomic neuropathy, much of the myocardial ischaemia in people with diabetes may be clinically silent (Chapter 3) until they present with an acute coronary syndrome (Chapter 4).

An evidence-based approach to reducing cardiovascular risk in people with diabetes is therefore necessary, involving:

- Treatment of blood glucose (Chapter 5)
- Treatment of hypertension (Chapter 5)
- Treatment of dyslipidaemia (Chapter 6)
- Treatment of existing cardiovascular disease using pharmacological and non-pharmacological means (Chapters 4, 7 and 8)
- Modification of lifestyle through improvements in diet, and physical activity (Chapter 9).

Several guidelines, based on this evidence, are now available. Polypharmacy seems an inevitable consequence, leading to potential problems with compliance and adherence, and implementation of these guidelines is a challenge for primary and secondary care alike (Chapter 10).

In this rapidly developing area, studies are being published at an increasing rate, and by the time this book is published there will be several new studies that will add important information. To paraphrase what my friend and former colleague, John Hinnie, says in Chapter 6, this book presents what is currently known about heart disease in diabetes, as well as possible treatment options, in a way that will allow the reader to integrate any future advances in knowledge into their clinical practice with ease.

Inevitably, when editing a book, there is a delay between the time the book is started, when the contributions arrive, and when the book is finally published. When this book was started I was a consultant in the Royal Alexandra Hospital, Paisley, and I am delighted that several friends and former colleagues have been able to contribute to this book. I thank all of the contributors for their patience and perseverance in producing stimulating and exciting material. My final thanks go to my wife Margaret, and sons Ben and Marc who have been patient and supportive as always.

Miles Fisher

Glasgow Royal Infirmary, Glasgow, UK

Insulin resistance, vascular endothelial dysfunction and cardiovascular risk in type 2 diabetes

Stephen J Cleland, John R Petrie and John MC Connell

Introduction

In the Banting lecture of 1988 Gerald Reaven introduced the concept of a 'metabolic syndrome' ('syndrome X') which included insulin resistance, glucose intolerance, hyperinsulinaemia, dyslipidaemia and hypertension.[1] He hypothesized that metabolic dysfunction might be causally linked to the cardiovascular features of this syndrome and proposed a number of putative mechanisms that might underlie the association. In the first part of this chapter, key points from Reaven's lecture will be expanded in the light of current knowledge. In the second part, the pivotal role of vascular endothelial dysfunction in syndrome X will be discussed, as well as more recent evidence suggesting possible mechanisms for the association of central obesity,

1

insulin resistance and type 2 diabetes with atherothrombotic complications, including coronary artery disease.

'Syndrome X'—the 1988 Banting lecture revisited

Insulin resistance

'In normal subjects there is a threefold variation between the most insulin-sensitive and most insulin-resistant.'

What is 'insulin resistance'?

Insulin is a peptide hormone which is secreted from pancreatic β-cells into the portal circulation in response to various stimuli, including glucose, free fatty acids and amino acids. One of its main roles is to facilitate cellular uptake and processing of these building blocks for storage as glycogen, triglycerides and protein. The main sites of peripheral glucose disposal are skeletal muscle (80%) and adipose tissue (5–10%). Stimulation of insulin receptors in these tissues results in a complex series of intracellular events, ultimately resulting in translocation of glucose transporter proteins (GLUT-4) to the cell surface and subsequent glucose uptake. Insulin also exerts an important influence on the liver, resulting in suppression of gluconeogenesis and stimulation of lipogenesis. In addition, it is an important modulator of cellular growth.

The nature of 'resistance' to the physiological actions of insulin is incompletely understood. There are several inherited syndromes of profound insulin resistance which commonly involve the insulin receptor itself. For example, in type A insulin resistance syndrome the defective insulin receptors cannot stimulate the intracellular cascade that promotes glucose uptake and metabolism. Although the resultant compensatory high insulin levels are unable to overcome the receptor defect which results in hyperglycaemia, they continue to exert growth effects, perhaps via an action on IGF-1 receptors, causing the syndrome's characteristic phenotypic features, including acanthosis nigricans. In this syndrome, and in the much commoner form of insulin resistance, the term is used rather loosely to imply diminished cellular glucose uptake and metabolism.

In the majority of cases of insulin resistance associated with type 2 diabetes or hypertension, the cause of resistance to insulin action is likely to be multifactorial involving both genetic and environmental influences. When insulin sensitivity is measured in apparently healthy subjects, this creates considerable (2–3-fold) variation in insulin responsiveness.[2] Insulin responsiveness is a continuous variable within a normal population so that the majority of subjects defined as insulin 'resistant' are still able to maintain normal glucose tolerance via compensatory hyperinsulinaemia. In a proportion of insulin resistant subjects there is an inadequate pancreatic compensatory response and impaired glucose tolerance ensues.

How is insulin resistance measured?

Quantification of insulin sensitivity in man requires measurement of glucose disposal: high insulin-mediated glucose disposal implies high sensitivity/low resistance and vice versa. Several techniques have been used to quantify this variable (Table 1.1). The 'gold standard' for the measurement is the hyperinsulinaemic euglycaemic clamp technique, in which a fixed rate of insulin is infused and the plasma glucose concentration is maintained at a constant level (i.e. 'clamped') by infusing 20% glucose at a variable rate. After 2–3 hours, a steady state is achieved when the rate of glucose infusion is equal to the rate of insulin-mediated glucose disposal. Thus, insulin sensitivity is

---

Table 1.1 Methods for measurement of insulin sensitivity

- Hyperinsulinaemic euglycaemia clamp
- Insulin suppression test
- Intravenous glucose tolerance test
- 'Area under curve' insulin during oral glucose tolerance test
- Fasting insulin resistance index

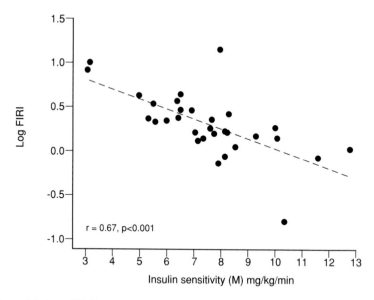

Figure 1.1 *Log$_{10}$ FIRI (fasting insulin resistance index: insulin × glucose/25) plotted against whole-body insulin sensitivity measured by the hyperinsulinaemic euglycaemic clamp technique in 31 subjects with normal glucose tolerance. (Adapted from reference 3.)*

expressed as mg glucose/kg body weight per minute ('M value'). Since the hyperinsulinaemic euglycaemic clamp technique is obviously impractical in large-scale studies, a surrogate index is often used as a simpler, more practical alternative: for example FIRI (fasting insulin resistance index), which equates to fasting [insulin] × fasting [glucose] divided by 25, has been shown to correlate well with clamp-derived M values (Fig. 1.1).[3]

Insulin resistance—a beneficial physiological response?
Metabolism is controlled by complex interaction of a number of mechanisms which allows for 'fine tuning' to environmental circumstances such as feeding, starvation and exercise. Changes in metabolism involve numerous short- and long-term endocrine mechanisms, including thyroid hormones, glucocorticoids, growth hormone and adrenergic activity. Immediate control is primarily dependent on

insulin and glucagon secreted from the pancreas. In this context, these other modulators of insulin signalling ensure optimum utilization and targeting of fuel delivery depending on circumstances. For example, if feeding occurs in a sedentary state, skeletal muscle insulin resistance combined with adipose tissue insulin sensitivity ensures that the energy ingested is directed to fat stores and away from muscle. If feeding occurs after exercise, increased muscle insulin sensitivity ensures restoration of energy stores used up in exercise. Teleologically, the insulin sensitivity of a given tissue can be conceptualized as a complex product of multi-dimensional metabolic control mechanisms acting at both systemic and local levels in order to ensure optimal processing of ingested energy in response to the prevailing environmental stressors.

Evolutionary role of insulin resistance

Insulin resistance may confer a positive survival advantage in times of stress and starvation by favouring incorporation of carbohydrate into adipose tissue. Unfortunately, such a mechanism that has evolved over millions of years may have adverse effects in a modern Westernized society, where diet is high in refined carbohydrate and saturated fat, and the ready availability of food is promoting an epidemic of obesity. Furthermore, levels of physical activity have been dramatically reduced resulting in a vicious circle of inactivity, obesity and insulin resistance (Fig. 1.2). This adverse effect of unhealthy lifestyle is amplified in migrant groups who have evolved in physical adversity but who move into a Westernized society.

Insulin resistance is an appropriate physiological response in certain circumstances of physiological stress, such as major trauma, sepsis, starvation, pregnancy and puberty, with the result that essential glucose substrate is diverted from muscle metabolism and priority given to energy storage, neural nutrition, growth and healing. Thus, in times of physical adversity, selective insulin resistance may confer an important survival advantage, which may explain its apparent prevalence in an ostensibly healthy population.[4]

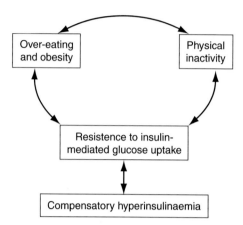

Figure 1.2 *Schematic diagram illustrating the 'vicious circle' linking unhealthy lifestyle (obesity and inactivity) with insulin resistance and compensatory hyperinsulinaemia.*

Insulin resistance, diabetes and cardiovascular disease

'It is likely that resistance to insulin-mediated glucose uptake is involved in the aetiology of type 2 diabetes, hypertension and coronary artery disease.'

The historical background

Over 70 years ago, Joslin noted that arteriosclerosis was the main cause of death in diabetic patients and he went on to suggest that obesity played an important role in this association.[5] In 1936, Himsworth described two distinct forms of diabetes, insulin 'sensitive' and 'insensitive', and initiated the concept of insulin resistance as a fundamental aetiological factor in the development of type 2 diabetes.[6] Twenty years later, Vague observed that central distribution of adiposity was a risk factor for diabetes and atherosclerosis, accounting for the higher prevalence of these conditions in males.[7] In 1966 Welborn et al demonstrated that patients with essential hypertension had elevated insulin levels, highlighting the link between dysfunctional insulin action and risk of cardiovascular disease.[8] In the 1970s, Reaven's group showed that type 2 diabetes is characterized by a reduction in insulin's ability to stimulate whole-body glucose uptake (insulin resistance).[9] Therefore, by the time Reaven gave the Banting lecture in 1988 on the 'Role of insulin resistance in human disease',[1] the notion that insulin resistance plays a key role in the aetiology of type 2 diabetes was well established and observational studies had already suggested that insulin resistance might be linked in some way with accelerated cardiovascular disease.

Epidemiological evidence

The risk of coronary artery disease is greatly increased in type 2 diabetes. In a study examining the 7-year incidence of myocardial infarction (MI), Haffner et al reported that the 10-year risk for a non-diabetic subject without previous MI was 3.5%; if a subject had previously had an MI, the risk of a further event was 18.8% (Fig. 1.3).[10] In contrast, in diabetic subjects without previous MI, the risk was comparable to that for a non-diabetic post-MI subject (20.2%), while

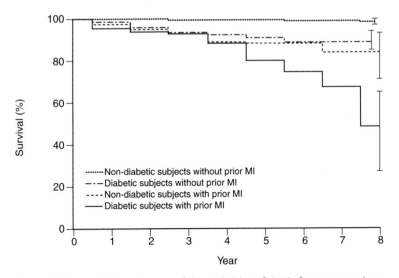

Figure 1.3 *Kaplan-Meier estimates of the probability of death from coronary heart disease in 1059 subjects with type 2 diabetes and 1378 non-diabetic subjects with and without prior myocardial infarction. MI denotes myocardial infarction. Bars indicate 95% confidence intervals. (From reference 10.)*

the risk of a second MI in a diabetic subject was 45%. Thus, diabetes that is characterized by insulin resistance and hyperinsulinaemia is associated with an accelerated risk of atherosclerosis.

In order to establish causality, a number of prospective epidemiological studies have sought to quantify the independent risk bestowed by increased glucose or insulin levels on incidence of cardiovascular events. It has been demonstrated in a meta-analysis that glucose levels are independently related to cardiovascular risk,[11] with the effect starting in the non-diabetic glucose range (<6.1 mmol/l) and rising exponentially within the diabetic glucose range. Furthermore, there appears to be a positive independent association between insulin levels and cardiovascular risk, although the relationship is relatively weak.[12–14] The strength of the relationship may be underestimated as fasting insulin levels are a poor surrogate for insulin resistance. Nonetheless, a small prospective study has suggested that insulin resistance is predictive of cardiovascular events,[15] although there has not been a well-designed, large-scale prospective study examining the relationship of insulin resistance with cardiovascular outcome. Two recent studies have reinforced the apparent link between insulin resistance and MI. First, British Indian Asian men with premature MI displayed insulin resistance, as did their first-degree healthy relatives.[16] Second, components of insulin resistance have been shown to predict the progress of atherosclerosis in non-grafted coronary arteries 5 years after coronary artery bypass surgery.[17]

Role of insulin resistance in the pathogenesis of type 2 diabetes

'The ability of the β-cell to compensate for resistance to insulin-stimulated glucose uptake plays a crucial role in determining the degree to which glucose homeostasis can be maintained.'

Insulin resistance and pancreatic β-cell function in diabetes

In the 12 years since Reaven's Banting lecture it has now become firmly established that the majority of patients with type 2 diabetes

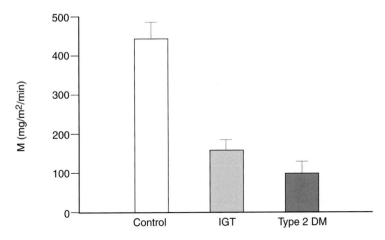

Figure 1.4 *Mean ± SE for whole-body insulin-mediated glucose uptake (M) during hyperinsulinaemic euglycaemic clamp studies. Subjects with normal glucose tolerance (white) were significantly more insulin sensitive than subjects with either impaired glucose tolerance (IGT, grey) or type 2 diabetes (black). (Adapted from reference 1.)*

and 'impaired glucose tolerance' (IGT) are insulin resistant. Reaven demonstrated that subjects with IGT or established diabetes had similar degrees of insulin resistance (Fig. 1.4) and, therefore, differences in glucose levels between the two groups must be determined by other factors. The main factor responsible for the progression from insulin resistance to IGT and, eventually, to diabetes is the ability of pancreatic β-cells to compensate for insulin resistance by secreting more insulin both in the fasting state and post-prandially. Diabetic patients with relatively low glucose levels have the highest insulin levels and the progressive increase in ambient glucose levels seen in type 2 diabetes is associated with a decline in plasma insulin concentration. Inability to sustain the hyperinsulinaemic state is associated with the development of severe hyperglycaemia (Fig. 1.5). Why then should pancreatic β-cells be unable to compensate for insulin resistance by increasing their capacity to secrete insulin, thereby preventing hyperglycaemia?

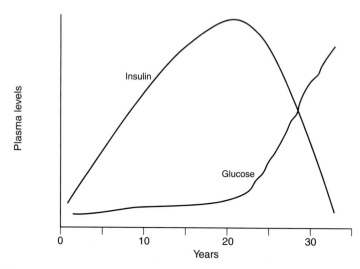

Figure 1.5 *Schematic diagram illustrating a typical time course of insulin and glucose levels in the context of underlying insulin resistance. Hyperglycaemia only supervenes when insulin secretion is no longer able to compensate.*

Insulin resistance and free fatty acid production

Reaven hypothesized that free fatty acid (FFA) metabolism was very sensitive to changes in circulating insulin levels. Inadequate insulin secretion in response to insulin resistance would elevate circulating FFA levels which, in turn, would cause hyperglycaemia. He argued that this could occur at two main sites—first, hepatic gluconeogenesis would increase and, second, muscle glucose utilization would decrease secondary to substrate competition from FFAs (Randle hypothesis). The final product would be hyperglycaemia due to a combination of increased glucose production and decreased glucose disposal. This concept has been the basis of a number of more recent studies suggesting that FFA release from central adipose stores may be of central importance not only in promoting metabolic dysfunction, but also in the process of vascular endothelial dysfunction and atherothrombosis.

Pancreatic β-cell toxicity

Recently, it has been suggested that an adverse lipid environment might play a key role in the process of pancreatic β-cell dysfunction.[18]

It is proposed that excessive cytosolic triglyceride stores in pancreatic β-cells result in increased production of oxygen free radicals by respiring mitochondria. Pancreatic β-cells have a much lower free radical scavenging capacity than most other tissues and they cannot adapt their level of anti-oxidant enzyme expression in response to chronic oxidative stress.[19] Despite initial efforts to overcome insulin resistance by increasing insulin production, β-cells may succumb to oxidative damage and eventually cell death. Once hyperglycaemia supervenes, this process is accelerated due to further glucose-mediated oxidative stress and other mechanisms of glucotoxicity[20] and a positive feedback cycle is initiated. There are also a number of other factors that may influence the susceptibility of β-cells to fail, including insulin gene expression and accumulation of islet cell amyloid, which may help to explain why many insulin resistant subjects do not go on to develop type 2 diabetes.

Insulin resistance and hypertension

'Abnormalities of glucose and insulin metabolism may play some role in the aetiology of high blood pressure in humans.'

Association of insulin resistance/hyperinsulinaemia with hypertension

An elevation in serum insulin concentrations in patients with essential hypertension was first noted over 30 years ago and a number of cross-sectional epidemiological studies have demonstrated an association between insulin levels and blood pressure (BP).[21] Whether hyperinsulinaemia is a cause, a consequence or an epiphenomenon in hypertension remains controversial, but the relationship is certainly not direct and simple. For example, chronic artificial elevation of serum insulin concentrations increases BP in rats,[22] has no effect in dogs[23] and lowers BP in man.[24] Patients with insulinomas do not tend to have hypertension.[25] Nevertheless, prospective studies have shown that individuals with hyperinsulinaemia have a higher risk of developing both hypertension[26] and coronary events.[14]

Studies using the hyperinsulinaemic euglycaemic clamp technique have demonstrated that hyperinsulinaemia occurs in hypertension as a compensatory response to reduced insulin-stimulated glucose uptake by skeletal muscle.[27,28] Insulin resistance is absent in secondary hypertension but present in normotensive offspring of essential hypertensive patients,[29] suggesting that it may precede the development of high blood pressure. It has been suggested that the relationship between insulin resistance and blood pressure may be confounded by obesity, as body mass index (BMI) has a strong association with both insulin resistance and hypertension.[30] Pooled analysis of insulin sensitivity data from 333 subjects from various European centres has recently demonstrated that both systolic and diastolic BP have a negative relationship with insulin sensitivity, even after adjustment for age, gender, BMI and fasting serum insulin concentration, i.e. the data are consistent with the hypothesis that the association between BMI and blood pressure is mediated by insulin sensitivity.[31]

Possible mechanisms linking insulin with blood pressure

Insulin has depressor peripheral vasodilator actions mainly in skeletal muscle vascular beds, probably by an endothelium-dependent mechanism, an action which will be discussed in more detail later. The hormone also has pressor effects mainly via stimulation of the sympathetic nervous system[32] and enhancement of renal sodium absorption.[33] The net physiological effect is a balance of pressor and depressor effects and maintenance of blood pressure. In pathophysiological states such as obesity, the balance may be disrupted by enhanced sympathetic activation in response to hyperinsulinaemia[34] together with 'blunting' of insulin-mediated vasodilation (vascular insulin resistance).[35] Indeed there is positron emission tomography evidence to suggest that insulin-stimulated muscle blood flow is impaired in lean patients with mild essential hypertension.[36] This result concurs with previous reports of a negative correlation between insulin-induced vasodilation and blood pressure using less sensitive techniques for measurement of blood flow.[37,38] Other authors have refuted these results[39] and it remains unclear whether blunting of insulin-mediated vasodilation contributes to hypertension in insulin-resistant states via increased peripheral vascular resistance. Thus, while there is undoubtedly a link between insulin resistance, hyperinsulinaemia and hypertension, the association may not be causal: instead it may reflect shared underlying pathophysiological abnormalities.

Association of dyslipidaemia with insulin resistance and hypertension

'Abnormalities of carbohydrate and lipoprotein metabolism are present in patients with hypertension and significant relationships exist between the various metabolic variables.'

Insulin resistance and the 'atherogenic lipid profile'

Abnormalities in lipid levels and lipoprotein profile which are characteristic of insulin resistance may play a key role in promoting atherothrombotic disease via increased oxidative stress. The major lipid changes found in insulin-resistant subjects and type 2 diabetic patients are hypertriglyceridaemia and reduced HDL-cholesterol.[40] Reaven's original description of Syndrome X identified these abnormalities, along with insulin resistance, glucose intolerance, hyperinsulinaemia and hypertension. The pathophysiological importance of this combination of high triglyceride and low HDL-cholesterol levels may be the resulting increased levels of small dense LDL-cholesterol, which causes damage to vascular endothelial cells via generation of oxygen free radicals.[41-44]

How might insulin resistance cause this atherogenic lipid profile? The most attractive hypothesis suggests that dysfunctional hepatic lipid processing plays a central role.[40,43] Abdominal obesity is closely related with insulin resistance. Decreased activity of lipoprotein lipase, and enhanced paracrine actions of cytokines (such as tumour necrosis factor α (TNFα), see later) in these adipose cells results in increased delivery of free fatty acids (FFAs) to the liver via the portal circulation. Consequently, there is increased hepatic secretion of triglyceride-rich very low density lipoprotein (VLDL) and apolipoprotein B. In addition, activity of hepatic lipase is increased. The result of this combination appears to be increased exchange of cholesteryl

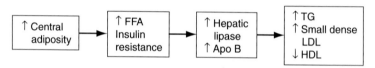

Figure 1.6 *Schematic diagram illustrating the causal association of central adiposity, insulin resistance and dyslipidaemia.*

esters from HDL/LDL to VLDL along with triglyceride from VLDL to HDL /LDL. This has two main adverse effects: first, production of atherogenic 'remnant particles' is increased[45] and, second, hydrolysis of accumulated triglyceride in LDL and HDL results in smaller denser particles[46] which are toxic to vascular endothelium (Fig. 1.6).

Post-prandial state, insulin resistance and atherogenesis

There is increasing recognition that metabolic disturbances in the post-prandial period may be of key importance in causing vascular damage. While this notion is not new,[47] more is now known about the inter-action of post-prandial carbohydrate and lipid metabolism with vascu-lar endothelial function and atherosclerosis. The atherogenic lipid profile associated with insulin resistance is exaggerated in the post-prandial period,[48,49] while post-prandial hyperglycaemia has additive effects on promotion of vascular oxidative stress.[50] The implication of this is that subjects with impaired glucose tolerance or diabetes, in the context of insulin resistance, have post-prandial glucose and lipid pro-oxidant factors exerting adverse effects on the vasculature. Of interest is a recent study demonstrating post-prandial dyslipidaemia in healthy first-degree relatives of diabetic patients in the absence of abnormal glucose tolerance,[51] indicating the potential of vascular damage long before the clinical presentation of metabolic disease.

Sedentary lifestyle as risk for cardiovascular disease

'Obesity and decreased physical activity have also been shown to be correlated with hyperinsulinaemia, glucose intolerance, increased plasma triglyceride concentration, decreased HDL-cholesterol concentration, and high blood pressure.'

Insulin resistance—an epidemic in Western society?

There is already evidence of a global epidemic of type 2 diabetes. Currently, there are 100 million patients worldwide; it has been predicted that this figure will double by the year 2020.[52] The notion that Western lifestyle is responsible for this epidemic is supported by the high prevalence of type 2 diabetes in migrant people groups such as South Asians, Aborigines and Polynesians.[53] For example, the prevalence of diabetes in South Asians aged 40–75 in the UK is 20–30%, compared with a prevalence in the indigenous population of 2–3%.[54] The fact that these same groups have a high incidence of cardiovascular disease supports the concept of common aetiological mechanisms linking insulin resistance with vascular dysfunction.

The importance of central obesity and physical inactivity

It is clear that abdominal obesity is closely related with other aspects of the insulin resistance syndrome and may play a key role in promoting the adverse atherogenic lipid profile as discussed above.[40] The cause of increase in coronary artery disease that occurs in association with central obesity is likely to be multi-factorial; as well as the adverse lipid changes resulting from increased free fatty acid load to the liver, other factors including hypertension, impaired glucose tolerance, associated defects in coagulation/fibrinolysis and elevations in inflammatory cytokines (discussed later) are likely to contribute. In addition, lack of physical activity may be pro-atherogenic, independent of the associated weight gain. In a recent study of human coronary artery endothelial function, significant improvements were noted after 4 weeks of aerobic exercise.[55] The most likely mechanism for this benefit is increased coronary flow causing stimulation of endothelial nitric oxide production.

Putative mechanisms linking dysfunctional carbohydrate and lipoprotein metabolism

'We propose that the relationship between insulin resistance, plasma insulin level and glucose intolerance is mediated to a significant degree by changes in ambient plasma free fatty acid concentration.'

15

Mechanisms of free fatty acid effects on insulin sensitivity

Reaven discussed putative mechanisms for FFA effects on hepatic gluconeogenesis and insulin sensitivity. It is assumed that FFAs reduce peripheral insulin sensitivity (mainly skeletal muscle) probably by substrate competition with glucose in the 'Randle cycle'. More recently, the use of nuclear magnetic resonance technology has suggested that FFAs primarily inhibit cellular glucose uptake with secondary reduction of both glucose oxidation and glycogen synthesis.[56] It may be that protein kinase C (PKC) is a key mediator of this effect.[57]

Emerging role of adipose tissue as an endocrine organ

Far from being a simple storage depot for fat, adipose tissue is emerging as a dynamic and integral player in metabolic control. Adipocytes secrete the 'adipostat' hormones leptin and TNFα. Leptin causes a down-regulation of food intake and an increase in energy expenditure via the hypothalamus,[58] as well as exerting peripheral effects on insulin action.[59] TNFα causes increased rates of lipolysis in adipose cells as well as interfering with insulin signalling in skeletal muscle.[60]

FFA effects on endothelial function

As well as adversely influencing insulin action, FFAs exert effects on vascular endothelial function. For example, FFA infusion caused blunting of endothelium-dependent leg vasodilation during insulin suppression.[61] Interestingly, this effect was reversed in the presence of insulin. This result has been confirmed by others[62] and is supported by a study in which the free fatty acid, oleic acid, was shown to inhibit nitric oxide synthase in endothelial cell culture.[63] In addition, it has recently been shown that endothelial dysfunction in obesity is associated with central distribution of adiposity, further supporting the role of central obesity as a cardiovascular risk factor.[64]

Thus, a reduction in insulin-stimulated glucose uptake and metabolism in skeletal muscle and adipose tissue (insulin resistance) is not only a risk factor for development of type 2 diabetes but is also associated with increased incidence of coronary artery disease. Reaven's observations in his 1988 Banting lecture fit with current data which suggest that there is a complex interaction among insulin action, obesity, circulating lipids and blood pressure which underlies this association. Central to the link between metabolic and vascular dysfunction is likely to be abnormal vascular endothelial function.

Type 2 diabetes, vascular endothelial dysfunction and mechanisms of atherothrombotic disease

Although Reaven's contribution has been important in understanding the link between diabetes and cardiovascular disease, recent evidence has shifted the emphasis from hyperinsulinaemia to vascular insulin resistance. It now appears likely that defective insulin action on vascular endothelial cells is a key intermediate mechanism of vascular dysfunction in insulin resistant conditions.

Vascular endothelial dysfunction

Overview of vascular endothelial function and role of nitric oxide (NO)
Cells of the endothelial monolayer produce a variety of mediators in response to a wide range of agonists. The emerging concept of vascular endothelial dysfunction as a crucial factor linking syndrome X with atherothrombotic disease has been described above. Here, we use the term 'endothelial dysfunction' specifically to refer to abnormal endothelial NO availability. This can represent either abnormal NO synthesis (e.g. reduced activity of endothelial nitric oxide synthase: eNOS) or increased NO quenching (e.g. by superoxide or other cellular free radicals). It is often assumed that defects in NO production equate with global dysfunction of other endothelial mechanisms, although there is very little direct supporting evidence.

Measurement of NO availability in vivo
Measurement of either stimulated or basal NO production is the 'gold standard' for assessment of endothelial function. A useful surrogate

17

measure is evaluation of endothelium-dependent limb blood flow. This can be assessed by a number of methods, the most commonly used being forearm venous-occlusion plethysmography. A number of different compounds have been infused via a limb artery to demonstrate local vasodilation via stimulation of endothelial NO production; these include acetylcholine, methacholine and bradykinin. In such protocols, it is important to study in parallel the effects of an endothelium-independent donor of NO (e.g. sodium nitroprusside) which is used as an experimental control to assess sensitivity of adjacent vascular smooth muscle to NO.

An alternative approach is to assess basal endothelial NO production. The most commonly used method for this in man is measurement of the vasoconstrictor response to a local infusion of N_G-monomethyl-L-arginine (L-NMMA), which is a stereospecific substrate inhibitor of eNOS. Vasoconstriction to L-NMMA in the human forearm is dose-dependent with maximal reduction in blood flow in the order of 30–40%.[65] Basal production of endothelial NO contributes significantly to the determination of resting blood flow. It is likely that this method of assessing endothelial function is more physiologically relevant since stimulation by pharmacological doses of agonists is artificial. It remains unclear whether L-NMMA has any other effects that may confuse interpretation of blood flow responses. It is common practice to use an experimental control which is usually the endothelium-independent vasoconstrictor, noradrenaline.

Microvascular versus macrovascular dysfunction

It is important to consider vessel size when examining the relationship between endothelial dysfunction and complications of type 2 diabetes. In general terms, it appears that insulin resistance has more of an impact on macrovascular function (e.g. coronary and cerebral circulation) while hyperglycaemia is more closely associated with microvascular abnormalities (e.g. renal and retinal microcirculation), although there is a clear overlap. In addition, little is known about the extent of capillary endothelial dysfunction in metabolic disease. Understanding the mechanisms underlying the associations between endothelial dysfunction and both insulin resistance and hyperglycaemia may ultimately explain why different patterns of microvascular and macrovascular complications occur in type 1 and type 2 diabetes.

Insulin resistance and endothelial dysfunction

Insulin's direct vascular action

It is now generally acknowledged that insulin has a direct vasodilator action on peripheral arterioles, mainly in skeletal muscle vascular beds. However, there is debate as to the physiological relevance of this effect[66] since significant vasodilation only occurs after 40–50 minutes of systemic insulin infusion at high physiological levels.[67] A more likely role for insulin in this context is as a chronically-acting regulator of blood flow in metabolically-active vascular beds. While this concept is controversial, it is teleologically attractive since it would be useful for insulin to direct fuel substrate to relevant tissues prior to stimulating cellular uptake, and it is supported by the demonstration of a positive association between insulin sensitivity and insulin-mediated vasodilation in man (Fig. 1.7).[68]

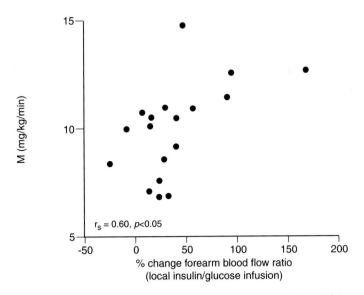

Figure 1.7 Whole-body insulin sensitivity (M) plotted against local insulin/glucose-mediated vasoreactivity in 18 healthy male volunteers. (Adapted from reference 68.)

Insulin resistance causes endothelial dysfunction?

There is accumulating evidence that insulin directly stimulates eNOS activity in vascular endothelial cells.[69–71] This is supported by human studies showing a positive association between the vasodilator action of

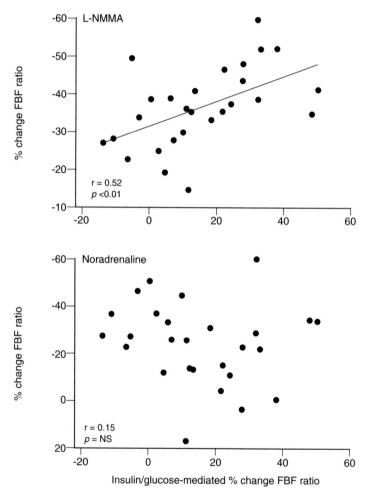

Figure 1.8. *Percentage change in forearm blood flow ratio in response to intra-arterial infusions of L-NMMA and noradrenaline plotted against local insulin/glucose-mediated vasodilation (percentage change in forearm blood flow ratio). Pooled correlation analysis (n = 27). (Adapted from reference 73.)*

insulin, which is NO-dependent, and basal endothelial function, both in healthy subjects and in patients with either hypertension or type 2 diabetes (Fig. 1.8).[72,73] It appears that this endothelial effect of insulin is mediated through a signalling pathway that involves activation of PI-3-kinase via phosphorylation of insulin receptor substrate. This mechanism also mediates glucose transport and metabolism in skeletal muscle, raising the possibility that a primary defect in proximal insulin signalling may be responsible for insulin resistance/metabolic dysfunction as well as abnormal endothelial function. This hypothesis has been supported in two animal models: first, defective endothelium-dependent vasorelaxation was demonstrated in mice lacking insulin receptor substrate-1[74] and, second, multiple defects in components of the insulin signalling pathway have been reported in vascular tissue of the insulin resistant obese Zucker rat.[75] Thus, 'vascular insulin resistance' may be a key intermediate mechanism that links metabolic and vascular dysfunction.

Endothelial dysfunction causes insulin resistance?

The alternative view is that dyfunctional vascular endothelium causes insulin resistance.[76] It is possible that reduced substrate delivery is rate-limiting for insulin-stimulated glucose uptake,[77] although this concept has been dismissed by a number of authors.[78–80] A recent study demonstrating insulin resistance in eNOS 'knockout' mice has been interpreted as supporting the role of decreased blood flow to skeletal muscle resulting in diminished glucose uptake,[81] but is also consistent with the alternative explanation that there is an interaction between NO and insulin signalling at the level of the skeletal myocytes, since there is increasing evidence that NO plays a key role in muscle metabolic control especially in the context of exercise.[82,83] There is evidence of expression of eNOS in skeletal muscle, and it is possible that vascular endothelial dysfunction in insulin resistant states may reflect more generalized dysfunction of NO pathways in insulin sensitive tissues.

Hyperglycaemia and endothelial dysfunction

Endothelial dysfunction in type 2 diabetes

Impairment of vascular endothelial function is a feature of type 2 diabetes.[84] Despite the suggestion that this is secondary to obesity/insulin resistance rather than hyperglycaemia per se,[85] significant endothelial dysfunction has been demonstrated in type 2 diabetic patients compared with age- and BMI-matched control subjects.[86] Coronary artery endothelial function has been shown to be impaired in type 2 diabetes[87] and LDL-cholesterol size has been shown to correlate with the degree of endothelial function in diabetes, supporting the notion that an atherogenic lipid profile might be a key intermediate mechanism.[88] However, while hyperglycaemia may contribute independently to endothelial dysfunction, it is unlikely to be the primary underlying cause since studies have shown that altered vascular function is present in insulin resistant states with normoglycaemia.[89,90]

Mechanisms of endothelial glucose toxicity

A number of mechanisms may contribute to endothelial dysfunction and promotion of the atherothrombotic process in the context of hyperglycaemia.[91–94]

Central to endothelial 'glucose toxicity' appears to be superoxide formation, PKC upregulation and advanced glycosylation end-product (AGE) formation. In summary, the intracellular $NAD(P)H:NAD^+$ ratio is increased by hyperglycaemia via increased glycolysis and elevation of sorbitol levels (via the aldose reductase pathway). This, in turn, promotes production of diacylglycerol and superoxide, both of which stimulate PKC. A number of adverse effects in vascular cells ensue including changes in gene expression affecting key proteins involved in cell membrane potential, extracellular matrix production and cell growth. Superoxide also promotes LDL oxidation, reacts with NO to form peroxynitrite which causes oxidative enzymic damage, stimulates nuclear factors which promote expression of cell adhesion molecules and activates the coagulation cascade. Formation of AGEs causes endothelial activation, activation of coagulation, increased levels of cytokines and adhesion molecules and increased oxidizability of lipoproteins. In addition to these adverse effects a number of other mechanisms have been proposed, including stimulation of vasoconstrictor prostanoids and quenching of intracellular NADPH resulting in further reductions in NO availability and free radical scavenging ability.

Thus, normal endothelial function is an important target for the toxic effects of chronic hyperglycaemia in addition to its better known effects on other tissues, although a number of factors involved in the atherothrombotic process are also directly affected.

Acute versus chronic glucose exposure: effects on endothelial dysfunction

There is much debate on the effect of glucose exposure on vascular endothelial function. Having just discussed the multiple putative mechanisms of glucose toxicity, the assumption would be that glucose would have a deleterious effect on endothelial function. However, there is a significant body of data, both in vivo and ex vivo, which suggests that acute exposure to glucose does not have the same effect as chronic hyperglycaemia. For example, while it was shown that exposure to hyperglycaemia for 6 hours results in impairment of endothelial function in one study,[95] hyperglycaemia was shown to cause dose-dependent vasodilation using similar techniques in another.[96] Effects of glucose on blood flow are not simply due to osmotic factors; D-glucose augmented insulin-mediated vasodilation in the forearm while L-glucose (metabolically-inactive stereoisomer) did not.[67] Studies of endothelial cell cultures have revealed an acute stimulatory effect of glucose on NO production,[97,98] although chronic exposure to glucose attenuates this.[99] It is becoming clear that glucose may have a stimulatory endothelial action on acute exposure and an inhibitory effect on more chronic exposure. This may help to explain the well-recognized phenomenon of increased microvascular blood flow and glomerular filtration rate in newly-diagnosed type 1 diabetes, with subsequent reductions in these parameters as the disease progresses.

Abnormalities of coagulation and fibrinolysis in insulin resistance

Insulin resistance and the thrombotic–fibrinolytic equilibrium

Abnormalities of coagulation and fibrinolysis are consistently associated with insulin resistance, although it is unclear whether the relationships are causal or influenced by a 'third factor'.[100,101] The three key molecules involved are plasminogen activator inhibitor 1 (PAI-1), von Willebrand factor (vWF) and fibrinogen. PAI-1 inhibits fibrinolysis; increased levels are associated with insulin resistance/hyperinsulinaemia,[102] type 2 diabetes,[103] myocardial infarction[104] and dyslipidaemia.[105] VWF is a pro-coagulant factor and plasma levels are generally interpreted as representing the extent of endothelial activation. VWF levels have been shown to correlate with insulin levels in population studies.[106] Fibrinogen is clearly a central component of the coagulation cascade and elevated levels are associated with hyperinsulinaemia and cardiovascular risk.[107,108] The relationship of fibrinogen with insulin resistance and endothelial dysfunction is complicated by the fact that it is also an acute-phase protein synthesized by the liver in response to circulating interleukin-6 (IL-6). The putative role of inflammation in cardiovascular disease and insulin resistance will be discussed in the next section.

Insulin resistance and platelet aggregation

In one study in newly-diagnosed type 2 diabetic patients significant platelet hyperaggregation was demonstrated in whole blood.[109] After control of blood glucose there was a significant reduction in platelet aggregability, suggesting that both hyperinsulinaemia and hyperglycaemia may influence aggregation mechanisms.[109] The role of hyperinsulinaemia and insulin resistance on platelet glucose transport and on the metabolic function of platelets is poorly understood. In one study, platelet aggregation was measured in healthy volunteers before and after intravenous insulin: aggregation was significantly reduced after insulin, suggesting that insulin may have important anti-aggregatory properties.[110] One group has used platelet-rich plasma (PRP) to study the relationship between insulin and platelet aggregability: first, an anti-aggregatory effect of insulin on platelet stimulation by collagen or ADP was shown in PRP from healthy volunteers.[111] Cyclic GMP (cGMP) production was also measured and it was concluded that insulin's anti-aggregatory effect was via a cGMP-dependent mechanism. This effect was significantly impaired in the insulin resistant states of obesity and type 2 diabetes[112] and, more recently, it was demonstrated that lean patients with type 2 diabetes exhibited normal insulin anti-aggregation,[113] suggesting that insulin resistance is the most important underlying mechanism for this effect rather than hyperglycaemia. These data indicate that platelet aggregability is increased in association with insulin resistance, and this may be an important factor in terms of predisposition to thrombotic vascular disease.

Insulin resistance, pro-inflammatory cytokines and endothelial dysfunction

Atherosclerosis—an inflammatory disease

Central to the formation of an atherosclerotic plaque is the involvement of the immune system in the form of monocyte-derived macrophages and activated T-lymphocytes.[114] Factors which have been proposed to induce or promote the inflammatory process in atherosclerosis include oxidized LDL particles, homocysteine, angiotensin II and infections (such as *Chlamydia pneumoniae* and *Helicobacter pylori*).[114] Circulating cytokines, including IL-6 and TNFα, are involved in mediating this inflammatory response. It is noteworthy that TNFα has been shown to induce both insulin resistance in skeletal muscle[115] and endothelial dysfunction;[116,117] IL-6 stimulates hepatic production of fibrinogen, a pro-coagulant factor; furthermore, CRP (a marker of inflammation) is associated with insulin resistance, obesity and cardiovascular risk markers[118] and has recently been shown to correlate with basal endothelial NO production.[119] As IL-6 and TNFα are secreted from abdominal adipose cells (see above), this has raised the question of whether central obesity is the primary abnormality accounting for the pro-coagulant and pro-inflammatory phenotype which is associated with the atherogenic lipid profile and which manifests as insulin resistance, endothelial dysfunction and, ultimately, atherothrombotic disease.[100,120,121]

Summary and conclusions

'It is likely that resistance to insulin-mediated glucose uptake is involved in the aetiology of type 2 diabetes, hypertension and coronary artery disease. Although this concept may seem outlandish at first blush, the notion is consistent with available experimental data.'

In 1988 Reaven described syndrome X, a common constellation of features including insulin resistance, glucose intolerance, hyperinsulinaemia, dyslipidaemia and hypertension. The concept of a common aetiological mechanism underlying obesity, type 2 diabetes and atherosclerosis was not new, but Reaven's 'hypothesis' served to stimulate a huge body of research in the subsequent years and our understanding of the mechanisms linking metabolic and vascular dysfunction is much clearer. Three major concepts have emerged from this work. First, the pivotal role of abdominal adipose tissue is becoming increasingly clear. Not only does the delivery of FFAs to the liver and peripheral tissues result in insulin resistance and vascular endothelial dysfunction but there is also increasing evidence that cytokines released from adipose cells contribute to the pro-coagulant and pro-inflammatory environment which predisposes to vascular atherothrombotic complications. Second, the adverse effects of hyperglycaemia on micro- and macrovascular function have been elucidated, and there is increasing awareness of the importance of glycaemic control in the prevention of vascular complications of diabetes. Third, the concept of vascular insulin resistance has emerged in which defective insulin action at the level of vascular endothelial cells may be a key mechanism underlying vascular dysfunction in insulin resistant states. It is of interest to note that Reaven has recently published data in this area showing a positive correlation between cGMP production and insulin sensitivity,[122] which is consistent with the notion of a functional link between insulin's metabolic and vascular actions.

In conclusion, the combination of central obesity, insulin resistance and hyperglycaemia is associated with high cardiovascular risk.

Further understanding of mechanisms linking metabolic and vascular dysfunction will result in identification of novel therapeutic targets with the ultimate aim of reducing cardiovascular morbidity and mortality in type 2 diabetes.

References

1. Reaven GM. Role of insulin resistance in human disease. Diabetes 1988;37:1595–607.
2. Hollenbeck C, Reaven GM. Variations in insulin-stimulated glucose uptake in healthy individuals with normal glucose tolerance. J Clin Endocrinol Metab 1987;64:1169–73.
3. Cleland SJ, Petrie JR, Morris AD et al. FIRI: a fair insulin resistance index? Lancet 1996;347:770.
4. Swinbur BA. The thrifty genotype hypothesis: how does it look after 30 years? Diabet Med 1996;13:695–9.
5. Joslin EP. Arteriosclerosis and diabetes. Ann Clin Med 1927;5:1061.
6. Himsworth H. Diabetes mellitus: a differentiation into insulin-sensitive and insulin-insensitive types. Lancet 1936;1:127–30.
7. Vague J. The degree of masculine differentiation of obesities: a factor determining predisposition to diabetes, atherosclerosis, gout, and uric calculous disease. Am J Clin Nutr 1956;4:20–34.
8. Welborn TA, Breckenridge A, Dollery CT et al. Serum insulin in essential hypertension and in peripheral vascular disease. Lancet 1966;1:1336–7.
9. Ginsberg H, Kimmerling G, Olefsky M, Reaven GM. Demonstration of insulin resistance in untreated adult onset diabetic subjects with fasting hyperglycaemia. J Clin Invest 1975;55:454–61.
10. Haffner SM, Lehto S, Ronnemaa T et al. Mortality from coronary heart disease in subjects with type 2 diabetes and in nondiabetic subjects with and without prior myocardial infarction. N Engl J Med 1998;339:229–34.
11. Coutinho M, Gerstein HC, Wang Y, Yusuf S. The relationship between glucose and incident cardiovascular events: a metaregression analysis of published data from 20 studies of 95,783 individuals followed for 12.4 years. Diabetes Care 1999;22:233–40.
12. Ruige JB, Assendelft WJJ, Dekker JM et al. Insulin and risk of cardiovascular disease: a meta-analysis. Circulation 1998;97:996–1001.
13. Pyorala M, Miettinen H, Laakso M, Pyorala K. Hyperinsulinemia predicts coronary heart disease risk in healthy middle-aged men: the 22-year follow-up results of the Helsinki Policemen Study. Circulation 1998;98:398–404.
14. Despres J-P, Lamarche B, Mauriege P et al. Hyperinsulinemia as an independent risk factor for ischemic heart disease. N Engl J Med 1996;334:952–7.

15. Yip J, Facchini FS, Reaven GM. Resistance to insulin-mediated glucose disposal as a predictor of cardiovascular disease. J Clin Endocrinol Metab 1998;83:2773–6.
16. Kooner JS, Baliga RR, Wilding J et al. Abdominal obesity, impaired nonesterified fatty acid suppression, and insulin-mediated glucose disposal are early metabolic abnormalities in families with premature myocardial infarction. Arterio Throm Vasc Biol 1998;18:1021–6.
17. Korpilahti K, Syvanne M, Engblom E et al. Components of the insulin resistance syndrome are associated with progression of atherosclerosis in non-grafted arteries 5 years after coronary artery bypass surgery. Eur Heart J 1998;19:711–19.
18. Bakker SJL, IJzerman RG, Teerlink T et al. Cytosolic triglycerides and oxidative stress in central obesity: the missing link between excessive atherosclerosis, endothelial dysfunction, and beta-cell failure? Atherosclerosis 2000;148:17–21.
19. Tiedge M, Lortz S, Drinkgern J, Lenzen S. Relation between antioxidant enzyme gene expression and antioxidative defense status of insulin-producing cells. Diabetes 1997;46:1733–42.
20. Yki-Jarvinen H. Glucose toxicity. Endocr Rev 1992;13:415–31.
21. Feskens EJM, Tuomilehto J, Stengaard JH et al. Hypertension and overweight associated with hyperinsulinaemia and glucose tolerance: a longitudinal study of the Finnish and Dutch cohorts of the Seven Countries Study. Diabetologia 1995;38:839–47.
22. Brands MW, Hildebrandt DA, Mizelle HL, Hall JE. Sustained hyperinsulinemia increases arterial pressure in conscious rats. Am J Physiol 1991;260:R764–8.
23. Brands MW, Mizelle HL, Gaillard CA et al. The hemodynamic response to chronic hyperinsulinemia in conscious dogs. Am J Hypertens 1991;4:164–8.
24. Heise T, Magnusson K, Heinemann L, Sawicki PT. Insulin resistance and the effect of insulin on blood pressure in essential hypertension. Hypertension 1998;32:243–8.
25. Fujita N, Baba T, Tomiyami T et al. Hyperinsulinaemia and blood pressure in patients with insulinoma. BMJ 1992: 304:1157.
26. Haffner SM, Valdez RA, Hazuda HP et al. Prospective analysis of the insulin-resistance syndrome (Syndrome X). Diabetes 1992;41:715–22.
27. Ferrannini E, Buzzigoli G, Bonadonna R et al. Insulin resistance in essential hypertension. N Engl J Med 1987;317: 350–7.
28. Lind L, Berne C, Lithell H. Prevalence of insulin resistance in essential hypertension. J Hypertens 1995;13:1457–62.
29. Beatty OL, Harper R, Sheridan B et al. Insulin resistance in offspring of hypertensive parents. BMJ 1993;307:92–6.
30. Jarrett RJ. In defence of insulin: a critique of syndrome X. Lancet 1992;340:469–71.

31. Ferrannini E, Natali A, Capaldo B et al. Insulin resistance, hyperinsu-linemia, and blood pressure: role of age and obesity. Hypertension 1997;30:1144–9.

32. Anderson EA, Balon TW, Hoffman RP et al. Insulin increases sympa-thetic activity but not blood pressure in borderline hypertensive humans. Hypertension 1992;19:621–7.

33. Ferrannini E, Natali A. Insulin resistance and hypertension: connections with sodium metabolism. Am J Kid Dis 1993;21:37–42.

34. Scherrer U, Randin D, Tappy L et al. Body fat and sympathetic nerve activity in healthy subjects. Circulation 1994;89:2634–40.

35. Laakso M, Edelman SV, Brechtel G, Baron AD. Decreased effect of insulin to stimulate skeletal muscle blood flow in obese man. A novel mechanism for insulin resistance. J Clin Invest 1990;85:1844–52.

36. Laine H, Knuuti MJ, Ruotsalainen U et al. Insulin resistance in essential hypertension is characterized by impaired insulin stimulation of blood flow in skeletal muscle. J Hypertens 1998;16:211–19.

37. Baron AD. Cardiovascular actions of insulin in humans. Implications for insulin sensitivity and vascular tone. Baillieres Clin Endocrinol Metab 1993;7:961–87.

38. Feldman RD, Bierbrier GS. Insulin-mediated vasodilation: impairment with increased blood pressure and body mass. Lancet 1993;342:707–9.

39. Hunter SJ, Harper R, Ennis CN et al. Skeletal muscle blood flow is not a determinant of insulin resistance in essential hypertension. J Hyper-tens 1997;15:73–7.

40. Brunzell JD, Hokanson JE. Dyslipidemia of central obesity and insulin resistance. Diabetes Care 1999;22:C10–13.

41. Reaven GM, Chen Y-D, Jeppesen J et al. Insulin resistance and hyper-insulinemia in individuals with small, dense, low density lipoprotein particles. J Clin Invest 1993;92:141–6.

42. Haffner SM, Mykkanen L, Robbins D et al. A preponderance of small dense LDL is associated with specific insulin, proinsulin and the compo-nents of the insulin resistance syndrome in non-diabetic subjects. Diabetologia 1995;38:1328–36.

43. Sattar N, Petrie JR, Jaap AJ. The atherogenic lipoprotein phenotype and vascular endothelial dysfunction. Atherosclerosis 1998;138:229–35.

44. Krauss RM. Atherogenicity of triglyceride-rich lipoproteins. Am J Cardiol 1998;81:13B–17B.

45. Ebenbichler CF, Kirchmair R, Egger C, Patsch JR. Postprandial state and atherosclerosis. Curr Opin Lipidol 1995;6:286–90.

46. Austin MA, Edwards KL. Small, dense low density lipoproteins, the insulin resistance syndrome and noninsulin-dependent diabetes. Curr Opin Lipidol 1996;7:167–71.

47. Zilversmit DB. Atherogenesis: a postprandial phenomenon. Circulation 1979;60:473–85.

48. Mero N, Syvanne M, Taskinen M-R. Postprandial lipid metabolism in diabetes. Atherosclerosis 1998;141:S53–5.
49. Mero N, Suurinkeroinen L, Syvanne M et al. Delayed clearance of postprandial large TG-rich particles in normolipidemic carriers of LPL Asn291Ser gene variant. J Lipid Res 1999;40:1663–70.
50. Ceriello A, Bortolotti N, Motz E et al. Meal-induced oxidative stress and low-density lipoprotein oxidation in diabetes: the possible role of hyperglycemia. Metab Clin Exp 1999;48:1503–8.
51. Axelsen M, Smith U, Eriksson JW et al. Postprandial hypertriglyceridemia and insulin resistance in normoglycemic first-degree relatives of patients with type 2 diabetes. Ann Intern Med 1999;131:27–31.
52. O'Rahilly S. Science, medicine, and the future. Non-insulin dependent diabetes mellitus: the gathering storm. BMJ 1997;314:955–9.
53. Rowley KG, Best JD, McDermott R et al. Insulin resistance syndrome in Australian Aboriginal people. Clin Exp Pharmacol Physiol 1997;24:776–81.
54. McKeigue PM, Marmot MG. Mortality from coronary heart disease in Asian communities in London. BMJ 1988;297:903.
55. Hambrecht R, Wolf A, Gielen S et al. Effect of exercise on coronary endothelial function in patients with coronary artery disease. N Engl J Med 2000;342:454–60.
56. Roden M, Price TB, Perseghin G et al. Mechanism of free fatty acid-induced insulin resistance in humans. J Clin Invest 1996;97:2859–65.
57. Griffin ME, Marcucci MJ, Cline GW et al. Free fatty acid-induced insulin resistance is associated with activation of protein kinase C theta and alterations in the insulin signaling cascade. Diabetes 1999;48:1270–4.
58. Haynes WG, Morgan DA, Walsh SA et al. Cardiovascular consequences of obesity: role of leptin. Clin Exp Pharmacol Physiol 1998;25:65–9.
59. Desvergne B, Wahli W. Peroxisome proliferator-activated receptors and nuclear control of metabolism. Endocr Rev 1999;20:649–88.
60. Hotamisligil GS, Peraldi P, Budavari A et al. IRS-1-mediated inhibition of insulin receptor tyrosine kinase activity in TNF-alpha- and obesity-induced insulin resistance. Science 1996;271:665–8.
61. Steinberg HO, Tarshoby M, Monestel R et al. Elevated circulating free fatty acid levels impair endothelium-dependent vasodilation. J Clin Invest 1997;100:1230–9.
62. deKreutzenberg SV, Crepaldi C, Marchetto S et al. Plasma free fatty acids and endothelium-dependent vasodilation: effect of chain-length and cyclooxygenase inhibition. J Clin Endocrinol Metab 2000;85:793–8.
63. Davda RK, Stepniakowski KT, Lu G, Ullian ME et al. Oleic acid inhibits endothelial nitric oxide synthase by a protein kinase C-independent mechanism. Hypertension 1995;26:764–70.
64. Arcaro G, Zamboni M, Rossi L et al. Body fat distribution predicts the degree of endothelial dysfunction in uncomplicated obesity. Int J Obes 1999;23:936–42.

65. Vallance P, Collier J, Moncada S. Effects of endothelium-derived nitric oxide on peripheral arteriolar tone in man. Lancet 1989;2:997–1000.
66. Yki-Jarvinen H, Utriainen T. Insulin-induced vasodilatation: physiology or pharmacology? Diabetologia 1998;41:369–79.
67. Ueda S, Petrie JR, Cleland SJ et al. The vasodilating effect of insulin is dependent on local glucose uptake: a double blind, placebo-controlled study. J Clin Endocrinol Metab 1998;83:2126–31.
68. Cleland SJ, Petrie JR, Ueda S et al. Insulin-mediated vasodilation and glucose uptake are functionally linked in humans. Hypertension 1999;33:554–8.
69. Zeng G, Quon MJ. Insulin-stimulated production of nitric oxide is inhibited by wortmannin: direct measurement in vascular endothelial cells. J Clin Invest 1996;98:894–8.
70. Aljada A, Dandona P. Effect of insulin on human aortic endothelial nitric oxide synthase. Metab Clin Exp 2000;49:147–50.
71. Kuboki K, Jiang Z-Y, Takahara N et al. Regulation of constitutive nitric oxide synthase gene expression in endothelial cells and in vivo. A specific vascular action of insulin. Circulation 2000;101:676–81.
72. Petrie JR, Ueda S, Webb DJ et al. Endothelial nitric oxide production and insulin sensitivity: a physiological link with implications for pathogenesis of cardiovascular disease. Circulation 1996;93:1331–3.
73. Cleland SJ, Petrie JR, Small M et al. Insulin action is associated with endothelial function in hypertension and type 2 diabetes. Hypertension 2000;35:507–11.
74. Abe H, Yamada N, Kuwaki T et al. Hypertension, hypertriglyceridemia, and impaired endothelium-dependent vascular relaxation in mice lacking insulin receptor substrate-1. J Clin Invest 1998;101:1784–8.
75. Jiang ZY, Lin Y-W, Clemont A et al. Characterization of selective resistance to insulin signaling in the vasculature of obese Zucker (fa/fa) rats. J Clin Invest 1999;104:447–57.
76. Pinkney JH, Stehouwer CDA, Coppack SW, Yudkin JS. Endothelial dysfunction: cause of the insulin resistance syndrome. Diabetes 1997;46:S9–13.
77. Baron AD. Hemodynamic actions of insulin. Am J Physiol Endocrinol Metab 1994;267:E187–202.
78. Utriainen T, Nuutila P, Takala T et al. Intact insulin stimulation of skeletal muscle blood flow, its heterogeneity and redistribution, but not of glucose uptake in non-insulin-dependent diabetes mellitus. J Clin Invest 1997;100:777–85.
79. Natali A, Bonadonna R, Santoro D et al. Insulin resistance and vasodilation in essential hypertension. Studies with adenosine. J Clin Invest 1994;94:1570–6.
80. Nuutila P, Raitakari M, Laine H et al. Role of blood flow in regulating insulin-stimulated glucose uptake in humans: studies using bradykinin,

[^{15}O]water, and [^{18}F]fluoro-deoxy-glucose and positron emission tomography. J Clin Invest 1996;97:1741–7.

81. Shankar RR, Wu Y, Shen H-Q et al. Mice with disruption of both endothelial and neuronal nitric oxide synthase exhibit insulin resistance. Diabetes 2000;49:684–7.

82. Hayashi T, Wojtaszewski JFP, Goodyear LJ. Exercise regulation of glucose transport in skeletal muscle. Am J Physiol Endocrinol Metab 1997;273:E1039–51.

83. Young ME, Radda GK, Leighton B. Nitric oxide stimulates glucose transport and metabolism in rat skeletal muscle in vitro. Biochem J 1997;322:223–8.

84. Williams SB, Cusco JA, Roddy M-A et al. Impaired nitric oxide-mediated vasodilation in patients with non-insulin-dependent diabetes mellitus. J Am Coll Cardiol 1996;27:567–74.

85. Steinberg HO, Chaker H, Leaming R et al. Obesity/insulin resistance is associated with endothelial dysfunction. Implications for the syndrome of insulin resistance. J Clin Invest 1996;97:2601–10.

86. Hogikyan RV, Galecki AT, Pitt B et al. Specific impairment of endothelium-dependent vasodilation in subjects with type 2 diabetes independent of obesity. J Clin Endocrinol Metab 1998;83:1946–52.

87. Nitenberg A, Paycha F, Ledoux S et al. Coronary artery responses to physiological stimuli are improved by deferroxamine but not by L-arginine in non-insulin-dependent diabetic patients with angiographically normal coronary arteries and no other risk factors. Circulation 1998;97:736–43.

88. Makimattila B, Liu M-L, Vakkilainen J et al. Impaired endothelium-dependent vasodilation in type 2 diabetes: relation to LDL size, oxidized LDL, and antioxidants. Diabetes Care 1999;22:973–81.

89. Tooke JE, Goh KL. Vascular function in Type 2 diabetes mellitus and pre-diabetes: the case for intrinsic endotheliopathy. Diabet Med 1999;16:710–15.

90. Caballero AE, Arora S, Saouaf R et al. Microvascular and macrovascular reactivity is reduced in subjects at risk for type 2 diabetes. Diabetes 1999;48:1856–62.

91. Stehouwer CDA, Lambert J, Donker AJM, Van HV. Endothelial dysfunction and pathogenesis of diabetic angiopathy. Cardiovasc Res 1997;34:55–68.

92. Koya D, King GL. Protein kinase C activation and the development of diabetic complications. Diabetes 1998;47:859–66.

93. King GL, Wakasaki H. Theoretical mechanisms by which hyperglycemia and insulin resistance could cause cardiovascular diseases in diabetes. Diabetes Care 1999;22:C31–7.

94. Laakso M. Hyperglycemia as a risk factor for cardiovascular disease in type 2 diabetes. Prim Care Clin Office Pract 1999;26:829–39.

95. Williams SB, Goldfine AB, Timimi FK et al. Acute hyperglycemia attenuates endothelium-dependent vasodilation in humans in vivo. Circulation 1998;97:1695–701.
96. Van Veen S, Frolich M, Chang PC. Acute hyperglycaemia in the forearm induces vasodilation that is not modified by hyperinsulinaemia. J Hum Hypertens 1999;13:263–8.
97. Sobrevia L, Nadal A, Yudilevich DL, Mann GE. Activation of L-arginine transport (system y+) and nitric oxide synthase by elevated glucose and insulin in human endothelial cells. J Physiol 1996;490:775–81.
98. Graier WF, Wascher TC, Lackner L et al. Exposure to elevated D-glucose concentrations modulates vascular endothelial cell vasodilatatory response. Diabetes 1993;42:1497–505.
99. Sobrevia L, Yudilevich DL, Mann GE. Elevated D-glucose induces insulin insensitivity in human umbilical endothelial cells isolated from gestational diabetic pregnancies. J Physiol 1998;506:219–30.
100. Yudkin JS. Abnormalities of coagulation and fibrinolysis in insulin resistance. Diabetes Care 1999;22:C25–30.
101. Schneider DJ. Acceleration of atherosclerosis by abnormalities in thrombosis and fibrinolysis associated with diabetes mellitus. Curr Opin Endocrinol Diabetes 1998;5:75–9.
102. Carmassi F, Morale M, Ferrini L et al. Local insulin infusion stimulates expression of plasminogen activator inhibitor-1 and tissue-type plasminogen activator in normal subjects. Am J Med 1999;107:344–50.
103. Gray RP, Yudkin JS, Patterson DL. Plasminogen activator inhibitor: a risk factor for myocardial infarction in diabetic patients. Br Heart J 1993;69:228–32.
104. Gray RP, Patterson DLH, Yudkin JS. Plasminogen activator inhibitor activity in diabetic and nondiabetic survivors of myocardial infarction. Arterio Thromb 1993;13:415–20.
105. Alessi MC, Peiretti F, Morange P et al. Production of plasminogen activator inhibitor 1 by human adipose tissue: possible link between visceral fat accumulation and vascular disease. Diabetes 1997;46:860–7.
106. Juhan-Vague I, Thompson SG, Jespersen J. Involvement of the hemostatic system in the insulin resistance syndrome: a study of 500 patients with angina pectoris. Arterio Thromb 1993;13:1865–73.
107. Landin K, Tengborn L, Smith U. Elevated fibrinogen and plasminogen activator inhibitor (PAI-1) in hypertension are related to metabolic risk factors for cardiovascular disease. J Intern Med 1990;227:273–8.
108. Schmidt MI, Duncan BB, Sharrett AR et al. Markers of inflammation and prediction of diabetes mellitus in adults (Atherosclerosis Risk in Communities study): a cohort study. Lancet 1999;353:1649–52.
109. Mandal S, Sarode R, Das S, Dash RJ. Hyperaggregation of platelets detected in whole blood platelet aggregometry in newly diagnosed non-insulin dependent diabetes mellitus. Am J Clin Pathol 1993;100:103–7.

110. Kahn NN, Bauman WA, Hatcher VB, Sinha AK. Inhibition of platelet aggregation and the stimulation of prostacyclin synthesis by insulin in humans. Am J Physiol 1993;265:H2160–7.

111. Trovati M, Massucco P, Mattiello L et al. Insulin increases guanosine-3′,5′-cyclic monophosphate in human platelets: a mechanism involved in the insulin anti-aggregating effect. Diabetes 1994;43:1015–19.

112. Trovati M, Mularoni EM, Burzacca S et al. Impaired insulin-induced platelet antiaggregating effect in obesity and in obese NIDDM patients. Diabetes 1995;44:1318–22.

113. Anfossi G, Mularoni EM, Burzacca S et al. Platelet resistance to nitrates in obesity and obese NIDDM, and normal platelet sensitivity to both insulin and nitrates in lean NIDDM. Diabetes Care 1998;21:121–6.

114. Ross R. The pathogenesis of atherosclerosis: a perspective for the 1990s. Nature 1993;362:801–9.

115. Peraldi P, Spiegelman B. TNF-alpha and insulin resistance: summary and future prospects. Mol Cell Biochem 1998;182:169–75.

116. Bhagat K, Collier J, Vallance P. Endothelial stunning following a brief exposure to endotoxin: a mechanism to link infection with infarction? Cardiovasc Res 1996;32:822–9.

117. Wang P, Ba ZE, Chaudry IH. Administration of tumour necrosis factor-alpha in vivo depresses endothelium-dependent relaxation. Am J Physiol 1994;266:H2535–41.

118. Yudkin JS, Stehouwer CDA, Emeis JJ, Coppack SW. C-reactive protein in healthy subjects: associations with obesity, insulin resistance, and endothelial dysfunction: a potential role for cytokines originating from adipose tissue? Arterio Thromb Vasc Biol 1999;19:972–8.

119. Cleland S J, Sattar N, Petrie JR et al. Endothelial dysfunction as a possible link between CRP levels and cardiovascular disease. Clin Sci 2000;98:531–5.

120. Byrne CD. Triglyceride-rich lipoproteins: are links with atherosclerosis mediated by a procoagulant and proinflammatory phenotype? Atherosclerosis 1999;145:1–15.

121. Vallance P, Collier J, Bhaga, K. Infection, inflammation and infarction: does acute endothelial dysfunction provide a link? Lancet 1997;349:1391–2..

122. Piatti PM, Monti LD, Zavaroni I et al. Alterations in nitric oxide/cyclic-GMP pathway in nondiabetic siblings of patients with type 2 diabetes. J Clin Endocrinol Metab 2000;85:2416–20.

chapter 2

Diabetic autonomic neuropathy and the cardiovascular system

Paul G McNally and Ian G Lawrence

Introduction

Cardiovascular autonomic neuropathy plays a major role in the increased morbidity and mortality in patients with diabetes. Cardiovascular disease accounts for about 70% of all deaths in people with diabetes,[1] and both sudden death and silent myocardial infarction have been attributed to cardiovascular autonomic neuropathy. Historically, cardiovascular autonomic neuropathy was thought to be a late complication of diabetes, but the advent of new non-invasive techniques has shown that autonomic changes often occur early in the course of the disease.

Using standard tests of autonomic function, a prevalence of cardiac autonomic neuropathy in diabetic patients of up to 20–40% has been reported.[2] Although most patients with abnormal autonomic function are asymptomatic, postural hypotension and cardiac complications are a major problem for some patients. Risk factors for cardiac autonomic neuropathy include hyperglycaemia, hypertension, dyslipidaemia, age, body mass index, smoking and physical fitness.[3] The potential role that cardiac autonomic dysfunction plays in sudden and unexpected death in young patients with type 1 diabetes has been highlighted.[4] Sudden death is a devastating complication, albeit rare. Nonetheless, most physicians dealing with patients affected by diabetes will be familiar with this scenario. The cause of unexpected and sudden death is ill defined, but evidence is beginning to accrue to implicate both cardiac autonomic dysfunction and concomitant hypoglycaemia. This chapter will review the aetiology, natural history and consequences of autonomic neuropathy and the cardiovascular system.

Aetiology of autonomic neuropathy

Poor metabolic control over long periods is the major factor precipitating autonomic nerve injury. The prevalence of abnormal autonomic function tests was shown to be significantly less in those patients in the intensive glycaemic control group of the Diabetes Control and Complications Trial.[5] The R–R interval variation was less abnormal in the intensively treated group of type 1 patients compared to conventionally treated (5% with abnormal results at around 4 to 6 years versus 9%, respectively—a 44% relative reduction). Tight glycaemic control not only influenced the development of abnormal results in those without abnormality at the onset (primary intervention group) but also in those with evidence of abnormal results at the outset (secondary intervention group; Fig. 2.1). The prevalence of autonomic neuropathy rises with duration of diabetes, in parallel with distal symmetrical neuropathy.[6] It is estimated that symptoms of autonomic neuropathy increase from 4% after 1 year of diabetes to around 28% after 5 years in patients with type 1 diabetes.[7] Some researchers have suggested an immunological basis for autonomic nerve injury in some patients with type 1 diabetes. Circulating autoantibodies against sympathetic ganglia and infiltration of these ganglia with immune cells have been documented.[8–13] However, the prevalence of autoantibodies to autonomic nervous tissue structures (to vagus nerve, sympathetic ganglia and adrenal medulla) in patients with type 1 diabetes failed to identify an association with the presence

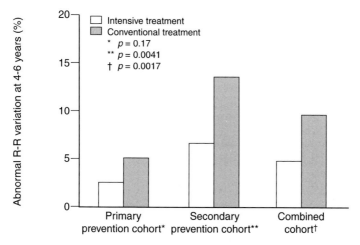

Figure 2.1 *Prevalence of abnormal R–R variation after 4 to 6 years of DCCT therapy. The intensive treatment group are shown in white, and the conventional treatment group in grey. *p = 0.17; **p = 0.0041; +p = 0.0017.*

of complications, including retinopathy, peripheral neuropathy and nephropathy.[12] Thus, this mechanism of injury is likely to play only a minor role, if any, for the majority of patients with autonomic neuropathy.

The prominent role of dysglycaemia has been recently highlighted in the pathogenesis of cardiovascular disease in a number of population studies.[14,15] Increased cardiovascular mortality has been demonstrated in non-diabetic subjects with either impaired glucose tolerance or fasting blood glucose levels in the upper normal range. A recent cross-sectional study in healthy adult volunteers demonstrated reduced autonomic function (using spectral analysis baroreflex sensitivity) associated with high normal fasting blood glucose levels.[15] However, this correlation was not significant after accounting for confounding factors. In contrast, a highly significant correlation was demonstrated between fasting insulin levels and autonomic dysfunction which was independent of other covariates.[15] It is possible that hyperinsulinaemia is a more important risk factor than hyperglycaemia in the early development of cardiovascular autonomic neuropathy.[16]

Others have shown that fasting hyperinsulinaemia more strongly predicts parasympathetic neuropathy in newly diagnosed type 2 diabetic patients than fasting blood glucose.[17] However, improved autonomic function has been demonstrated in patients who achieved improved glycaemic control over a year.[18] Further studies are required to examine the role of hyperinsulinaemia and cardiovascular autonomic neuropathy in type 2 diabetes, and therapeutic interventions such as the thiazolidinedione agents whose actions include reducing hyperinsulinaemia.

Natural history of cardiac autonomic neuropathy

Although autonomic dysfunction can be detected in up to 40% of patients with diabetes, only a small percentage will have symptoms attributable to the neuropathy. Patients with symptomatic autonomic neuropathy have a poor prognosis.[19–21] It has been recognized for several decades that patients with cardiac autonomic neuropathy secondary to diabetes sometimes die a sudden and unexpected death without an obvious cause apparent at autopsy.[20,21] Page and Watkins described 12 cases of cardiorespiratory arrests occurring in eight young patients aged between 31 and 41 years with diabetes and severe autonomic neuropathy.[20] No evidence of myocardial infarction, cardiac arrhythmia or hypoglycaemia was present at the time of arrest. Instead, they suggested that the arrests were precipitated by a defective respiratory rather than cardiovascular reflex pathway. In most of these cases, some interference with respiration was documented, either by anaesthetic agents, drugs or intrinsic lung disease. This led them to suggest that normal respiratory reflexes were impaired in diabetic autonomic neuropathy, although little evidence supports this hypothesis in the literature. Catterell et al reported that apnoea, hypopnoea and oxygen desaturation during sleep are no more common in patients with diabetes and significant autonomic neuropathy than in patients with diabetes of the same age without autonomic neuropathy.[22] Although other groups have reported breathing abnormalities in patients with diabetes and autonomic neuropathy, most studies were not rigorously controlled for natural variation in sleep patterns.[23,24] In patients with progressive autonomic failure with multiple system atrophy (Shy-Drager syndrome), there is an increased incidence of sleep apnoea, but in contrast to patients with diabetes, these patients have evidence of central autonomic neuropathy.[25] It seems unlikely that the unexplained deaths of patients with diabetes and autonomic neuropathy are due to disorders of breathing during sleep.

Ewing and colleagues described the natural history of autonomic neuropathy occurring in 73 patients who presented with symptoms suggestive of autonomic failure, including postural hypotension, intermittent diarrhoea, hypoglycaemic unawareness, sweating abnormalities, gastric fullness and impotence.[21] Mortality was found to be substantially greater (53%) in those with abnormal tests of autonomic neuropathy, compared to patients with normal tests at the outset (15%) over a 5-year period. Five out of 26 deaths from the total group were described as sudden and unexpected cardiorespiratory deaths, occurring in most without a history of ischaemic heart disease or an obvious cause at autopsy. A more recent study of 237 patients with type 1 diabetes revealed a 23% mortality over a 5-year period in those with autonomic neuropathy.[26]

The presence of autonomic neuropathy is associated with and may contribute to the development of other diabetes-related complications. The prevalence and severity of autonomic neuropathy increases with developing nephropathy. Abnormal cardiovascular reflex tests are more common in patients with macroalbuminuria compared to normoalbuminuria.[27,28] Patients with microalbuminuria also show abnormalities in vagal function and sympathovagal balance.[29,30] Subtle changes in blood pressure occur, consisting of a reversal of the circadian rhythm in systolic blood pressure. Patients with type 1 diabetes display a lower nocturnal fall in systolic blood pressure than those without autonomic dysfunction.[31] Alterations in the diurnal pattern of urine output and sodium excretion have also been described in patients with diabetic autonomic neuropathy. Higher levels of urinary albumin and sodium excretion occur in patients with type 1 diabetes, possibly due to abnormal renal haemodynamic neural control.[32] Finally, it has been proposed that diabetic autonomic neuropathy may be a risk factor for the development of proliferative retinopathy via functional abnormalities in retinal blood flow.[33]

Postural hypotension

On assuming an upright posture blood pools in the legs, leading to a fall in blood pressure, and is associated with a 20–50% fall in cardiac output. Maintenance of a normal blood pressure on standing involves afferent impulses from baroreceptors and efferent sympathetic impulses to the heart and blood vessels. This reflex arc increases sympathetic vasoconstrictor tone in the peripheral and splanchnic circulations and leads to a reflex tachycardia. Both sympathetic and parasympathetic nervous pathways are involved in this mechanism. Postural hypotension is defined as a fall in systolic blood pressure of greater than 30 mm Hg. Studies in patients with diabetes show that it is a relatively uncommon finding.[34] Symptoms vary from feeling dizzy on standing to loss of consciousness. In clinical practice very few patients are severely disabled by postural symptoms. The falls in systolic blood pressure do not necessarily correlate with the severity of symptoms reported by the patient, and management can prove difficult. Patients should be advised to change posture slowly and to exercise leg muscles before standing. Therapeutic agents associated with postural hypotension should be withdrawn. Agents including fludrocortisone[35,36] and non-steroidal anti-inflammatory drugs may need to be taken to promote sodium and water retention. Attention must be paid to potential side-effects including hypokalaemia, fluid overload and supine hypertension. Some patients benefit from wearing support stockings. Occasionally, the use of midodrine, an alpha-adrenergic agonist, in doses of 2.5 to 10 mg has proved beneficial.[37]

Sudden and unexpected death in diabetes

Little is known about the extent of the problem. Tattersall and Gill[38] investigated sudden and unexplained deaths occurring in patients with type 1 diabetes under the age of 50 years over a 12-month period in 1989 in the UK. The study was initiated following the debate surrounding the use of human insulin and whether there might be a link between human insulin and sudden death in patients. Information was ascertained from a variety of sources including autopsy, medical records and staff, and relatives. A total of 50 cases of sudden death were identified during this period, of which five had a definite cause of death, eleven were attributable to deliberate self-harm and six to ketoacidosis. Of the 24 remaining deaths there were two cases of profound hypoglycaemic brain damage, leaving 22 patients in which the cause of death remained unexplained. These patients were aged 12–43 years and were reported to be in good health and in many cases had retired to bed, only to be found dead the following morning. Interestingly, most were sleeping alone at the time of death and there was little to suggest a seizure, as in virtually all cases they were found in an undisturbed bed. Three-quarters of deaths occurred during the nightime, with a history of one or more nocturnal episodes of severe hypoglycaemia in the preceding 6 months reported in 14 cases. In most cases the cause of death was attributed to hypoglycaemia, although with little or no evidence. In a cohort of patients developing type 1 diabetes under the age of 17 years in Leicestershire, UK, between 1940 and 1989, a total of six sudden and unexplained deaths were observed out of a total of 44 deaths occurring in 850 patients.[39] Other case reports and groups elsewhere have similarly described sudden and unexplained death in type 1 patients.[4,40,41]

Mortality and QT interval prolongation

In view of the documented association of cardiac autonomic neuropathy and sudden death, attention has focused on the electrophysiology of the cardiac cycle in patients with diabetes. The QT interval has commanded much interest, as abnormalities in this component of cardiac cycle are known to be associated with sudden death in two distinct conditions, the long QT syndrome and sudden infant death syndrome.[42] Subsequently, reports appeared in the literature demonstrating that QT interval prolongation did occur in patients with cardiac autonomic neuropathy secondary to diabetes.[43–49] In a cross-sectional evaluation of 3250 patients with type 1 diabetes from the EURODIAB IDDM complication study the QTc interval was assessed in one lead (V_5) and it was demonstrated that QTc was independently related to gender, age, $HbA1_C$ and blood pressure.[49]

Ewing and co-workers demonstrated that changes in QT interval length with duration of diabetes parallel changes in autonomic function and, more importantly, diabetic subjects with autonomic neuropathy who subsequently die have longer QT intervals than those who survive.[50] More specifically, in diabetic patients with clinical autonomic neuropathy, QT interval prolongation has been demonstrated and it has been proposed that it may have a role in sudden cardiac death in these patients.[45,50] Similarly, a long-term follow-up of type 1 diabetic patients with hypertension and diabetic nephropathy found that QT interval was an important risk marker for mortality, and furthermore that sudden and unexpected deaths occurred only in patients with a maximal QT interval equal to or above $450\,\mathrm{ms}^{-1}$.[51,52] It is important to note that QT interval prolongation may also occur secondary to myocardial injury inducing abnormalities in cardiac repolarization, which also increase the risk of ventricular arrhythmias developing.[53]

The interlead variability of QT interval, also known as QT dispersion, has also been proposed as a measure of arrhythmic risk in a number of settings.[54] QT dispersion relates to a variety of factors including possible underlying ischaemia, left ventricular dilatation, left ventricular hypertrophy, myocardial fibrosis and autonomic neuropathy. However, few data exist about the role of the autonomic nervous system and dispersion of the QT interval. In a study of 13 patients with diabetic nephropathy it was demonstrated that severe autonomic neuropathy is associated with increased QT dispersion,[55] although many of these patients had evidence of coronary heart disease and other cardiac problems that could have been responsible for the observed increase in QT dispersion. However, in a recent study of the Dundee UKPDS participants, QT interval and QTc dispersion were shown to be accurate predictors of cardiac death in patients with newly diagnosed type 2 diabetes (patients with overt cardiac disease having been excluded).[56] Indeed, recent studies suggest that QTc dispersion is a better predictor of mortality in type 2 diabetes than maximum QTc duration.[56,57] Sawicki and colleagues have speculated that autonomic neuropathy and subsequent sympathetic imbalance leading to QTc max prolongation is of greater importance in type 1 diabetes, whereas in type 2 diabetes focal myocardial ischaemia or fibrosis increasing the QTc dispersion is more important.[57]

Assessment of cardiovascular autonomic neuropathy

The early identification of diabetic autonomic neuropathy is clinically important in view of the associated high mortality. Assessment of cardiac autonomic neuropathy may be evaluated using a battery of relatively simple, bedside, non-invasive cardiovascular reflexes, which require active co-operation of the patient (Table 2.1).[2] Using these simple bedside tests, autonomic neuropathy is found in 20–40% of unselected patients with diabetes. These tests involve the measurement of heart rate changes induced by manoeuvres that affect vagal and sympathetic influences of the heart and systemic vascular resistance (Fig. 2.2). These tests include determining the ratio of maximum to minimum heart rate variation during deep breathing (I/E ratio), the ratio of maximum to minimum R–R interval during the Valsalva manoeuvre, the heart rate response to standing (30:15 ratio) and the blood pressure response to standing and sustained hand grip.

Valsalva manoeuvre
Subjects are asked to undertake a forced expiration at 40 mm Hg for 15 seconds into a mouthpiece connected to a pressure-monitoring device,

Table 2.1 Bedside tests of cardiovascular autonomic function

Test	Normal response	Abnormal response
Heart-rate variation during deep breathing		
■ Maximum–minimum (bpm)	>15	<10
Heart-rate increase on standing		
■ 15 s after standing (bpm)	>15	<12
■ 30:15 ratio	>1.04	<1.00
Heart-rate during Valsalva		
■ Maximum:minimum ratio	>1.21	<1.10
Postural fall in systolic BP		
■ 2 min after standing (mm Hg)	<10	>30
Diastolic rise in BP after sustained handgrip (30% of maximum) for up to 5 min (mm Hg)	>16	<10

such as a mercury sphygmomanometer. The mean ratio of the maximum to minimum R–R interval during the manoeuvre for three consecutive manoeuvres is defined as the Valsalva ratio. The Valsalva manoeuvre consists of four phases. Phase 1 is a short-lasting increase in heart rate and systolic blood pressure, after taking a deep breath before blowing. Phase 2 occurs as intrathoracic pressure rises during forced expiration. During this phase cardiac output falls due to a reduction in venous return, leading to a fall in blood pressure and increase in heart rate. Phase 3 occurs after release of the strain, producing a further fall in blood pressure. Finally, phase 4 occurs when intrathoracic pressure falls after release of the strain, leading to an increase in venous return and

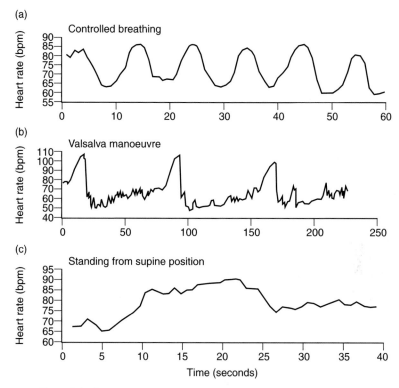

Figure 2.2 *Cardiovascular reflex tests for detecting autonomic neuropathy (bpm = beats per minute).*

increase in cardiac output. The increased cardiac output is forced into a vascular system that is constricted, leading to an increase in blood pressure and a reflex bradycardia. This manoeuvre assesses the parasympathetic (phase 4) and sympathetic (phase 2) arms of the autonomic nervous system as well as the whole of the baroreflex mechanism. The heart-rate change during the Valsalva manoeuvre (the Valsalva ratio) is greater than 1.21 in normal and less than 1.20 in abnormal subjects.

Heart-rate response to standing

Standing from a supine position results in a predominantly parasympathetically mediated response in heart rate. There is a rapid increase in heart rate on standing, peaking around the fifteenth beat after assuming an upright posture. Subsequently, a relative bradycardia ensues that is maximal around the thirtieth beat. The maximal heart-rate peak is predominantly mediated by withdrawal of vagal tone, although enhanced sympathetic outflow to the sinus node also contributes to this response. The test is performed by asking the patient to stand from the supine position, with the electrocardiogram recording continuously. The ratio of the longest R–R interval (around the thirtieth beat after standing) to the shortest R–R interval is expressed as the 30:15 ratio. The heart-rate increase on standing is normally greater than 15 beats per minute, with the 30:15 ratio being greater than 1.04 in normal subjects and less than 1.00 in abnormal cases.

Heart-rate response to deep breathing

Heart rate continually varies in normal healthy subjects, mostly with respiration. Normally, heart rate accelerates during inspiration and decelerates during expiration (sinus arrhythmia), with these fluctuations under cardiac parasympathetic control. In patients with cardiac parasympathetic neuropathy heart rate variability decreases. The test is performed by asking the subject to breathe deeply and evenly at six breaths per minute for one minute (breathing in for 5 seconds and out for 5 seconds). The maximum and minimum heart rate during the cycles is calculated and the differences during three successive cycles are averaged. The normal response is for a heart-rate variation during deep breathing of greater than 15 beats per minute, with less than 10 beats per minutes representing an abnormal response.

Blood pressure response to standing

On assuming an upright posture blood pools in the legs, leading to a fall in blood pressure. A reflex tachycardia, and peripheral and splanchnic vasoconstriction rapidly correct this fall in blood pressure. Both sympathetic and parasympathetic nervous pathways are involved in this mechanism. The test is performed by measuring the blood pressure with the patient supine and one minute after standing. A fall in systolic pressure exceeding 30 mm Hg is abnormal, invariably causing postural symptoms.

Blood pressure response to sustained handgrip

Isometric exercise raises blood pressure by stimulating sympathetic efferent pathways and is assessed by sustaining a handgrip of one-third of maximum voluntary contract for 3 to 4 minutes using a handgrip dynamer. Blood pressure is measured each minute and the difference between diastolic blood pressure before starting and just before release of the handgrip is taken as a measure of the response. A normal response is a rise above 16 mm Hg in diastolic pressure from just before release of the hand grip. A rise of less than 10 mm Hg is regarded as an abnormal result.

These tests have been and are widely used in clinical practice. Age-adjusted normal ranges have been produced.[2] However, the sensitivity of these tests is a major limitation.[58] It has been assumed that the tests of heart rate variability were tests of parasympathetic function and blood pressure responses sympathetic function. As shown above, the Valsalva manoeuvre represents the combined effects of all aspects of the autonomic system. Therefore, more sensitive techniques, using power spectral analysis of heart rate variability, have evolved in recent times to help identify cardiac autonomic neuropathy, and also provide an assessment of the relative vagal and sympathetic components of the cardiac cycle.[59,60] Using these new techniques, baro-receptor–cardiac reflex sensitivity, a measure of cardiac autonomic function, may be calculated to assess cardiac autonomic function in patients with diabetes.[61,62]

Baroreflex sensitivity

The baroreceptors are located at the carotid sinus and are stimulated by stretch of the arterial walls, which is caused by a rise in arterial pressure. Stimulation of the carotid sinus leads to a slowing of heart rate and peripheral vasodilatation, both actions reducing the blood pressure. Baroreflex sensitivity was originally measured in humans by monitoring the rise in systolic blood pressure and the lengthening of the R–R interval, in response to alpha-adrenoreceptor stimulation by phenylephrine. Thus baroreflex sensitivity is calculated by measuring the changes in the R–R interval, which are produced in reflex to acute pharmacological-induced changes in blood pressure.[63,64] The initial studies required arterial cannulation for the measurement of changes in blood pressure responses, but this limitation has been overcome by the non-invasive measurement of beat-to-beat blood pressure, using a computer-based system incorporating a device called the Finapres.[65] This device uses a modified version of the volume clamp method and reliably records beat-to-beat blood pressure non-invasively from a digital artery, allowing data recording up to 30 minutes. The administration of pharmacological agents to assess the baroreflex sensitivity has the theoretical disadvantage of altering the viscoelastic properties of the aorta and thus potentially influencing indirectly baroreflex sensitivity.[66] The more recent approach using the Finapres has been validated against intra-arterial recordings and the slope of the regression line between systolic blood pressure and pulse interval changes is taken as an index of baroreflex sensitivity.[67] The Finapres can be used to measure baroreflex sensitivity using several methods, including during phase IV of the Valsalva manoeuvre, time domain analysis and power spectral analysis.[68]

To help clarify the extent and nature of cardiac autonomic dysfunction in diabetes, we investigated a group of 30 patients with type 1 diabetes. Power spectral analysis of heart rate variability was used in order to identify individual contributions to heart rate and blood pressure variability made by the sympathetic and parasympathetic nervous system, and compared to the standard bedside tests of autonomic function.[69] Thirty control subjects were matched for age, sex and systolic blood pressure to the type 1 patients and autonomic function was assessed using both spectral analysis and the five standard tests of autonomic function. None of the subjects or patients had any evidence of autonomic neuropathy as assessed by the standard tests. However, spectral analysis of heart rate variability revealed significant abnormalities in cardiac autonomic function. Power spectral analysis was able to demonstrate that there were

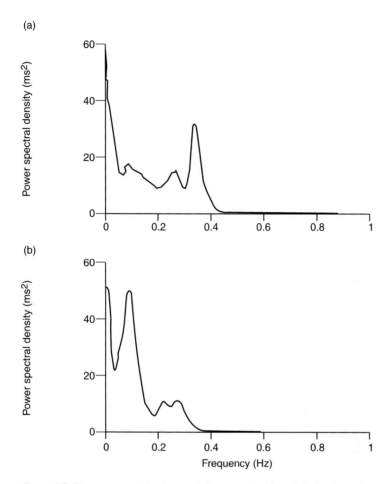

Figure 2.3 *Power spectral density graph for control subjects (a) showing a low-frequency band (0.02–0.035 Hz). Power spectral density graph for type I diabetic subjects; (b), matched for age and systolic blood pressure to the control subjects, showing a significant reduction in the high frequency band (parasympathetic tone).*

significant reductions in the absolute values of low frequency (predominantly sympathetic tone) and high frequency (parasympathetic tone) powers in the patients with diabetes compared to the control group (Fig. 2.3). The ratio of the low-frequency to high-frequency power, which is a measure of sympathovagal balance,[70,71]

49

was significantly higher in the diabetic population and implies a relative sympathetic predominance in this group. Similar sympathetic predominance has already been associated with increased mortality in patients after acute myocardial infarction.[72–76] In the ATRAMI study, post-myocardial infarction mortality was significantly higher in the group of patients with a low baroreflex sensitivity, consistent with altered autonomic balance in favour of sympathetic tone.[76] Impairment of parasympathetic function leading to a relative overactivity of the sympathetic nervous system is considered to be the underlying reason for elevated mortality, thus increasing the risk of ventricular arrhythmias. Vagal activity plays an important protective role in the prevention of malignant ventricular arrhythmias. Thus, it is conceivable that susceptibility to sudden death in patients with diabetes is the result of an increased risk of developing ventricular arrhythmias from overactivity of the sympathetic nervous system relative to parasympathetic tone. This hypothesis gains support from clinical studies which demonstrate the powerful secondary preventative effects of beta-blockers in patients with diabetes after myocardial infarction (see page 56).[77] Evidence of sympathetic overactivity also comes from studies that have reported raised plasma noradrenaline levels in patients with poorly controlled diabetes.[78] In patients with symptomatic diabetic autonomic neuropathy and no evidence of ischaemic heart disease, abnormal ventricular systolic function has been also demonstrated by radionucleotide techniques.[79] Similarly, in type 1 patients with poor metabolic control, echocardiographic evidence of abnormal left ventricular function can be demonstrated and is associated with adrenergic hypersensitivity.[80]

Baroreflex sensitivity derived from the resting heart rate and systolic blood pressure data was also significantly reduced in the patients with diabetes studied, even in those patients of 5 years or less duration.[69] A low baroreflex sensitivity was directly related to duration of diabetes ($p < 0.001$), and inversely related to average glycated haemoglobin ($p < 0.05$). Interestingly, a significant inverse relationship was shown to exist between left ventricular mass and baroreflex sensitivity in type 1 patients with diabetes.[81] Abnormalities of baroreflex sensitivity in rats have been associated also with an increase in left ventricular mass independent of blood pressure.[82] This increase in left ventricular mass index might be secondary to relative sympathetic overactivity. In other clinical settings, increased left ventricular mass has been associated with risk of sudden death.[83,84] Thus the use of spectral analysis methods enabled the detection of a significant abnormality of autonomic function in a group of young asymptomatic insulin patients with type 1 diabetes that went undetected using the traditional tests of autonomic function, suggesting an abnormality of parasympathetic function. These autonomic abnormalities in cardiac autonomic neuropathy have also been reported in children with diabetes, in some cases from the first year after diagnosis, using power spectral analysis.[85,86] An increased prevalence of autonomic nerve dysfunction is evident in adolescent patients with microalbuminuria and in this group may prove to be a marker for those at higher risk of early renal complications.[87] Similarly, a study of middle aged patients with longstanding type 1 diabetes complicated by microalbuminuria demonstrated impaired baroreflex sensitivity compared to their normoalbuminuric counterparts.[88]

Earlier studies investigating the circadian rhythm of sympathovagal balance in patients with diabetes have found evidence of an increase in sympathetic activity in the morning and a relative decrease in parasympathetic tone during the night.[89] An increase in cardiovascular events during night time is reported in patients with type 2 diabetes, raising the possibility that the alterations in sympathovagal activity, in favour of sympathetic overactivity, may be in part responsible.[90] Thus, it is interesting to speculate that the increased incidents of sudden death in type 1 patients[38,91,92] could be due to abnormal baroreflex sensitivity promoting an increase in left ventricular mass and hence, an increased risk of sudden cardiac death. Nonetheless, we recently described a sudden and unexpected death in a 31-year-old man with type 1 diabetes who had normal left ventricular mass, but in whom the baroreflex sensitivity was extremely low.[4] Also, it is possible that nocturnal hypoglycaemia (see below) increases the sympathetic tone, over and above the increased sympathovagal balance demonstrated in diabetes, and hence has a proarrhythmic effect. In patients with type 1 diabetes, we have shown QTc interval prolongation and baroreflex sensitivity to be inversely related.[93] This supports the proposed association between autonomic neuropathy and cardiac repolarization,[43–49] although others have been unable to confirm such a relationship.[94–96] However, a recent meta-analysis has demonstrated that autonomic failure was 2.26 times (95% CI 1.90–2.70) more likely to be present in diabetic patients with than in patients without QTc prolongation.[97] It is thus plausible that the abnormalities in autonomic function induced by diabetes lead to prolongation of cardiac repolarization, and that this abnormality of cardiac repolarization increases the risk of developing malignant ventricular arrhythmias.

Alternative methods to assess cardiovascular autonomic neuropathy

The myocardial uptake of meta-iodobenzylguanidine (MIBG) is a technique that allows evaluation of cardiac sympathetic neuropathy by measuring post-ganglionic presynaptic noradrenergic uptake. Radio-iodinated MIBG serves as an analogue of noradrenaline and shares the same uptake and storage mechanisms without being metabolized. It can be used to image organs, such as the heart, which are rich in sympathetic innervation. Significant reductions in MIBG uptake have been reported in patients with type 1 diabetes and symptomatic autonomic neuropathy.[98] However, the sensitivity of the technique is debatable. Studies in patients with normal bedside tests of autonomic function have also reported abnormal MIBG scans,[99] although as indicated above, the sensitivity of bedside testing of autonomic injury is suspect. Abnormal ventricular function is also associated with abnormalities in MIBG scanning, further compromising the validity of this method of assessing autonomic cardiovascular function.

Effect of hypoglycaemia on cardiac function

In normal humans hypoglycaemia provokes an intense haemodynamic response.[100] In the patient with diabetes and concomitant macrovascular disease the cardiovascular stress of hypoglycaemia may have serious or even fatal consequences.[101] Although some of the deaths associated with severe hypoglycaemia are a direct result of neuroglycopenic injury to the brain, it is possible that a significant proportion of hypoglycaemia-induced sudden deaths are caused by cardiovascular events precipitated by the physiological stress as a consequence. Anecdotal cases report the pro-arrhythmic affect of hypoglycaemia.[102–104] A variety of arrhythmias are reported, including an increase in ectopic foci of atrial, ventricular and nodal origins. Atrial fibrillation was first described during experimental hypoglycaemia in non-diabetic patients with heart disease,[105] and was observed during insulin shock therapy for schizophrenia.[106] In patients with diabetes and coronary heart disease, atrial fibrillation has been described during experimentally induced hypoglycaemia[104] and case reports of documented atrial fibrillation occurring during accidental hypoglycaemia in diabetic patients with and without overt clinical evidence of heart disease.[105–107] In most cases the cardiac rhythm returned spontaneously to sinus rhythm rapidly with the correction of hypoglycaemia. Few serious arrhythmias have been recorded, but Judson and Hollander[108] described an episode of transient ventricular tachycardia during experimental hypoglycaemia in a non-diabetic patient with coronary heart disease, which spontaneously reverted to sinus rhythm. There are no reported episodes of sustained ventricular tachycardia or fibrillation occurring in diabetic patients during hypoglycaemia in the literature, however, development of malignant arrhythmias secondary to hypoglycaemia remains a possible mechanism of sudden death. One study has found an increase in the QTc interval during experimentally-induced hypoglycaemia,[109] making it possible that nocturnal hypoglycaemia further prolongs the QTc and increases the risk of developing malignant ventricular arrhythmias. Furthermore, a fatal cardiac arrest is described in a 56-year-old man with type 1 diabetes following acute hypoglycaemia, presumed secondary to a malignant ventricular arrhythmia.[110] Paradoxically, acute *hyperglycaemia*

53

has also been shown to produce significant increments of QTc and QTc dispersion in normal subjects, with endogenously released insulin apparently playing a minor role.[111] Nevertheless, attention thus far has focused upon hypoglycaemia, and in particular nocturnal hypoglycaemia.[112]

There are several potential mechanisms whereby hypoglycaemia may increase the sympathetic drive with consequent secretion of catecholamines promoting an increase in ectopic activity.[113] Acute hypoglycaemia is associated with a fall in serum potassium, which may provoke or pre-dispose to cardiac arrhythmias. Insulin has a direct inotropic effect on the myocardium and might directly promote atrial ectopic activity. The heart uses glucose as a substrate and it is possible that the arrhythmia might be provoked by localized glucopenia affecting the myocardium or conducting tissue. Furthermore, an arrhythmia might occur secondary to myocardial ischaemia.

Sudden death: potential therapeutic interventions

Tight glycaemic control and attention to other vascular risk factors is likely to reduce the risk of cardiac autonomic dysfunction, although the risk of hypoglycaemia may be increased.[5] However, agents that augment intrinsic cardiac parasympathetic activity might confer a beneficial effect. One group of drugs, angiotensin converting enzyme (ACE) inhibitors, has recently been shown not only to improve mortality in heart failure, but also to improve heart rate variability, baroreflex sensitivity and QT dispersion in heart failure.[114] Furthermore, it has recently been demonstrated that the ACE inhibitor quinopril administered over a 3-month period to patients with diabetic autonomic neuropathy increased parasympathetic activity as measured using heart rate variability.[115] Other studies in normotensive men and patients with congestive heart failure have shown that therapy with ACE inhibitors may increase vagal and decrease sympathetic tone.[116] These effects were attributed to an increase in efferent vagal tone through baroreflex sensitivity, haemodynamic and symptomatic improvement and reduction of angiotensin II levels. The failure to demonstrate an improvement with trandolapril in patients with type 1 and type 2 diabetes may relate to the use of insensitive techniques in the assessment of autonomic neuropathy.[117]

Beta-blockers are also associated with a significant reduction in mortality in diabetes[77] and have a beneficial effect in patients with idiopathic QT interval prolongation.[118] This protective action may relate to a direct reduction in sympathetic overactivity and/or an increase in vagal tone, both of which occur with beta-blocker therapy,[119] as well as a reduction in arrhythmias[120] (Table 2.2). This beneficial effect is evident only with agents without intrinsic sympathomimetic activity (metoprolol,[121] timolol[122] and propranolol[123]) and not with those with intrinsic sympathomimetic activity (pindolol[124]). Similarly, certain drugs which increase heart rate variability are associated with a beneficial effect on survival and sudden cardiac death (ACE inhibitors[113]), while others have a detrimental effect by decreasing heart rate variability (class Ic anti-arrhythmic agents[125]). Intervention studies are urgently required in patients with diabetes and cardiac autonomic neuropathy to assess the potential benefit of both ACE inhibitors and beta-blocker therapy on baroreflex sensitivity and sympathovagal balance, as well as longer term studies to assess mortality.

Conclusions

Autonomic neuropathy affecting the cardiovascular system has important implications for patients with diabetes mellitus. More sensitive techniques to assess cardiac autonomic function have revealed that many patients of short duration of diabetes already have abnormalities of neural control. Recent evidence implicates a role for cardiac autonomic dysfunction promoting a shift towards sympathetic activity, which in turn increases the risk of left ventricular hypertrophy, malignant ventricular arrhythmias and sudden death.

Table 2.2 The effect of therapeutic agents on cardiac function, mortality and sudden death

Therapeutic drug	Actions	Effects on mortality and sudden death
Beta-blockers (without intrinsic sympathomimetic activity)	↑ HRV ↓ Sympathetic activity ↑ Vagal tone[117] ↓ Arrhythmias[118]	Metoprolol ↓ post-MI SCD by 40%[121] Timolol ↓ incidence of SCD post-MI by 44%[122] Propranolol ↓ post-MI SCD by 28%[123]
Beta-blockers (with intrinsic sympathomimetic activity)	↓ HRV[123]	↑ Mortality in diabetic patients[125]
ACE inhibitors	↑ Vagal tone ↓ Sympathetic tone ↑ HRV, BRS and QT dispersion[115-117]	↓ Mortality in patients with CCF and post MI[11]
Class Ic antiarrhythmic agents (flecainide, encainide)	↓ HRV[125]	↑ Mortality in patients post-MI[125]

HRV, heart rate variability; MI, myocardial infarction; SCD, sudden cardiac death; BRS, baroreceptor sensitivity; CCF, congestive cardiac failure. (Adapted from D Aronson, Diabetologia 1997;40:476–481.)

References

1. Laakso M. Hyperglycaemia and cardiovascular disease in type 2 diabetes. Diabetes 1999;48:937–42.
2. Ewing DJ, Martyn CN, Young RJ et al. The value of cardiovascular autonomic function tests: a ten-year experience in diabetes. Diabetes Care 1985;8:491–8.
3. Björnholt JV, Erikssen G, Aaser E et al. Fasting blood glucose: an underestimated risk factor for cardiovascular death. Results from a 22 year follow-up of healthy non-diabetic men. Diabetes Care 1999;22:45–9.
4. Lawrence IG, Weston PJ, Bennett MA et al. Is impaired baroreflex sensitivity a predictor or cause of sudden death in insulin-dependent diabetes mellitus. Diabet Med 1997;14:82–5.
5. The Diabetes Control and Complications Trial research Group. The effect of intensive diabetes therapy on measures of autonomic nervous system function in the Diabetes Control and Complications Trial. Diabetologia 1998;41:416–23.
6. Lluch I, Hernandez A, Real JT et al. Cardiovascular autonomic neuropathy in type 1 diabetic patients with and without peripheral neuropathy. Diabetes Res Clin Pract 1998;42:35–40.
7. Canal N, Comi G, Saibene V et al. The relationship between peripheral and autonomic neuropathy in insulin-dependent diabetes: a clinical and instrumental evaluation. In: Canal N, Pozza G, eds. Peripheral Neuropathies. Elsevier, Amsterdam, 1978:247–55.
8. Duchen LW, Anjorin A, Watkin PJ, Mackay AD. Pathology of autonomic neuropathy in diabetes mellitus. Ann Int Med 1980;92:301–3.
9. Guy RJC, Richards F, Edmonds ME, Watkins PJ. Diabetic autonomic neuropathy and iritis: an association suggesting an immunological cause. BMJ 1984;289:343–5.
10. Brown FM, Watts M, Rabinow SL. Aggregation of subclinical of autonomic nervous system dysfunction and autoantibodies in families with type 1 diabetes. Diabetes 1991;40:1611.
11. Zanone MM, Peakman M, Purewal T et al. Autoantibodies to nervous tissue structures are associated with autonomic neuropathy in type 1 diabetes mellitus. Diabetologia 1993;36:564–9.
12. Ejskjaer N, Arif S, Dodds W et al. Prevalence of autoantibodies to autonomic nervous tissue structures in type 1 diabetes mellitus. Diabet Med 1999;7:544–9.
13. Muhr-Becker D, Ziegler AG, Druschky A et al. Evidence for specific autoimmunity against sympathetic and parasympathetic nervous tissues in type 1 diabetes mellitus and the relation to cardiac autonomic dysfunction. Diabet Med 1998;15:467–72.
14. Gerstein HC, Yusuf S. Dysglycaemia and risk of cardiovascular disease. Lancet 1996;347:949–50.

15. Watkins LL, Surwit RS, Grossman P, Sherwood A. Is there a glycemic threshold for impaired autonomic control? Diabetes Care 2000;23:826–30.
16. Sima AAF. Does insulin play a role in cardiovascular autonomic regulation? Diabetes Care 2000;23:724–5.
17. Toyry JP, Niskanen LK, Mantysaari MJ et al. Occurrence, predictors and clinical significance of autonomic neuropathy in NIDDM: ten year follow-up from the diagnosis. Diabetes 1996;45:308–15.
18. Vanninen E, Uusitupa M, Lansimies E et al. Effect of metabolic control on autonomic function in obese patients with newly diagnosed type 2 diabetes. Diabet Med 1993;10:66–73.
19. Watkins PJ. Diabetic autonomic neuropathy. N Engl J Med 1990;322:1078–9.
20. Page McBN, Watkins PJ. Cardio-respiratory arrest and diabetic autonomic neuropathy. Lancet 1978;i:14–16.
21. Ewing DJ, Campbell IW, Clarke BF. The natural history of diabetic and autonomic neuropathy. Quart J Med 1980;193:95–108.
22. Catterell JR, Calverley PMA, Ewing DJ et al. Breathing, sleep, and autonomic neuropathy. Diabetes 1984;33:1025–7.
23. Guilleminault C, Briskin JG, Greenfield MS, Silvestri R. The impact of autonomic nervous system dysfunction on breathing during sleep. Sleep 1981;4:263–78.
24. Rees PJ, Prior JG, Cochrane GM, Clarke TJH. Sleep apnoea in diabetic patients with autonomic neuropathy. J R Soc Med 1981;74:192–5.
25. Lockwood AH. Shy-Drager syndrome with abnormal respiration and anti-diuretic hormone release. Arch Neurol 1976;33:292–5.
26. Sampson MJ, Wilson S, Karagiannis P et al. Progression of diabetic autonomic neuropathy over a decade in insulin-dependent diabetics. Quart J Med 1990;75:635–46.
27. Zander EZ, Schulz B, Heinke P et al. Importance of cardiovascular autonomic dysfunction in IDDM subjects with diabetic nephropathy. Diabetes Care 1989;12:259–64.
28. Wirta OR, Pasternack AI, Mustonen JT et al. Urinary albumin excretion rate is independently related to autonomic neuropathy in type 2 diabetes mellitus. J Int Med 1999;245:329–35.
29. Molgaard H, Christensen PD, Hermansen K et al. Early recognition of autonomic dysfunction in microalbuminuria: significance for cardiovascular mortality in diabetes mellitus? Diabetologia 1994;37:788–96.
30. Rutter MK, McComb JM, Brady S, Marshall SM. Autonomic neuropathy in asymptomatic subjects with non-insulin-dependent diabetes mellitus and microalbuminuria. Clin Auto Res 1998;8:251–7.
31. Spalone V, Gambardella S, Maiello MR et al. Relationship between autonomic neuropathy, 24-hour blood pressure profile and nephropathy in normotensive IDDM patients. Diabetes Care 1994;17:578–84.

32. Nakano S, Uchida K, Ishii T et al. Association of nocturnal rise in plasma alpha-atrial natriuretic peptide and reversed diurnal blood pressure rhythm in hospitalised normotensive subjects with non-insulin-dependent diabetes mellitus. Eur J Endocrinol 1994;131:184–90.

33. Krowlewski AS, Barzilay J, Warram JH et al. Risk of early-onset proliferative retinopathy in IDDM is closely related to cardiovascular autonomic neuropathy. Diabetes 1992;41:430–7.

34. Purewal TS, Watkins PJ. Postural hypotension in diabetic autonomic neuropathy: a review. Diabet Med 1995;12:192–200.

35. Campbell IW, Ewing DJ, Clarke BF. 9-alpha fludrocortisone in the treatment of postural hypotension in diabetic autonomic neuropathy. Diabetes 1975;24:381–4.

36. Campbell IW, Ewing DJ, Clarke BF. Therapeutic experience with fludrocortisone in diabetic postural hypotension. BMJ 1976;1:872–4.

37. McTavish D, Goa Kl. Midodrine: a review of its therapeutic use in orthostatic hypotension and secondary hypotensive disorders. Drugs 1989;38:757–77.

38. Tattersall RB and Gill GV. Unexplained deaths of type 1 diabetic patients. Diabet Med 1991;8:49–58.

39. McNally PG, Raymond NT, Burden ML et al. Trends in mortality of childhood-onset insulin-dependent diabetes mellitus in Leicestershire 1940–91. Diabet Med 1995;12:961–6.

40. Sartor G, Nvstron L, Dedahlqvist G. The Swedish Childhood Diabetes Study: a seven fold decrease in short-term mortality? Diabet Med 1990;8:18–21.

41. Joner G, Patrick S. The mortality of children with type 1 (insulin-dependent) diabetes mellitus in Norway 1973–88. Diabetologia 1991;34:29–32.

42. Schwartz PJ. Sympathetic imbalance and cardiac arrhythmias. In: Randall WC, ed. Nervous Control of Cardiovascular Function. Oxford University Press, Oxford, 1984:225–52.

43. Khan JK, Sisson JC, Vinik AI. QT interval prolongation and sudden cardiac death in diabetic autonomic neuropathy. J Clin Endocrinol Metab 1987;64:751–4.

44. Bellevere F, Ferri M, Guarani L et al. Prolonged QT interval in diabetic autonomic neuropathy: a possible role in sudden cardiac death? Br Heart J 1988;59:379–83.

45. Ewing DJ, Neilson JMM. QT interval length in diabetic autonomic neuropathy. Diabet Med 1990;7:23–6.

46. Gonin JM, Kadrofske MM, Schmaltz S et al. Corrected QT interval prolongation as diagnostic tool for assessment of cardiac autonomic neuropathy in diabetes mellitus. Diabetes Care 1990;13:68–71.

47. Chambers JB, Samson MJ, Sprigings DC, Jackson G. QT prolongation on the electrocardiogram in diabetic autonomic neuropathy. Diabet Med 1990;7:105–10.

48. Veglio M, Chinaglia A, Borra M, Perin PC. Does abnormal QT prolongation reflect autonomic dysfunction in diabetic patients? QTc interval measure firstly standardised tests in diabetic autonomic neuropathy. Diabet Med 1995;12:302–6.

49. Veglio M, Borra M, Stevens LK et al. The relation between QTc interval prolongation and diabetic complications. The EURODIAB IDDM Complication Study Group. Diabetologia 1999;42:68–75.

50. Ewing DJ, Boland O, Neilson JMM et al. Autonomic neuropathy, QT interval lengthening, and unexpected deaths in male diabetic patients. Diabetologia 1991;34:182–5.

51. Sawicki PT, Dahne R, Bender R, Berger M. Prolonged QT interval as a predictor of mortality in diabetic nephropathy. Diabetologia 1996;39:77–81.

52. Sawicki PT. Mortality in diabetic nephropathy: the importance of the QT interval. Nephrol Dial Transplant 1996;11:1514–15.

53. Towbin JA. New revelations about the long-QT syndrome. N Engl J Med 1995;333:384–5.

54. Higham PD, Campbell RWF. QT dispersion. Br Heart J 1994:71:508–10.

55. Kirvela M, Yli-Hankala A, Lindgren L. QT dispersion and autonomic function in diabetic and non-diabetic patients with renal failure. Br J Anaesth 1994;73:801–4.

56. Naas AA, Davidson NC, Thompson C et al. QT and QTc dispersion are accurate predictors of cardiac death in newly diagnosed non-insulin dependent diabetes: cohort study. BMJ 1998;316:745–6.

57. Sawicki PT, Kiwitt S, Bender R, Berger M. The value of QT dispersion for identification of total mortality risk in non-insulin-dependent diabetes mellitus. J Intern Med 1998;243:49–56.

58. Parati G, Pomidossi G, Ramirez AJ et al. Variability of the haemodynamic responses to laboratory tests employed in assessment of neural cardiovascular regulation in man. Clin Sci 1985;69:533–40.

59. Akselrod S, Gordon D, Ubell FA et al. Power spectrum analysis of the heart rate fluctuation: a quantitative probe of beat-cardiovascular control. Science (Wash DC) 1981;213:220–2.

60. Pomeranz B, Macauley RJB, Caudill MA et al. Assessment of autonomic function in humans by heart rate spectral analysis. Am J Physiol 1985;248:H151–3.

61. Bennett T, Hosking DJ, Hampton JR. Baroreflex sensitivity and responses to the Valsalva manoeuvre in subjects with diabetes mellitus. J Neurol Neurosurg Psychiatry 1976;39:178–83.

62. Ferrer NT, Kennedy WR, Sahinen F. Baroreflexes in patients with diabetes mellitus. Neurology 1991;41:1462–6.

63. Bristow A, Honour AJ, Pickering GW et al. Diminished baroreflex sensitivity in high blood pressure. Circulation 1969;39:48–54.

64. Gribbin S, Pickering TG, Sleight P, Peto R. Effect of age and blood pressure on baroreflex sensitivity in man. Circ Res 1971;29:424.

65. Molhoek GP, Wessling KH, Settels JJ. Evaluation of the Penaz servo-plethsmo-manometer for the continuous non-invasive measurement of finger blood pressure. Basic Res Cardiol 1984;79:598–609.
66. Kirscheim HR. Systemic arterial baroreceptor reflexes. Pharmcol Rev 1976;56:100–76.
67. Omboni S, Parati G, Frattola A et al. Spectral and sequence analysis of finger blood pressure variability: comparison with analysis of intra-arterial recordings. Hypertension 1993;22:26–33.
68. Dawson SL, Robinson TG, Youde JH et al. The reproducibility of cardiac baroreceptor activity assessed non-invasively by spectral sequence techniques. Clin Auton Res 1997;7:279–84.
69. Weston PJ, James MA, Panerai R et al. Abnormal baro-receptor-cardiac reflex sensitivity is not detected by conventional tests of autonomic function in patients with insulin dependent diabetes mellitus. Clin Sci 1996;91:59–64.
70. Pagani M, Lombardi F, Guzzetti S et al. Power spectral analysis of heart rate and arterial pressure variability as a marker of sympatho-vagal interactions in man and conscious dog. Circ Res 1996;59:178–93.
71. Bernardi L, Ricordi L, Lazzari P et al. Impaired circadian modulation of sympatho-vagal activity in diabetes. Circulation 1992;86:1443–52.
72. Bigger JT, Kleiger RE, Fleiss JL et al. Multi-centre post-infarction research group: components of heart rate variability measured during healing of acute myocardial infarction. Am J Cardiol 1988;61:205–15.
73. Farrell TG, Odemuyiw A, Bashir Y. Prognostic value of baroreflex sensitivity testing after myocardial infarction. Br Heart J 1992;67:129–37.
74. Bigger JT, Fleiss JL, Steinmann RC et al. Frequency domain measures of heart rate variability and mortality after myocardial infarction. Circulation 1992;85:164–71.
75. Billman G, Schwartz PJ, Stone HL. Baroreceptor reflex control of heart rate; a predictor of sudden cardiac death. Circulation 1982;66:874–80.
76. La Rovere MT, Bigger JT, Marcus FI et al for the ATRAMI investigators. Baroreflex sensitivity and heart-rate variability in prediction of total cardiac mortality after myocardial infarction. Lancet 1998;351:478–84.
77. Kjecshus J, Gilpin E, Cali G et al. Diabetic patients on beta-blockers after myocardial infarction. Eur Heart J 1990;11:43–50.
78. Eckberg DL, Harkins SW, Fritch JM et al. Baroreflex control of the plasma norepinephrine and heart period in healthy subjects in diabetic patients. J Clin Invest 1986;78:366–74.
79. Zola B, Khan JF, Juni JE, Vinik AI. Abnormal cardiac function in diabetic patients with autonomic neuropathy in the absence of ischaemic heart disease. J Clin Endocrinol Metab 1986;63:208–14.
80. Maraud L, Ginn H, Roudaut R et al. Echocardiographic study of left ventricular function in type 1 diabetes mellitus: hypersensitivity of beta-adrenergic stimulation. Diabetes Res Clin Pract 1991;11:161–8.

81. Weston PJ, Panerai RB, McCullough A et al. Assessment of barorecep-tor-cardiac reflex sensitivity using time domain analysis in patients with IDDM and the relation to left ventricular mass index. Diabetologia 1996:39:1385–91.

82. Minami N, Head GA. Relationship between cardiovascular hypertrophy and cardiac baroreflex function in spontaneously hypertensive and stroke-prone rats. J Hypertens 1993;11:523–33.

83. Koren MJ, Devereux RB, Casale PN et al. Relation of left ventricular mass and geometry to morbidity and mortality in uncomplicated essential hypertension. Ann Intern Med 1991;114:345–52.

84. McLenachan JM, Henderson E, Morris KI, Dargie HJ. Ventricular arrhyth-mias in patients with hypertensive left ventricular hypertrophy. N Engl J Med 1987;317:787–92.

85. Rollins MD, Jenkins JG, Carson DJ et al. Power spectral analysis of the electrocardiogram in diabetic children. Diabetologia 1992;35:452–5.

86. Wawryk AM, Bates DJ, Couper JJ. Power spectral analysis of heart rate variability in children and adolescents with IDDM. Diabetes Care 1997;20:1416–21.

87. Clarke CF, Eason M, Reilly A et al. Autonomic nerve function in adoles-cents with Type 1 diabetes mellitus: relationship to microalbuminuria. Diabet Med 1999;16:550–4.

88. Lefrandt JD, Hoogenberg K, Van Roon AM et al. Baroreflex sensitivity is depressed in microalbuminuric type 1 diabetic patients at rest and during sympathetic manoeuvres. Diabetologia 1999;42:1345–9.

89. Bernardi L, Ricordi L, Lazzari P et al. Impaired circadian modulation of sympathovagal activity in diabetes. A possible explanation for altered temporal onset of cardiovascular disease. Circulation 1992;86:1443–52.

90. Faba S, Azzopardi J, Muscat H, Fenech FF. Absence of circadian varia-tion in the onset of acute myocardial infarction in diabetic subjects. Br Heart J 1995;74:370–2.

91. Sartor G, Dahlquist G. Short-term mortality in childhood-onset insulin dependent diabetes mellitus: a high frequency of unexpected deaths in bed. Diabet Med 1995;12:607–11.

92. Thordarson H, Sorvik O. Dead in bed syndrome in young diabetic patients in Norway. Diabet Med 1995;12:782–7.

93. Weston PJ , Glancy JM, McNally PG et al. Can abnormalities of ventric-ular repolarisation identify insulin dependent diabetic patients at risk of sudden cardiac death? Heart 1997;78:56–60.

94. Jermendy G, Toth L, Voros P et al. Cardiac autonomic neuropathy and QT interval length. A follow up study in diabetic patients. Acta Cardiol 1991;46:189–200.

95. Lo SS, Sutton MS, Leslie RD. Information on type 1 diabetes mellitus and QT interval from identical twins. Am J Cardiol 1993;72:305–9.

96. Bravenboer B, Hendriksen PH, Oey LP et al. Is the corrected QT inter-

val a reliable indicator of severity of diabetic autonomic neuropathy? Diabetes Care 1993;16:1249–53.

97. Whitsel EA, Boyko EJ, Siscovick DS. Reassessing the role of QTc in the diagnosis of autonomic failure among patients with diabetes. Diabetes Care 2000;23:241–7.

98. Mantysaari M, Kuikka J, Mustonen J et al. Noninvasive detection of cardiac sympathetic nervous dysfunction in diabetic patients using (I123) meta-iodobenzylguanidine. Diabetes 1992;41:1069–75.

99. Murata K, Sumida S, Murashima S et al. A novel method for the assessment of autonomic neuropathy in type 2 diabetic patients: a comparative evaluation of 123I-MIBG myocardial scintigraphy and power spectral analysis of heart-rate variability. Diabet Med 1996;13:266–72.

100. Fisher BM, Gillen G, Hepburn DA et al. Cardiac responses to acute insulin-induced hypoglycemia in humans. Am J Physiol 1990;258: H1775–9.

101. Fisher BM, Heller SR. Mortality, cardiovascular morbidity and possible effects of hypoglycaemia on diabetic complications. In: Freir BM, Fisher BM, eds. Hypoglycaemia in Clinical Diabetes. John Wiley & Sons, Chichester, 1999:167–86.

102. Collier A, Matuse DM, Young RJ, Clarke BF. Transient atrial fibrillation precipitated by hypoglycaemia: 2 case reports. Postgrad Med J 1987; 63:895–7.

103. Baxter MA, Garewal C, Jordan R et al. Hypoglycaemia in atrial fibrillation. Postgrad Med J 1990;66:981.

104. O'Deh M, Oliven A, Bassan H. Transient atrial fibrillation precipitated by hypoglycaemia. Ann Emerg Med 1990;19:565–7.

105. Schaffer H, Bucka E, Friedlander K. Uber die Einwirkung des Insulins und der Hypoglykamie auf das menschliche Herz. Zeitschrift Gesamte Exp Med 1927;57:35–67.

106. Goldman D. The electrocardiogram in insulin shock. Arch Intern Med 1940;66:93–108.

107. Strouse S, Soskin S, Kaz LN, Rubinfeld SH. Treatment of older diabetic patients with cardiovascular disease. J Am Med Assoc 1932;98:1703–6.

108. Judson WE, Hollander W. The affects of insulin-induced hypoglycaemia in patients with angina pectoris. Before and after intravenous hexamethonium. Am Heart J 1956;52:198–209.

109. Marques JLB, George E, Peacey SR et al. Altered ventricular repolarization during hypoglycaemia in patients with diabetes. Diabet Med 1997;14:648–54.

110. Frier BM, Barr StCG, Walker JD. Fatal cardiac arrest folowing acute hypoglycaemia in a diabetic patient. Pract Diabetes Int 1995;12:284.

111. Marfella R, Nappo F, De Angelis L et al. The effect of acute hyperglycaemia on QTc duration in healthy man. Diabetologia 2000;43:571–5.

112. Weston PJ, Gill GV. Is undetected autonomic dysfunction responsible

for sudden death in type 1 diabetes mellitus? The 'dead in bed' syndrome revisited. Diabet Med 1999;16:626–31.

113. Leak D, Starr P. Mechanism of arrhythmias during insulin induced hypoglycaemia. Am Heart J 1962;63:688–91.

114. Yee KM, Struthers AD. Can drug effects on mortality and heart failure be predicted by any surrogate markers. Eur Heart J 1997;18:1860–4.

115. Kontopoulos AG, Athyros VG, Didangelos TP et al. Effect of chronic quinapril administration on heart rate variability in patients with diabetic autonomic neuropathy. Diabetes Care 1997;20:355–61.

116. Binkley PF, Haas GJ, Starling RC et al. Sustained augmentation of parasympathetic tone with angiotensin converting enzyme inhibition in patients with congestive heart failure. J Am Coll Cardiol 1993;21:655–61.

117. Malik RA, Williamson S, Abbott C et al. Effect of angiotensin-converting-enzyme (ACE) inhibitor trandolapril on human diabetic neuropathy: randomised double-blind controlled trial. Lancet 1998;352:1978–81.

118. Schwarz PJ. Idiopathic long QT syndrome. Progress and questions. Am Heart J 1985;2:399–411.

119. Molgaard H, Mickley H, Pless P et al. Effects of metoprolol on heart rate variability in survivors of acute myocardial infaction. Am J Cardiol 1993;71;1357–9.

120. Kennedy HL, Brooks MM, Barker AH et al for the CAST investigators. Beta-blocker therapy in the cardiac arrhythmia suppression trial. Am J Cardiol 1994;74:674–80.

121. Olsson G, Wikstrand J, Warnold I et al. Metoprolol-induced reduction in postinfarction mortality: pooled results from five double-blind randomized trials. Eur Heart J 1992;13:28–32.

122. The Norwegian Multicenter Study Group. Timolol-induced reduction in mortality and reinfarction. N Engl J Med 1981;304:801–7.

123. β-Blocker Heart Attack Trial Research Group. A randomized trial of propranolol in patients with acute myocardial infarction. Mortality results. J Am Med Assoc 1982;247:1707–14.

124. Australian and Swedish Pindolol Study Group. The effect of pindolol on the two year mortality after complicated myocardial infarction. Eur Heart J 1983;4:367–75.

125. The Cardiac Arrhythmia Suppression Trial (CAST) investigators. Preliminary report: effect of encainide and flecainide on mortality in a randomized trial of arrhythmia suppression after myocardial infarction. N Engl J Med 1989;321:406–12.

chapter 3

Silent myocardial ischaemia in people with diabetes

Iain Findlay

Introduction

The high incidence of unrecognized or silent myocardial infarction in people with diabetes has been recognized for some time.[1] Almost half of all acute myocardial infarctions that occur in diabetic patients are asymptomatic. The mortality rate approaches 50%.[2] In the mid-1980s, there was significant research interest in what was termed 'silent myocardial ischaemia' (SMI) and its relevance to those with coronary heart disease (CHD). It was identified at an early stage that silent myocardial ischaemia was more prevalent in certain diabetic populations. This led to a number of other significant discoveries concerning the relationship between SMI and hypertension, autonomic dysfunction, and nervous system activity and CHD. Collectively, these findings increased hope that the detection of such asymptomatic myocardial ischaemia might point to a group of diabetic patients in which aggressive medical therapy or revascularization could be usefully targeted.

Historical background

The identification of SMI can be traced back to 1974 when Stern and Tzivoni used the (then) innovative technique of 24-hour ambulatory

ECG recording (later known as Holter monitoring) in ambulant subjects.[3] They recorded the development of ST segment depression that was unaccompanied by anginal pain. In 1977 Schang and Pepine confirmed these findings in patients with CHD when they noted that transient asymptomatic ST segment depression occurred during daily activities.[4] This discovery led to a mushrooming of interest in Holter monitoring and the term silent myocardial ischaemia became established in the literature.

Between the late 1980s and early 1990s there was an increased interest in the benefits of screening for coronary heart disease, which fostered further interest in SMI. As an example, the TROSMO study screened almost 30 000 subjects for evidence of cardiovascular disease.[5] In this study, a subgroup of approximately 300 men and 300 women was examined in greater detail for evidence of exercise-induced silent ischaemia. The incidence of SMI was small, and importantly a positive correlation was noted between the presence of SMI and hypertension in men.

Diabetes was not specifically examined as a possible risk factor for SMI in this population. However, since hypertension is strongly associated with diabetes, studies attempting to determine whether

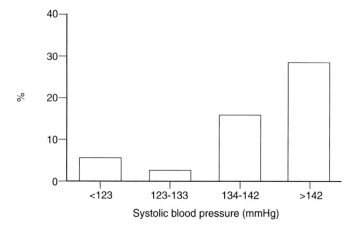

Figure 3.1 *Prevalence of silent ischaemia in the diabetes group according to quartiles of the ambulatory systolic blood pressure (n = 152).*

silent ischaemia is more common in people with diabetes must take account of co-existing hypertension, which is known to be strongly associated with ECG changes. This has been demonstrated by many studies, for example the Reykjavik study, where in the absence of any other manifestations of coronary disease, asymptomatic ST T wave changes on resting ECG were associated with twice the expected subsequent mortality.[6]

Silent myocardial ischaemia in people with diabetes

Hospital-based studies

In 1985, Chiariello and colleagues reported one of the earliest applications of ambulatory ECG monitoring in people with diabetes.[7] They determined the frequency of asymptomatic transient ST segment change during ambulatory ECG monitoring in 51 type 2 diabetic patients, 70 non-diabetic patients with proven coronary disease and 40 non-diabetic patients with no evidence of overt coronary disease. The majority of the 51 diabetic patients (75%) had evidence of coronary disease, and 37% had evidence of previous myocardial infarction. Episodes of SMI (as judged by the presence of asymptomatic ST segment depression) were significantly more common than symptomatic episodes. The incidence of asymptomatic myocardial ischaemia was twice as common in people with diabetes as in non-diabetic patients with coronary artery disease. This was despite the fact that overt CHD was present in only 75% of people with diabetes. The proportion of asymptomatic versus symptomatic episodes was higher in the diabetic group. It was not reported whether both groups had comparable levels of hypertension.

In 1987, Chipkin and colleagues determined the frequency of pain during ischaemia in patients with or without diabetes during exercise treadmill testing.[8] To be eligible for inclusion in the study, patients had to have a positive exercise test with exercise-induced ST segment depression of at least 2 mm. They examined over 3000 exercise tests

67

and 211 patients had tests that satisfied their inclusion criteria. Diabetes was present in 12% of patients, and hypertension was more common in diabetic subjects. In contrast to the findings of Chiariello, no difference was found in the frequency of SMI in patients with or without diabetes. This may be because the diabetic and non-diabetic subjects were reasonably comparable as a result of the inclusion criteria. In this study, 50% of patients underwent cardiac catheterization and although there was a tendency for patients with diabetes to have significantly more triple vessel disease, the extent of the coronary disease was similar in diabetic and non-diabetic patients. Furthermore, the extent of disease was similar in those with and without SMI whether diabetic or non-diabetic, as was the incidence of hypertension.

Callaham et al further broadened the knowledge of SMI in people with diabetes by performing a retrospective study of 1747 unselected, predominantly male patients referred for exercise testing to a veteran administration hospital.[9] The researchers were particularly interested in whether age, presence of myocardial infarction or diabetes influenced the prevalence of silent myocardial ischaemia. In this study group there were 180 diabetic patients, 93 of whom had type 1 diabetes. SMI occurred with equal frequency in diabetic and non-diabetic patients. Overall, SMI was present in two-thirds of all ischaemic episodes. The prevalence of silent ischaemia was directly related to age in both groups. In this study, SMI did not carry a higher risk of death. The presence of ST segment depression during treadmill testing was associated with a significantly higher overall 2-year mortality rate compared with those without ST segment depression. This occurred irrespective of whether or not this was associated with angina.

Dellborg and colleagues used coronary angioplasty as a model to look at SMI.[10] It was established that individuals exhibited classical ST segment elevation without pain during occlusion of a coronary artery, particularly on subsequent balloon inflations. This was termed 'preconditioning'. Dellborg found that painless ST segment elevation was more common during angioplasty in people with diabetes.

The Asymptomatic Cardiac Ischaemic Pilot (ACIP) study was an international randomized trial to compare three treatment strategies aimed at abolishing silent and symptomatic ischaemia.[11] There were 558 patients, of whom only 77 had diabetes. To be considered for screening the patients had to have an ischaemic exercise test and ischaemia during 48-hour Holter monitoring. In addition they had to have angiographic evidence of coronary artery disease suitable for revascularization. Thus these were well-characterized patients, typical of the patient with well-established CHD. The researchers examined whether patients with diabetes had significantly more episodes of SMI during exercise testing and Holter monitoring than non-diabetic patients. They examined the magnitude of any differences and their relationship, if any, to the severity of coronary disease in diabetic and non-diabetic patients.

Multi-vessel disease was more frequent in people with diabetes, being present in 87% of cases versus 74% in the non-diabetic patients. During the qualifying exercise test and 48-hour Holter ECG, diabetic patients did not have a higher prevalence of SMI than non-diabetic patients. Alhough the diabetic group had more extensive and diffuse CHD, they tended to have less measurable ischaemia, less total ischaemic time per day and time per episode and less maximum depth of ST segment depression during 48-hour ambulatory ECG. Furthermore, no differences were noted in the severity of ischaemia during treadmill testing. The results from the ACIP study differ from Chiariello, who reported twice the incidence of asymptomatic ischaemia in patients with diabetes compared with non-diabetic patients with CHD, during Holter monitoring.[7]

Chiariello and Indolfi commented on the ACIP study finding that SMI was no more common in diabetic than in non-diabetic subjects.[12] They suggested that caution should be used in applying the ACIP data to a general population of people with diabetes. Presumably they were concerned that clinicians would not regard looking for SMI as useful because of the ACIP findings. There was little unusual in the characteristics of the diabetic subjects in the ACIP study to suggest they were atypical in the amount of SMI that they displayed. In fact, analysis of the data suggests that they might be more likely to display SMI than the non-diabetic subjects as they were significantly more hypertensive and less likely to have been prescribed a beta-blocker. Both of these features would have been expected to increase the incidence of SMI in the patients with diabetes. The absence of an increase in SMI in this study further weakens any argument that diabetic patients with angina are more likely to exhibit SMI than non-diabetic patients.

The findings of the ACIP study are supported by the CASS registry, which compared 113 patients with diabetes and 1321 non-diabetic patients.[13] This study showed that the people with diabetes had more severe CHD but that the prevalence of exercise-induced SMI was similar in both groups, being present during exercise testing in 40% of diabetic subjects and 33% of non-diabetic subjects.

Similar rates of SMI during treadmill testing were found by Naka et al, who compared the prevalence of SMI in 132 diabetic patients and 140 non-diabetic patients.[14] Silent ST segment depression was noted in just fewer than 33% in both groups, although coronary artery disease was present in 39% of diabetic versus 18% of non-diabetic patients.

Thus, in the main, these relatively large hospital-based studies do not support the contention that SMI is more common in diabetic patients with CHD.

Community-based studies

These may not apply to people with diabetes who have not progressed to the stage of referral to hospital. May et al examined 240 diabetic patients (aged 40 to 70) from a community sample of residents from the Danish Municipality of Horsens.[15] The study included 178 people with diabetes (approximately 20% of all registered people with diabetes in this municipality), 50% of whom were on treatment with insulin. They compared 97 diabetic subjects in the younger half of the group (mean age 51) with age- and sex-matched non-diabetic control subjects. This younger diabetic cohort differed from controls in that they were heavier and had higher blood pressures (mean 24 hour BP 129/78 versus 122/76 mm Hg).

Based on a definition of SMI as being ST segment depression of 1 mm on either exercise ECG or Holter ECG occurring without anginal pain, the incidence of SMI in all people with diabetes was 13.5%. In the younger diabetic cohort with matched controls, the prevalence was 11.4% compared with 6.4% in control subjects. Thus, SMI was twice as common in people with diabetes compared with controls. While there was no association between gender and type of diabetes, there was a strong correlation between elevated systolic blood pressure and SMI in the diabetic group. No predictive value could be shown for any other study variables. This study further emphasizes the importance of the relationship between hypertension and SMI. It also provided a convincing case that hypertension must be taken into account before any conclusions are drawn about the incidence of SMI in diabetic versus non-diabetic subjects.

In another community-based study, Koistinen and colleagues attempted to assess the prevalence of asymptomatic myocardial ischaemia in diabetic subjects and to correlate this with the presence or absence of coronary artery disease.[16] They invited 338 diabetic patients who were members of the Oulu Local Diabetic Association in Finland, of these, 170 were not willing to participate but 136 were both eligible and willing to participate. There were 72 patients with type 1 diabetes (33 women with a mean age of 46) and 64 patients with type 2 diabetes (19 women with a mean age of 49). The patients in the study group were aged between 35 and 60 and had a duration of diabetes of more than 5 years. They had no symptoms or clinical evidence of ischaemic heart disease and were not taking lipid-lowering medication, neither did they have severe renal disease or any type of disease that would contra-indicate performing a maximal exercise test. The control group was drawn from clients of the Occupational Health Service of Oulo University Central Hospital and the State Occupational Health Service. The researchers invited 145 subjects, of whom 80 were willing to be studied.

All subjects underwent maximal exercise electrocardiography and exercise thallium tomographic imaging, plus 24-hour ECG Holter monitoring. The patients were referred for cardiac catheterization if they showed signs of myocardial ischaemia. Fifteen diabetic patients and five control subjects were taking beta-blocker medication, which was stopped 2 days before the examination. Forty (29%) people with diabetes and four (5%) controls had positive stress tests. Coronary angiography was performed on 34 of the 40 patients with diabetes and in all four control subjects. Only 12 of the 34 diabetic patients had significant coronary disease and 15 had absolutely normal epicardial coronary arteries. Controls who were required to undergo coronary angiography because of a suggestion of ischaemia on one of the non-invasive tests had evidence of significant coronary disease.

This study emphasizes the fact that silent myocardial ischaemia on non-invasive testing is not specific for coronary artery disease. The study also shows a striking incidence of significant coronary disease in asymptomatic subjects with coronary disease being present in 9% of the population. Thus while in relatively non-selected hospital-based patients there is little evidence to support the contention that SMI is more common in people with diabetes, in community based studies reported to date this seems convincingly so.

Silent myocardial ischaemia and autonomic dysfunction

If the hypothesis that SMI is more common in people with diabetes is accepted as demonstrated by the Danish municipality study,[15] and given that autonomic dysfunction is also common during diabetes, it is pertinent to examine whether these phenomena are also linked.

Hume and colleagues designed a study to show whether an abnormal exercise ECG in diabetic patients without cardiac symptoms was more common in patients with diabetic peripheral neuropathy.[17] They studied 30 diabetics with and 30 diabetics without neuropathy. Autonomic neuropathy was present in 14. The frequency of a positive exercise tolerance test (ETT) or SMI was 27% in those with peripheral neuropathy versus 20% (p = ns) in those without, and 36% in those with autonomic neuropathy. Thus there was no evidence to support the contention that diabetic neuropathy was associated with SMI, but a strong suggestion that this might be the case for those with autonomic dysfunction.

Langer and colleagues looked at the prevalence of silent myocardial ischaemia in 58 male diabetic patients aged from 35 to 75 who had no symptoms of angina or other clinical evidence of coronary artery disease.[18] The patients were drawn from those attending a hospital diabetic clinic, and they underwent five tests of autonomic function (see Chapter 2):

■ Valsalva manoeuvre
■ Heart rate response to deep breathing
■ Heart rate response to standing
■ Blood pressure response to standing
■ Blood pressure response to sustained handgrip.

The researchers defined autonomic dysfunction as an abnormal response to at least two of the five autonomic function tests. The prevalence of this in non-diabetic subjects is less than 2%. In addition, the pain threshold or tolerance was assessed by electrical stimulation to the volar surface of both forearms. Myocardial ischaemia was detected by a standard exercise test, ambulatory Holter and ECG monitoring and exercise thallium 201 scintigraphy. Silent myocardial ischaemia was present in 10 of the 58 subjects.

The principal new findings of the study were a 17% prevalence of silent myocardial ischaemia in a selected cohort of asymptomatic diabetic men and a significantly greater frequency of silent myocardial ischaemia among subjects with than without autonomic dysfunction (36% versus 5%). The study also demonstrated that there was a similar pain threshold and tolerance to pain in patients with or without silent myocardial ischaemia. In patients with autonomic dysfunction there was an elevated pain threshold, suggesting that subclinical peripheral neuropathy may also be present in patients with autonomic dysfunction.

The authors concluded that the clinical implication of the study was that a lack of symptoms in diabetic men, especially those with autonomic dysfunction, is not an adequate guide to the presence or absence of myocardial ischaemia.

Researchers from the London Chest Hospital and the Newham Hospital in London provided further insights into the connections between SMI and autonomic dysfunction. In 1990, Ambepityia and colleagues examined the hypothesis that SMI was caused by a specific impairment of the sensory innervation of the heart.[19] They examined the 'anginal perceptual threshold', defined as the time taken from the onset of ST segment depression to the appreciation of chest pain during treadmill testing. The study group comprised 32 patients with diabetes and 36 non-diabetic control subjects, all with typical exertional angina. The groups were well matched for age, sex, smoking, hypertension, duration of angina, previous myocardial infarction and anti-anginal therapy. ST segment depression occurred almost 2 minutes earlier in diabetic subjects compared to non-diabetic control subjects (111 versus 216 seconds, $p < 0.005$). This implies that the diabetic patients had more severe CHD but, despite this, the time to experience angina after the onset of ischaemia was a mean of 23 seconds longer in diabetic patients compared to non-diabetic control patients. Thus, despite having earlier onset and more prolonged ischaemia, angina took longer to develop in patients with diabetes.

The group then carried out autonomic function tests that consisted of the Valsalva manoeuvre, heart rate and blood pressure response to standing and deep breathing plus assessments of median nerve motor and sensory function. In the diabetic patients there was evidence of a greater prevalence of abnormal responses during Valsalva, deep breathing and assessment of the maximal/minimal difference in heart rate. A higher number of significant abnormalities of median nerve sensory function were also noted in diabetic subjects compared with non-diabetic subjects. In both diabetic and non-diabetic patients, those who exhibited a heart rate response to Valsalva below the normal range showed marked prolongations of the anginal perceptual threshold. The authors postulated that in people with diabetes the prolongation of the anginal perceptual threshold was associated with an autonomic neuropathy involving the sensory innervation of the heart. This was a previously unrecognized feature of diabetic neuropathy and, if true, represented a significant new finding.

The ACIP study did not reproduce the findings of Ambepityia et al[19] that the anginal perceptual threshold was prolonged in people with diabetes. In the ACIP study, 60% of patients in both diabetic and non-diabetic groups experienced angina during the exercise test. The time to onset of 1 mm ST segment depression and the onset of angina was similar in both groups.[11]

The London researchers later examined the relationships between angina, diabetes, somatic pain threshold and autonomic function.[20] In this study, the investigators attempted to determine whether diabetic patients with prolonged anginal perceptual thresholds also exhibited reduced sensitivity to other painful stimuli, and whether these reactions were associated with an autonomic neuropathy.

The somatic pain threshold was measured by time taken to experience pain during the inflation of a sphygmomanometer cuff. The diabetic group (n = 19) had a longer anginal perceptual threshold when compared with control patients (n = 25) with coronary heart disease (138 seconds versus 34 seconds). In the diabetic patients this prolonged anginal perceptual threshold correlated positively with a prolonged somatic pain threshold (r = 0.5, $p < 0.03$). In these patients the prolonged anginal perceptual threshold did not correlate with abnormalities of heart rate response to Valsalva. There was a weak but significant relationship between somatic pain threshold and abnormalities of heart rate response to Valsalva. The authors concluded that in patients whose perception of angina is impaired there is also evidence of a heightened somatic pain threshold and that this is associated with subclinical autonomic neuropathy. Alhough this finding is useful, mechanisms underlying these patterns remain unknown.

Marchant et al investigated in more detail the role of subclinical neuropathy in patients with SMI.[21] Tests of autonomic function and heart rate variability were carried out in both diabetic patients (n = 22) and non-diabetic patients (n = 30) with proven coronary disease, exercise induced ST segment depression on treadmill testing and stable angina. Diabetic patients with a history of microvascular complications were excluded. Thirty-six subjects experienced angina during the treadmill test, leaving 16 patients to compose the SMI group. Patients in this latter group were twice as likely to be diabetic than non-diabetic.

Indices of autonomic function in the symptomatic (angina and ST depression) and SMI groups (no angina but ST depression) were compared. It was demonstrated that there were significant differences between the groups in the supine/standing heart rate ratio. However, this was not evident in other measures of autonomic function such as the Valsalva ratio, heart rate variation during deep breathing, decrease in systolic pressure during change in posture or increase in difference in diastolic pressure during handgrip. Furthermore, heart rate variability was not different in those with symptomatic myocardial ischaemia or SMI. A further subanalysis identified that abnormalities in the supine to standing heart rate ratio were evident only in diabetic patients with SMI. They were absent in diabetic patients with angina or non-diabetic patients with angina or SMI. The study's conclusion that diabetic patients with exertional SMI had evidence of significant autonomic impairment compared with symptomatic patients was based on subgroup analysis with small numbers and their conclusions must be regarded with caution. This conclusion and the authors' suggestion that subclinical autonomic neuropathy is an important cause of SMI in patients with diabetes require support from other studies.

Such support came from a retrospective review of 5 years of exercise tests by Murray and colleagues from Sligo in Ireland.[22] They examined 1653 exercise tests for evidence of ST segment depression; 247 were electrically positive and of these 29 occurred in diabetic patients and 218 in non-diabetic patients. SMI, defined as ST segment depression in the absence of anginal symptoms, occurred in 69% of the diabetic patients versus 35% of non-diabetic control subjects. In the diabetic group those with SMI had a significantly increased incidence of microvascular complications (70% versus 22%, $p < 0.05$). On the basis of these results, the authors went on to examine prospectively with positive exercise tests 30 diabetic patients who were being investigated for coronary artery disease. The patients also underwent extensive autonomic function testing. Anginal pain occurred during exercise testing in 12 of the 30 patients, while the remaining 18 had SMI.

A severe autonomic neuropathy was present in 11 of 18 of those with SMI versus only 1 of 12 with anginal pain during exercise. The authors concluded that SMI on exercise testing is common among patients with diabetes mellitus and is frequently associated with severe autonomic dysfunction. A further notable finding from this study was that SMI on exercise testing was associated with a longer duration of diabetes and higher incidence of macrovascular complications. No mention was made of the incidence of hypertension in these patients.

In 1991, further evidence to support the role of autonomic dysfunction in SMI in people with diabetes was provided by O'Sullivan et al.[23] These authors investigated the prevalence of SMI by Holter monitoring in 41 diabetic patients, 17 of whom had significant autonomic neuropathy and 24 had normal autonomic function. The two groups were matched for risk factors for coronary artery disease and history of angina pectoris. Close examination of the risk factor profile shows that while group differences were not significant, those with autonomic dysfunction were more likely to be cigarette smokers and to have a family history of CHD, hypertension, previous myocardial infarction and, importantly, a longer duration of diabetes with an increased number of complications. The prevalence of SMI in those with autonomic dysfunction was 65% as opposed to only 4% in those without autonomic dysfunction. The authors concluded that the results were consistent with autonomic neuropathy preventing the development of anginal pain, thereby obscuring the presence of coronary heart disease. They also suggested that 24-hour ambulatory ECG monitoring may identify a subgroup of diabetic patients who have myocardial ischaemia and to whom treatment should then be offered.

In 1993 an investigation of the possibility of screening and the complexities of the mechanisms influencing SMI in people with diabetes was undertaken by Hikita et al.[24] They looked at the usefulness of assessing plasma beta-endorphin levels, pain threshold and autonomic function in patients with exercise induced SMI. The study group comprised 110 patients who had an electrically positive exercise test, of whom 15 were diabetic and 95 non-diabetic. All 15 diabetic patients and 49 of the non-diabetic patients exhibited SMI, while the remaining 46 non-diabetic patients had ST segment depression with anginal symptoms. Plasma beta-endorphin levels were measured before and during exercise. Pain threshold was assessed by electric skin stimulation tests. Autonomic function was assessed by the mean of the standard deviations of all normal sinus R–R intervals during successive 5-minute recording periods over the 24-hour period. There was a significantly greater increase in plasma beta-endorphin during exercise in non-diabetic patients with SMI when compared with diabetic patients (all of whom exhibited SMI). The authors suggest that the absence of pain in non-diabetic patients may be due to release of this endogenous painkiller. The significantly lower level of beta-endorphin in the diabetic patients suggests that the absence of angina may be due to a different mechanism. The authors postulate that a diabetic neuropathy may have affected the autonomic pain fibres in the heart and resulted in the absence of angina.

The mechanism by which autonomic system abnormalities could lead to SMI has begun to be gleaned using newer imaging techniques. Langer et al evaluated cardiac sympathetic innervation in 23 normal subjects and 65 asymptomatic diabetic patients by measuring the uptake of metaiodobenzylguanidine (MIBG) by dual isotope imaging.[25] MIBG is a noradrenaline analogue that is taken up by sympathetic nerve endings in the heart and it offers non-invasive quantitative assessment of cardiac autonomic function. Abnormalities in the myocardial uptake are related to sympathetic denervation in the context of left ventricular damage after myocardial infarction or dysfunction in patients with cardiomyopathy or in those with the long QT syndrome.[26–34]

The hypothesis of the study was that greater uptake abnormalities would be present with increasing degrees of autonomic dysfunction reflecting sympathetic denervation. Entry criteria were strict. In order to enter the study patients had to exhibit SMI during ambulatory ECG monitoring or exercise testing. Furthermore, patients passing this entry criterion had to exhibit abnormalities during exercise sestamibi imaging carried out in conjunction with the MIBG imaging. In this instance, SMI was defined as the presence of a reversible sestamibi myocardial perfusion defect in patients with ST segment depression on Holter monitoring or during stress testing. Patients did not have evidence of myocardial damage or dysfunction that might have resulted in abnormalities of the sympathetic nerve endings.

All medication capable of interfering with the assessment of autonomic function, including beta-blockers, calcium antagonists or any sympatholytic drugs, was withheld for 48 hours before testing. Autonomic function was assessed by five standard measures:

- Valsalva
- Deep breathing
- Heart rate response to standing
- Blood pressure response to standing
- Sustained handgrip.

Autonomic dysfunction was judged to be present if there was an abnormal response to two or more tests.

Sixty-five diabetic patients took part in the study and 71% of these had autonomic dysfunction defined as an abnormal response to at least two manoeuvres. SMI was evident in 21 of the 65 diabetic patients The authors reported that 'a striking difference' was present in the extent of MIBG uptake abnormalities in diabetic subjects compared with normal subjects after corrections were made for differences in sestamibi perfusion defects (i.e. areas of myocardial ischaemia). In those diabetic subjects with clinically significant autonomic dysfunction there were significantly greater abnormalities of MIBG uptake than in those diabetic subjects without autonomic dysfunction. The authors concluded:

'In contrast to normal subjects, diabetic patients have evidence of a significant reduction in MIBG uptake, most likely on the basis of autonomic dysfunction. Furthermore, diabetic patients with silent myocardial ischaemia have evidence of a diffuse abnormality in MIBG uptake, suggesting that abnormalities in pain perception may be linked to sympathetic denervation.'

Circadian rhythms

It is established that there are two peaks of myocardial ischaemia: in the waking hours and around early evening. These times correspond to an increase in rates of myocardial infarction. Morning wakening is associated with an increase in sympathetic tone and withdrawal of vagal tone. The resultant increase in myocardial work consequent upon the increase in heart rate and blood pressure is associated with an increased incidence of myocardial infarction.

Zarich and colleagues carried out ambulatory ECG monitoring in 60 diabetic patients with proven coronary artery disease.[35] Like most investigators, they found that ischaemia during daily activities was predominantly asymptomatic. Thirty-eight patients (two-thirds) exhibited ambulatory ischaemia and only 9% of episodes were associated with anginal pain. In keeping with the literature, the peak incidence of ischaemia occurred between 6 am and noon, compared with the other three 6-hourly quarters.

Autonomic nervous system testing was carried out in 25 of the patients with ambulatory ischaemia. Those patients with little or no autonomic dysfunction ($n = 15$) demonstrated the expected peak incidence of SMI between 6 and noon. The remainder, with moderate to severe autonomic dysfunction, did not show this morning peak and episodes of ischaemia occurred randomly throughout the day. The abolition of this morning peak with significant autonomic dysfunction is further suggestive evidence of the importance of the autonomic nervous system and its influence on the development and appreciation of myocardial ischaemia.

Risks of silent myocardial ischaemia in people with diabetes

If angina is viewed as a warning that an important mass of the myocardium is ischaemic, then a lack of perception of anginal pain could lead to harmful consequences akin to the damage that peripheral neuropathy can bring to the limbs. If, however, the development of ST segment depression occurs as an earlier sign of ischaemia, reflecting lesser amounts of ischaemic muscle, then the risk would be less than that associated with painful ischaemia, particularly if the episodes were brief in duration.

Evidence that myocardial dysfunction is greater in symptomatic myocardial ischaemia was provided by Nihoyannopoulos et al.[36] Their findings indicated that both symptomatic and asymptomatic ischaemia were associated with regional myocardial dysfunction. Painful ischaemia was associated with significantly more exercise induced left ventricular dysfunction than painless ischaemia. The authors suggested that there are many factors other than the extent of ischaemic myocardium that could account for the presence or absence of symptoms. These could include individual variations in pain threshold, possible problems with pain perception due to visceral neuropathy, as in diabetes mellitus, previous MI, bypass surgery or simply defective perception of painful stimuli.[37,38]

Nihoyannopoulos' findings indicated that the absence of pain made it possible for people with diabetes to continue to stress their myocardium and allow a greater mass of muscle to become ischaemic than would normally occur if pain were present. This would logically be expected to increase the risk of myocardial damage or cardiac rhythm instability. Thus SMI could carry the potential for increased risk, the opposite of what might be expected if it were only to reflect a lesser ischaemic muscle mass.

Clinical support for the hypothesis that SMI carries enhanced risk to the patient continues to be debated in the literature. In patients with CHD, Chiariello and Indolfi[12] state 'Numerous studies have demonstrated that the presence of silent myocardial ischaemia during exercise testing of AECG monitoring predicts adverse clinical outcome and poor survival'. In contrast, Mickley contends that 'ambulatory monitoring is of little practical value in the clinical management of unselected patients with stable angina'.[39] Extensive research into stable angina has produced differing results, with as many studies suggesting that patients who exhibit SMI are at risk of future death or myocardial infarction as do not.[39–47]

In the Malmo study, which was a prospective population study, men born in Malmo in 1914 underwent ambulatory ECG recording in 1982 to 1983.[48] For the study, 622 men were invited, representing a random 50% of all eligible men. Five hundred men were examined; 462 underwent ambulatory ECG monitoring and had a satisfactory recording made, and of these 394 were followed up after exclusion of atrial fibrillation and use of digoxin. Ninety-eight men demonstrated at least one episode of horizontal or downsloping ST segment depression (25%).

Three and a half years after the initial examination 8.7% of the men were dead. The incidence of fatal or non-fatal myocardial infarction in those with no SMI and no history of CHD was 2.3%. In those with SMI but no history of CHD this incidence was increased 4-fold. In those with a history of coronary disease this risk increased 16-fold compared to those with no SMI and no history of CHD.

This relative risk is greater than that generally reported and is probably explained by the age of the subjects (mean age 68). It is likely that this is an underestimate of the risk associated with asymptomatic ST segment depression in this age group as the study group as a whole had a lower mortality than those who declined to participate.

The Lipid Research Clinics Mortality Follow-up Study looked at the outcome of asymptomatic subjects with and without a positive exercise test.[49] At 8 years, after adjustment for age, a positive ETT was associated with a 4-fold increase in mortality. The study included 31 diabetic patients with a positive test and 211 with a negative test. Mortality was 23% versus 4%, respectively. Mortality in non-diabetic patients was 10% versus 1%. Thus while the numbers are small this also strongly supports the view that SMI induced by treadmill testing carries a poor outlook and in this case particularly so in diabetic patients.

Hume and colleagues reported similar results, and noted a high rate of adverse events over a 4-year follow-up, with four of 14 patients with SMI developing clinical CHD versus only one of 16 with negative ETT or no SMI.[17]

In patients with chronic stable angina the prognostic significance of SMI, alone and in relation to ischaemia during exercise, was assessed in 686 patients (475 men) taking part in the Angina Prognosis Study In Stockholm (APSIS).[47] Study subjects were followed up for a median 40 months. During this time, 29 patients died of cardiovascular causes, 27 had a non-fatal myocardial infarction and 89 underwent revascularization. Patients who died of a cardiovascular cause had more episodes and longer median duration of ST segment depression than patients without events. In a multivariate Cox model including sex, history of previous myocardial infarction, hypertension and diabetes, the duration of ST segment depression independently predicted cardiovascular death. When exercise testing was included, SMI during Holter monitoring carried additional prognostic information only in those patients with strongly positive ETTs. Thus, in patients with stable angina pectoris, SMI during Holter monitoring showed independent prognostic importance regarding cardiovascular death. Treatment reduced SMI, but the short-term treatment effects did not significantly influence prognosis.

In contrast, the TIBET study showed that the recording of ischaemic events in 48-hour Holter monitoring failed to predict hard or hard plus soft endpoints in patients with chronic stable angina.[50] This was a large, randomized, double-blind parallel group study of atenolol, nifedipine and their combination, in 682 men and women with a diagnosis of chronic stable angina who were not being considered for surgery. Patients were assessed with ambulatory ECG monitoring off treatment and after 6 weeks of randomized treatment and were followed up for 2 years on average. The hard endpoints were cardiac death, non-fatal myocardial infarction and unstable angina; soft endpoints were coronary artery bypass surgery, coronary angioplasty and treatment failure. The study showed no evidence of an association between the presence, frequency or total duration of ischaemic events on Holter monitoring, either on or off treatment, and the main outcome measures.

It is possible that discrepancies regarding the significance of SMI reported in various studies may relate, in part, to how it is detected, whether by Holter or treadmill. For instance, the ACIP investigators studied the relationship between treadmill-exercise-induced SMI and ambulatory ECG monitoring of SMI in patients with chronic stable CHD.[51] They found that the two modalities differed in the extent to which they provided useful prognostic information. There was a statistically significant relationship between ambulatory ECG monitoring and exercise testing in that exercise test could predict which patient was likely to exhibit ambulatory ECG ischaemia. The magnitude of ischaemia identified by each was not directly comparable. This suggests that different mechanisms may be responsible for the inducement of ischaemia. Exercise-induced ischaemia appears to have occurred at a higher heart rate than that detected during ambulatory ECG monitoring, suggesting that variations in coronary tone might be important in the latter.

Important evidence concerning the significance of SMI in people with diabetes was reported from the Coronary Artery Surgery Study (CASS) register.[52] This pivotal study laid the framework for the treatment of patients with coronary artery disease. The investigators looked at four groups of patients in a subanalysis.[13] All subjects had documented coronary artery disease and were followed up for 6 years. These groups were as follows:

Group 1: 45 diabetic patients with ischaemic ST segment depression during exercise tests who did not develop anginal chest pain (silent exercise-induced myocardial ischaemia patients).

Group 2: 37 diabetic patients with both ischaemic ECG change and chest pain (symptomatic ischaemic patients).

Group 3: 31 diabetic patients who developed neither ST segment depression nor chest pain during exercise testing (patients with no ischaemia).

Group 4: 429 patients who did not have diabetes but who did have SMI as group 1 during exercise testing (controls).

Survival was worst amongst the diabetic patients with SMI (group 1) who had a 6-year survival of 59%. In those with silent and symptomatic ischaemia (group 2) survival was 66%, while for those with no evidence of ischaemia (group 3) survival was 93%. There were only weak non-significant correlations between survival, the extent of disease and left ventricular function. Notably, when diabetic patients with SMI were compared with non-diabetic patients with SMI, 6-year survival for the medically treated patients was significantly lower in the diabetic patients.

The authors concluded that the lack of symptoms recorded in the diabetic patients with myocardial ischaemia may be related to diffuse sympathetic denervation. One explanation of this may be that an ineffective warning system failed to alert patients to the development of an unstable coronary syndrome. Alternatively, it may reflect a sudden death associated with an autonomic dysfunction.

This is not to say that we can use the conclusions from this study to recommend coronary surgery for people with diabetes who are found to have asymptomatic SMI during screening by either exercise or Holter monitoring. The numbers in this study were small and the authors do not seem to correct for the extent of CHD. Also, it is not clear what caused the patients in the study group to progress to angiography. It cannot be assumed that they were truly asymptomatic patients with SMI at all times. It has to be acknowledged that these patients may have had SMI during that classifying exercise test but were symptomatic at other times. It is possible that individuals may have a painless ST segment depression one day, but a painful ST segment depression on another. This is why the run-in phase of trials of anti-anginal drug therapy usually has at least two but usually three exercise tests to confirm a patient's stability.

There are few long-term follow-up studies of asymptomatic myocardial ischaemia in diabetic patients. One study from Beijing followed up 39 patients with type 2 diabetes for an average of just over 4 years.[53] The duration of diabetes ranged from 10 to 24 years. No patient had clinical evidence of coronary artery disease and all had a normal 12-lead ECG. They were compared with 31 healthy controls. Asymptomatic ST depression on Holter monitoring was recorded in 16 (41%) diabetic patients, but was not present in any of the controls.

During the 4-year follow-up, 14 of the diabetic patients developed myocardial infarction. There was a striking difference in the incidence of myocardial infarction in diabetic patients with SMI (10 of 16), versus diabetic patients without SMI (4 of 23) ($p < 0.005$). In total seven of the diabetic patients died, which represents a very high mortality rate over such a short period. No mention is made of degree of glycaemic control or control of other risk factors. Indeed, it may be that these patients were not representative as they had particularly poorly controlled diabetes.

The results of these studies make it difficult to make strong recommendations about searching for and treating SMI, and doubly so in people with diabetes as there is a lack of randomized trials. In general, no randomized study could be identified that answers effectively whether the detection and subsequent treatment of asymptomatic myocardial ischaemia improves survival. Also, no study of the revascularization of patients with truly asymptomatic myocardial ischaemia (that is asymptomatic during normal living activities, not during a stress test) was found. If a strategy of reducing asymptomatic myocardial ischaemia via medical therapy in patients with symptomatic coronary disease has not shown convincing definite benefit,[54] then it is unlikely that a positive result would be obtained by suppressing asymptomatic myocardial ischaemia by anti anginal therapy in totally asymptomatic patients.

It is conceivable that screening for asymptomatic myocardial ischaemia in certain people with diabetes might produce further refined risk and allow more targeted therapy. This might include those with micro-albuminuria. In the study by Rutter and colleagues, SMI was present in 65% of those with micro-albuminuria versus 40% of those without micro-albuminuria.[55] Blood pressure was significantly higher in those with micro-albuminuria (161/85 mm Hg versus 150/83 mm Hg). Since hypertension is strongly associated with asymptomatic ECG changes and ST segment depression during daily activities, the first strategy that should be employed in those patients might be aggressive antihypertensive therapy. The recent Heart Outcomes Prevention Evaluation (HOPE) study suggests that an ACE inhibitor would be most appropriate,[56] although if an anti-ischaemic benefit was desired, beta-blockers may be preferable (see Chapter 5).

Conclusions

In community-based studies SMI is more common in people with diabetes than in non-diabetic subjects. In hospital-based studies of patients with CHD the picture is the opposite, with little or no evidence that this is the case. The reason for this difference must lie in the different populations studied. It may be as simple as the fact that SMI lies in the continuum from no ischaemia to symptomatic ischaemia and reflects an intermediate severity of CHD. People with diabetes are further down the road to significant CHD. Once symptoms develop and patients reach the hospital service SMI is so common that the differences between diabetic patients and non-diabetic patients cease to exist or are so minimized as to be difficult to detect. None of the studies have addressed the reproducibility of SMI and it is interesting that SMI has a low specificity for CHD in the population studies.

None of the studies address effectively whether people with diabetes should be screened for asymptomatic myocardial ischaemia. Most practising cardiologists have a lower threshold for investigating people with diabetes, based on the belief that they have more severe coronary disease and a defective warning system. In the light of the ACIP study, it may be that we should re-evaluate this stance, although it is likely that this practice will continue until, if ever, larger clinical trials address this problem. In those diabetic patients with evidence of autonomic dysfunction it seems justified to screen aggressively for SMI. However, since screening for early autonomic dysfunction is not part of routine diabetic practice this presents a problem identifying those to be screened. An argument could be made that it might be simpler to use Holter monitoring for SMI as a means of screening for autonomic dysfunction.

The relevance of SMI to clinical practice in both non-diabetic and diabetic patients, symptomatic or otherwise, is still a contentious issue. The Malmo study and the Lipid Research Council Follow-Up Study present strong evidence for the adverse outcome in normal subjects with SMI, either on treadmill or on Holter monitoring. If it were demonstrated that aggressive treatment, such as revascularization of asymptomatic patients, offered significant improvements in survival, then a case could be made for screening and treating all patients exhibiting this. However, there is scant existing evidence that coronary revascularization is of proven benefit under these circumstances. What is now known is that statin therapy reduces mortality from CHD in high-risk asymptomatic populations [57] (see Chapter 6). People with diabetes form a high-risk group of patients in whom aggressive medical therapy is warranted, even in the absence of anginal symptoms. They are at such high risk that a strong case could be made for aspirin and lipid-lowering therapy to be available to these patients irrespective of the presence of SMI, obviating the need to search for it. However, the current recommendation would be to use a CHD risk calculator to see if the patient reached the 3% per annum risk of CHD (see Chapter 6).

The best case for using the detection of SMI as a therapeutic tool is made in relation to people with diabetes with evidence of autonomic dysfunction and it is reasonable to screen these patients for evidence of SMI. A poor exercise test or prolonged or frequent episodes of SMI would justify coronary angiography.

People with diabetes have a higher incidence of unrecognized myocardial infarction. The uncovering of this is likely to become more common with the increasing availability of ECGs in primary care and with more effective and formalized diabetic shared care. The clinician has two non-invasive techniques to evaluate these patients. Unless the patient has autonomic dysfunction then exercise testing, rather than 24-hour ambulatory ECG monitoring, is probably the correct approach since the prognostic content of the stress ECG is well worked out.

References

1. Garcia MJ, McNamara PM, Gordon T, Kannel WB. Morbidity and mortality in diabetics in a general population. Sixteen year follow-up experience in the Framingham study. Diabetes 1970;19:375.

2. Faerman I, Faccio E, Milie J et al. Autonomic neuropathy and painless myocardial infarction in diabetic patients. Histologic evidence of their relationship. Diabetes 1977;26:1147–58.

3. Stern S, Tzivoni D. Early detection of silent ischaemic heart disease by 24-hour electrocardiographic monitoring of active subjects. Br Heart J 1974;36:481–6.

4. Schang SJ, Pepine CJ. Transient asymptomatic ST segment depression during daily activity. Am J Cardiol 1977;39:396–402.

5. Lochen ML. The Tromso study: the prevalence of exercise-induced silent myocardial ischaemia and relation to risk factors for coronary heart disease in an apparently healthy population. Eur Heart J 1992;13:728–31.

6. Sigurdsson E, Sigfusson N, Sigvaldason H, Thorgeirsson G. Silent ST-T changes in an epidemiologic cohort study—a marker of hypertension or coronary heart disease, or both: the Reykjavik study. J Am Coll Cardiol 1996;27:1140–7.

7. Chiariello M, Indolfi C, Cotecchia MR et al. Asymptomatic transient ST changes during ambulatory ECG monitoring in diabetic patients. Am Heart J 1985;110:529–34.

8. Chipkin SR, Frid D, Alpert JS et al. Frequency of painless myocardial ischemia during exercise tolerance testing in patients with and without diabetes mellitus. Am J Cardiol 1987;59:61–5.

9. Callaham PR, Froelicher VF, Klein J et al. Exercise-induced silent ischaemia: age, diabetes melllitus, previous myocardial infarction and prognosis. J Am Coll Cardiol 1989;14:1175–80.

10. Dellborg M, Emanuelsson H, Swedberg K. Silent myocardial ischemia during coronary angioplasty. Cardiology 1993;82:325–34.

11. Caracciolo EA, Chaitman BR, Forman SA et al. Diabetics with coronary disease have a prevalence of asymptomatic ischemia during exercise tread-mill testing and ambulatory ischemia monitoring similar to that of nondi-abetic patients. An ACIP database study. Circulation 1996:93:2097–105.

12. Chiarello M, Indolfi C. Silent myocardial ischemia in patients with diabetes. Circulation 1996;93:2089–91.

13. Weiner DA, Ryan TJ, Parsons L et al. Significance of silent myocardial ischemia during exercise testing in patients with diabetes mellitus: a report from the Coronary Artery Surgery Study (CASS) Registry. Am J Cardiol 1991;68:720–34.

14. Naka M, Hiramatsu K, Aizawa T et al. Silent myocardial ischemia in patients with non-insulin-dependent diabetes mellitus as judged by treatmill exercise testing and coronary angiography. Am Heart J 1992;123:46–53.

15. May O, Arildsen H, Damsgaard EM, Mickley H. Prevalence and predic-tion of silent ischaemia in diabetes mellitus: a population-based study. Cardiovasc Res 1997;34:241–7.

16. Koistinen MJ. Prevalence of asymptomatic myocardial ischaemia in diabetic subjects. BMJ 1990;301:92–5.

17. Hume L, Oakley GD, Bouton AJ et al. Asymptomatic myocardial ischaemia in diabetes and its relationship to diabetic neuropathy: an exercise electrocardiography study in middle-aged diabetic men. Diabetes Care 1986;9:384–8.

18. Langer A, Freeman MR, Josee RG et al. Detection of silent myocardial ischemia in diabetes mellitus. Am J Cardiol 1991;67:1073–8.

19. Ambepityia G, Kopelman PG, Ingram D et al. Exertional myocardial ischemia in diabetes: a quantitative analysis of anginal perceptual threshold and the influence of autonomic function. J Am Coll Cardiol 1990;15:72–7.

20. Umachandran V, Ranjadayalan K, Ambepityia G et al. The perception of angina in diabetes: relation to somatic pain threshold and autonomic function. Am Heart J 1991;121:1649–54.

21. Marchant B, Umachandran V, Stevenson R et al. Silent myocardial ischemia: role of subclinical neuropathy in patients with and without diabetes. J Am Coll Cardiol 1993;22:1433–7.

22. Murray DP, O'Brien T, Mulrooney R, O'Sullivan DJ. Autonomic dysfunction and silent myocardial ischaemia on exercise testing in diabetes mellitus. Diabet Med 1990;7:580–4.

23. O'Sullivan JJ, Conroy RM, MacDonald K et al. Silent ischaemia in diabetic men with autonomic neuropathy. Br Heart J 1991;66:313–15.

24. Hikita H, Kurita A, Takase B et al. Usefulness of plasma beta-endorphin level, pain threshold and autonomic function in assessing silent myocardial ischemia in patients with and without diabetes mellitus. Am J Cardiol 1993;72:140–3.

25. Langer A, Freeman MR, Josse RG, Armstrong PW. Metaiodobenzylguanidine imaging in diabetes mellitus: assessment of cardiac sympathetic denervation and its relation to autonomic dysfunction and silent myocardial ischemia. J Am Coll Cardiol 1995;25:610–8.

26. Henderson EB, Kahn JK, Corbett JR et al. Abnormal I-123 metaiodobenzylguanidine myocardial washout and distribution may reflect myocardial adrenergic derangement in patients with congestive cardiomyopathy. Circulation 1988;78:1192–9.

27. Schofer J, Spielmann R, Schuchert A et al. Iodine-123 meta-iodobenzylguanidine scintigraphy: a noninvasive method to demonstrate myocardial adrenergic nervous system disintegrity in patients with idiopathic dilated cardiomyopathy. J Am Coll Cardiol 1988;12:1252–8.

28. Merlet P, Valette H, Dubois-Rande JL et al. Prognostic value of cardiac metaiodobenzylguanidine imaging in patients with heart failure. J Nucl Med 1992;33:471–7.

29. Rabinovitch MA, Rose CP, Rouleau JL et al. Metaiodobenzylguanidine [131I] scintigraphy detects impaired myocardial sympathetic neuronal transport function of canine mechanical-overload heart failure. Circ Res 1987;61:797–804.

30. Minardo JD, Tuli MM, Mock BH et al. Scintigraphic and electrophysiological evidence of canine myocardial sympathetic denervation and reinnervation produced by myocardial infarction or phenol application. Circulation 1988;78:1008–19.
31. Stanton MS, Tuli MM, Radtke NL et al. Regional sympathetic denervation after myocardial infarction in humans detected noninvasively using I-123 metaiodobenzyiguanidine. J Am Coll Cardiol 1989;14:1519–26.
32. Dae MW, Herre JM, O'Connell JW et al. Scintigraphic assessment of sympathetic innervation after transmural versus nontransmural myocardial infarction. J Am Coll Cardiol 1991;17:1416–23.
33. McGhie AI, Corbett JR, Akers MS et al. Regional cardiac adrenergic function using I-123 meta-iodobenzylguanidine tomographic imaging after acute myocardial infarction. Am J Cardiol 1991;67:236–42.
34. Gohl K, Feistel H, Weikl A et al. Congenital myocardial sympathetic dysinnervation (CMSD)—a structural defect of idiopathic long QT syndrome. Pacing Clin Electrophysiol 1991;14:1544–53.
35. Zarich S, Waxman S, Freeman RT et al. Effect of autonomic nervous system dysfunction on the circadian pattern of myocardial ischaemia in diabetes mellitus. J Am Coll Cardiol 1994;24:956–62.
36. Nihoyannopoulos P, Marsonis A, Joshi J et al. Magnitude of myocardial dysfunction is greater in painful than in painless myocardial ischemia: an exercise echocardiographic study. J Am Coll Cardiol 1995;25:1507–12.
37. Droste C, Roskamm H. Experimental pain measurement in patients with asymptomatic myocardial ischemia. J Am Coll Cardiol 1983;1:940–5.
38. Glazier JJ, Chierchia S, Brown MJ, Maseeri A. Importance of generalized defective perception of painful stimuli as a cause of silent myocardial ischemia in chronic stable angina pectoris. Am J Cardiol 1986;58:667–72.
39. Mickley H. Silent myocardial ischaemia. Br J Cardiol 1996;3:39–40.
40. Rocco MB, Nabel EG, Campbell S et al. Prognostic importance of myocardial ischaemia detected by ambulatory monitoring in patients with stable coronary artery disease. Circulation 1988;78:877–84.
41. Tzivoni D, Weisz G, Gavish A et al. Comparison of mortality and myocardial infarction rates in stable angina pectoris with and without ischemic episodes during daily activities. Am J Cardiol 1989;63:273–6.
42. Deedwania PC, Carbajai EV. Silent ischemia during daily life is an independent predictor of mortality in stable angina. Circulation 1990;81:748–56.
43. Mulcahy D, Parameshwar J, Holdright D et al. Value of ambulatory ST segment monitoring in patients with chronic stable angina: does measurement of the 'total ischaemic burden' assist with management? Br Heart J 1992;67:47–52.
44. Quyyumi A, Panza JA, Diodati JG et al. Prognostic implications of myocardial ischemia during daily life in low risk patients with coronary artery disease. J Am Coll Cardiol 1993;21:700–8.

45. Gandhi MM, Wood DA Lampe FC. Characteristics and clinical significance of ambulatory myocardial ischemia in men and women in the general population presenting with angina pectoris. J Am Coll Cardiol 1994;23:74–81.
46. Mulcahy D, Knight C, Patel D et al. Detection of ambulatory ischaemia is not of practical clinical value in the routine management of patients with stable angina. Eur Heart J 1995;16:317–24.
47. Forslund L, Hjemdahl P, Held C et al. Prognostic implications of ambulatory myocardial ischemia and arrhythmias and relations to ischemia on exercise in chronic stable angina pectoris (the Angina Prognosis Study In Stockholm [APSIS]). Am J Cardiol 1999;84:1151–7.
48. Hedblad B, Juul-Moller S, Svensson K et al. Increased mortality in men with ST segment depression during 24 h ambulatory long-term ECG recording. Results from prospective population study 'Men born in 1914' from Malmo, Sweden. Eur Heart J 1989;10:149–58.
49. Gordon DJ, Ekelund LG, Karon JM et al. Predictive value of the tolerance test for mortality in North American men: The Lipid Research Clinics Mortality Follow-up Study. Circulation 1986;74:252–61.
50. Dargie HJ, Ford I, Fox KM. Total Ischaemic Burden European Trial (TIBET). Effects of ischaemia and treatment with atenolol, nifedipine SR and their combination on outcome in patients with chronic stable angina. The TIBET Study Group. Eur Heart J 1996;17:104–12.
51. Stone PH, Chaitman, BR, McMahon, RP et al. Asymptomatic Cardiac Ischaemia Pilot (ACIP) Study. Relationship between exercise-induced and ambulatory ischemia in patients with stable coronary disease. Circulation 1996;94:1537–44.
52. Coronary Artery Surgery Study (CASS) Principal Investigators and Associates. Coronary Artery Surgery Study (CASS): a randomized trial of coronary artery bypass surgery. Survival data. Circulation 1983;68:939–50.
53. Li C, Cui J, Qio Y. Follow-up of asymptomatic myocardial ischemia in patients with diabetes mellitus. Chin Med Sci 1993;8:118–20.
54. Davies RF, Goldberg AD, Forman S et al. Asymptomatic Cardiac Ischemia Pilot (ACIP) Study two-year follow up: outcomes of patients randomized to initial strategies of medical therapy versus revascularisation. Circulation 1997;95:2037–43.
55. Rutter MK, McComb JM, Brady S, Marshall SM. Silent myocardial ischemia and microalbuminuria in asymptomatic subjects with non-insulin-dependent diabetes mellitus. Am J Cardiol 1999;83:27–31.
56. Heart Outcomes Prevention Evaluation (HOPE) Study Investigators. Effects of ramipril on cardiovascular and microvascular outcomes in people with diabetes mellitus: results of the HOPE study and MICRO-HOPE substudy. Lancet 2000;355:253–59.
57. Shepherd J, Cobbe SM, Ford I et al. Prevention of coronary heart disease with pravastatin in men with hypercholesterolemia. West of Scotland Coronary Prevention Study Group. N Engl J Med 1995;333:1301–307.

chapter 4

Myocardial infarction and acute coronary syndromes in diabetes

Miles Fisher

Introduction

Myocardial infarction is the most serious expression of coronary heart disease. The mortality from acute myocardial infarction is high, and almost half of the deaths occur immediately or before the patient has a chance to reach hospital. Over the last 20 years the prospects have been greatly improved for patients who survive long enough to reach hospital, and the widespread use of thrombolytic agents and powerful pharmacological interventions has significantly reduced the in-hospital mortality from acute myocardial infarction. Nevertheless, the mortality from acute myocardial infarction in people with diabetes remains twice that of the non-diabetic population, and an optimal management plan is an imperative.

Recent attention has widened from simply focusing on myocardial infarction to other acute coronary syndromes, including non-Q myocardial infarction and unstable angina. There are few specific published data on diabetes in the other acute coronary syndromes, but many published studies have included significant numbers of patients with diabetes, so some general comments are possible.

Epidemiology and prognosis

The publication by Haffner et al. of data based on a defined Finnish population has been described in Chapter 1.[1] The incidence of myocardial infarction was examined in a defined geographical population in people with diabetes compared with non-diabetic control subjects. Diabetic patients *without* previous myocardial infarction had as high a risk of myocardial infarction as non-diabetic patients *with* previous myocardial infarction. The mortality in diabetic patients without previous infarction was similar to that of non-diabetic patients with previous myocardial infarction, and was even higher in diabetic patients with prior myocardial infarction (Chapter 1, Fig. 1.3).

The prevalence of diabetes among patients with myocardial infarction admitted to hospital coronary care units varies between 6 and 30%,[2,3] and most of these patients have type 2 diabetes. In addition to patients with previously diagnosed diabetes, many patients with acute myocardial infarction have previously undiagnosed diabetes, based on persisting hyperglycaemia and a raised glycated haemoglobin at the time of admission.[4]

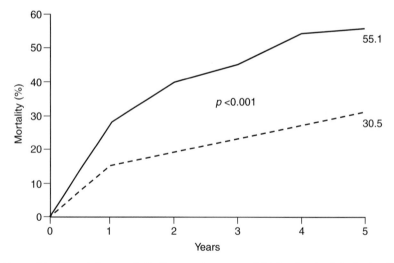

Figure 4.1   Cumulative mortality from acute myocardial infarction in diabetic (——) and non-diabetic (- - -) individuals. (Reproduced from reference 5.)

Studies performed before[5] and after[6] the introduction of thrombolytic therapy have demonstrated that the mortality of myocardial infarction in people with diabetes is double that of non-diabetic patients. This worse mortality affects both the early mortality and long-term mortality, and after 5 years up to three-quarters of diabetic patients hospitalized with myocardial infarction are dead[5] (Fig. 4.1).

Pathophysiology

There are several possible explanations for the increased mortality following myocardial infarction in people with diabetes (Table 4.1).[7] Firstly the underlying coronary might be more severe. There might

---

Table 4.1 Possible explanations for the increased mortality following myocardial infarction in people with diabetes

Severity of coronary artery lesions
- More severe, extensive and diffuse

Other structural abnormalities
- Specific heart disease of diabetes ('diabetic cardiomyopathy') causing diastolic or systolic dysfunction
- Diabetic autonomic neuropathy

Prothrombotic tendency
- Decreased fibrinolytic activity (increased PAI 1)
- Increased platelet aggregation
- Increased coagulation factors

Metabolic abnormalities
- Decreased insulin production
- Increased insulin resistance
- Increased metabolism of free fatty acids
- Impaired myocardial glucose utilization

be an adverse influence due to concomitant diabetic autonomic neuropathy or the specific heart disease of diabetes ('diabetic cardiomyopathy'). The prothrombotic tendency that is well described in people with diabetes may favour re-infarction, and the abnormal metabolic milieu following the infarction may be particularly disadvantageous in people with diabetes who are insulin resistant.

Many studies have been performed at post mortem or in patients with stable angina during coronary arteriography. Post mortem studies included patients who had died from cardiovascular and from other causes, and demonstrated that coronary artery disease was more severe and diffuse in people with diabetes. However, few studies have specifically examined patients who died following myocardial infarction. More recently, angiography has been performed in the acute situation to examine the efficacy of thrombolytic therapy. The Thrombolysis and Angioplasty in Myocardial Infarction (TAMI) study group performed angiography approximately 90 minutes after initiation of thrombolytic therapy.[8] Patients with diabetes had more extensive coronary disease, as defined by the number of vessels with at least one stenosis, with 66% of diabetic patients having multi-vessel disease compared with 46% of those without diabetes. Diabetic patients also had more diffuse coronary disease, as indicated by a mean of 3.4 diseased segments in patients with diabetes compared to 2.9 diseased segments in non-diabetic patients.

Studies that measure traditional cardiac enzyme release or estimate the infarct size using an ECG scoring system have demonstrated a similar infarct size in people with diabetes, and the increased mortality does not appear to be related to a larger size of infarction.[9]

Autonomic neuropathy

Several factors can impair autonomic function in people with diabetes, including diabetic neuropathy, increasing age and coronary heart disease itself. Many myocardial infarctions in people with diabetes are clinically silent or painless,[10,11] leading to delays in hospitalization and initiation of treatment that may reduce the efficacy of thrombolytic therapy. Indeed, many diabetic patients present too late for this life-saving therapy. It has been suggested that previous silent infarction may be present in up to 40% of patients with diabetes at the time they present with their first clinically recognized myocardial infarction.[2] Others have suggested that age rather than diabetes may be a more important contribution to silent infarction,[12] and the theory that silent infarction is indeed more common in people with diabetes has recently been challenged.[13] Some of these silent infarctions may be related to autonomic neuropathy,[14] which may occur in nearly half of all diabetic patients with coronary heart disease,[15] and abnormalities of autonomic function are very common in diabetic patients following myocardial infarction.[16]

Diabetic autonomic neuropathy may cause systolic and diastolic dysfunction, and sympathovagal imbalance has been associated with a poor prognosis following myocardial infarction in non-diabetic subjects, independent of left ventricular dysfunction. Many patients with diabetes have diminished vagal activity, causing a relative increase in sympathetic activity.

Diabetic cardiomyopathy
A detailed description of the evidence for a specific heart disease of diabetes or so-called 'diabetic cardiomyopathy' is beyond the scope of this chapter.[17,18] Indirect support for the possible influence of microangiopathy affecting the heart following myocardial infarction

---

Table 4.2 Complications of myocardial infarction that are increased in patients with diabetes

- Congestive cardiac failure
- Cardiac rupture
- Cardiogenic shock
- Atrioventricular and intraventricular conduction abnormalities
- Sudden death
- Re-infarction
- Increased case fatality

has come from a couple of small studies from Scotland and Malta.[19,20] In both studies, diabetic patients with retinopathy were more likely to die or develop cardiac failure following infarction than patients without retinopathy. Other increased complications of myocardial infarction in people with diabetes are detailed in Table 4.2.

Treatment of myocardial infarction in people with diabetes

Following myocardial infarction in people with diabetes, a number of measures are now available which may help to reduce the mortality rate (Table 4.3). These can be broken down into measures that are given immediately, and conventional secondary preventive measures. Secondary preventive measures are described in greater detail in Chapter 7.

Table 4.3 Possible treatments for myocardial infarction in people with diabetes

---

Immediate measures
- Aspirin
- Thrombolysis/fibrinolysis
- Immediate percutaneous coronary intervention (PCI)
- Intravenous insulin
- Beta-adrenoreceptor blockers/ACE inhibitors

Secondary prevention of myocardial infarction
- Aspirin
- Beta-adrenoreceptor blockers
- ACE inhibitors
- Subcutaneous insulin
- Lipid reduction with statins, gemfibrozil
- Cardiac rehabilitation

Aspirin

Treatment with aspirin causes a significant reduction in the morbidity and mortality of acute myocardial infarction in non-diabetic patients,[21] and the early administration of aspirin to patients with suspected myocardial infarction is now part of routine clinical care. In the Second International Study of Infarct Survival (ISIS-2), the mortality was reduced by 23% in non-diabetic subjects who received short-term aspirin 160 mg, but in diabetic patients the mortality did not differ between those who received aspirin and the placebo group.[21]

The large meta-analysis performed by the Antiplatelet Trialists' Collaboration included 29 trials in high risk patients with separate information on diabetes status.[22] The rate of cardiovascular events including myocardial infarction was reduced from 22% to 18% in people with diabetes, and from 16% to 13% in non-diabetic subjects (Figure 4.2). Because of the high number of cardiovascular events in people with diabetes the absolute benefit of aspirin therapy is greater

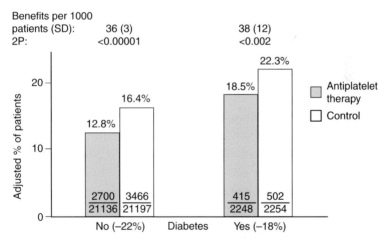

Antiplatelet Trialist's Collaboration, 1994

Figure 4.2 Benefits of aspirin on cardiovascular events in diabetic and non-diabetic subjects. (Data from reference 22, figure reproduced from reference 33.)

than in non-diabetic subjects.[23] It has been suggested that because of an increased turnover of platelets in people with diabetes, a 300 mg dose of aspirin may be required to suppress the synthesis of thromboxane A2.[24] The Hypertension Optimal Treatment (HOT) trial is described in Chapter 5. In the HOT study patients also received 75 mg of aspirin or placebo in addition to the trial anti-hypertensive therapy; patients who received aspirin 75 mg had a significant reduction in cardiovascular events. It was reported that the relative benefit was about the same in patients with diabetes, although the specific data were not provided.[25] The optimal dose of aspirin has yet to be identified in patients with diabetes, but the consensus is that a large initial dose should be administered as quickly as possible to diabetic patients with acute myocardial infarction.

Thrombolysis

The principal pathology at the time of acute myocardial infarction is thrombosis superimposed on a ruptured atheromatous plaque. Thrombolytic therapy aims to dissolve the thrombus to restore patency, and improve survival by reducing the amount of damaged myocardium, so maintaining cardiac function. In deciding whether to use this treatment, the benefits must be compared to potential side effects, particularly the risk of haemorrhage. Not all patients treated with thrombolytic therapy have successful reperfusion, and some patients with initial successful reperfusion subsequently sustain a re-occlusion of the diseased artery. Early studies confirmed that the mortality of acute myocardial infarction was reduced by thrombolytic therapy in diabetic patients as well as in non-diabetic patients. The Fibrinolytic Therapy Trialists' Collaborative Group performed a meta-analysis of studies containing over 40 000 patients, around 10% of whom had diabetes. They showed that the relative reduction in mortality after treatment with thrombolytic agents was similar in diabetic and non-diabetic subjects, but that a great number of lives could be saved in the diabetic subjects because of the higher overall mortality.[26] The proportional reduction in mortality with thrombolytic therapy was slightly, although non-significantly, greater among the diabetic patients studied, and the absolute benefit of treatment was greater among diabetic patients. In diabetic subjects 37 lives were saved for every 1000 treated, whereas in non-diabetic subjects 15 lives were saved per 1000 treated (Figure 4.3).

An initial small study that assessed reperfusion by the time to peak release of creatine kinase-MB isoenzyme suggested impaired reperfusion in diabetic patients after thrombolytic therapy.[27] Another small study using 'clinical parameters of reperfusion' also suggested a lower frequency of reperfusion in thrombolysed diabetic patients than in non-diabetic subjects.[20] Larger angiographic studies, however, have demonstrated a similar patency rate at 90 minutes following thrombolytic therapy in diabetic and non-diabetic individuals.[28,29] The TAMI study group showed that the initial patency rates were 71% in patients with diabetes and 70% in those without diabetes. A second angiogram was performed at 7 to 10 days, and showed a similar re-occlusion rate at 12% in the diabetic group and 11% in the non-diabetic group.[7]

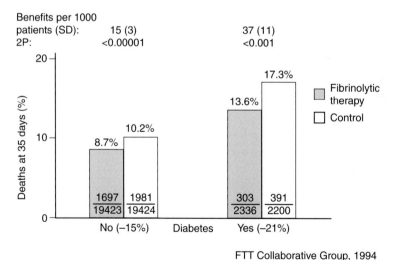

Figure 4.3 Effects of fibrinolytic therapy on mortality in the 35 days following myocardial infarction in diabetic and non-diabetic subjects. (Data from reference 26, figure reproduced from reference 33.)

Similar data were described by the GUSTO-I angiographic investigators, with patency rates of 70% in patients with diabetes and 67% in those without diabetes, and re-occlusion rates of 9% and 5% respectively (p = non-significant).[29]

Thrombolytic agents have been demonstrated to be safe in the diabetic population, with no significant increase in the incidence of serious bleeding complications or stroke.[28–31] Initial fears about the safety of thrombolysis in patients with retinopathy have proved to be unfounded and the indications and contraindications for thrombolysis in diabetic patients should be the same as in non-diabetic subjects.[32,33] Unfortunately, thrombolysis continues to be underused in people with diabetes because of the erroneous fear of retinal haemorrhage.[20,34]

Although meta-analysis of large studies has proven the benefit of thrombolysis in people with diabetes compared to placebo, there are insufficient data comparing different thrombolytic agents in people with diabetes to enable firm conclusions to be drawn about the most effective agent. Studies are presently being undertaken to compare different thrombolytic agents when combined with glycoprotein IIb/IIIa antagonists to identify the optimum pharmacological reperfusion treatment following myocardial infarction.

Primary angioplasty for acute myocardial infarction

The prevention of myocardial damage is the main goal of all reperfusion therapies for patients with acute myocardial infarction. Initial studies perfused thrombolytic therapy directly into the coronary circulation, but were superceded by the systemic administration of aspirin or thrombolytic therapy via the oral and intravenous route respectively. Primary percutaneous coronary intervention (PCI) has the theoretical advantage over systemic thrombolytic therapy in that it allows more complete restoration of the arterial lumen. This should decrease the area of myocardial necrosis and degree of myocardial dysfunction, and therefore improve overall prognosis. The avoidance of systemic thrombolysis should also reduce the risk of haemorrhagic complications. A meta-analysis of the results of 10 randomized trials confirmed the advantage of primary PTCA over thrombolytic therapy.[35] A small subgroup analysis from one study has confirmed that primary angioplasty is better than thrombolysis in people with diabetes.[36] In another study a comparison of direct PCI in diabetic and non-diabetic subjects has shown that the mortality at 30 days and one year was increased in the diabetic patients, and the left ventricular ejection fraction before discharge was lower in the diabetic patients.[37] Similar findings were obtained when PCI was used to treat non-ST segment elevation myocardial infarction.[38]

Recently, attempts have been made to reduce the high incidence of dissection of the intima, re-occlusions and restenosis of the artery by combining PTCA with coronary stenting plus glycoprotein IIb/IIIa blockade. A study of 140 patients, 20% of whom had diabetes, demonstrated that coronary stenting plus abciximab was associated with a better degree of myocardial salvage and a better clinical outcome than thrombolysis with a tissue plasminogen activator, alteplase.[39]

Data from national registries in the US and France have shown that in routine clinical practice the advantages of primary PCI for myocardial infarction disappeared because of delays in the start of intervention.[40,41] The limited availability of interventional cardiology, combined with the cost, will mean that this form of treatment will not be universally applicable as a treatment for myocardial infarction for the foreseeable future.

Other aspects of the use of PCI as a treatment for ischaemic heart disease in people with diabetes are discussed in Chapter 8.

Blood glucose control following myocardial infarction

The metabolic consequences of acute myocardial infarction include the release of adrenaline, glucagon and other counter-regulatory hormones. In patients with established diabetes this counter-regulatory hormonal release can cause significant hyperglycaemia and may precipitate metabolic decompensation. The release of counter-regulatory hormones leads to relative insulin resistance in the myocardium, and this favours the utilization of free fatty acids which may have deleterious effects on the myocardium following myocardial infarction (Table 4.1).

Prior to the publication of the Diabetes Mellitus Insulin Glucose Infusion in Acute Myocardial Infarction (DIGAMI) study the blood glucose was controlled at the time of myocardial infarction by intermittent subcutaneous insulin or intravenous glucose–insulin–potassium infusion. A low-dose insulin infusion regimen was found to be simple, safe and effective at lowering the blood glucose from a mean of 15 mmol/l on entry to the coronary care unit to a mean of 8 mmol/l at 12 hours,[42] but this had no effect on mortality.[43]

A small study from Dundee demonstrated a reduction in mortality in a group of 29 patients admitted in one year compared with a historical control of 33 patients who were treated the previous year.[44] This study was heavily criticised because of the use of a historical control, and the small number of subjects, and attempts to replicate the results in a larger, multi-centre, randomized, control trial were unsuccessful.[45]

DIGAMI

The DIGAMI study has re-awakened interest in methods of controlling blood glucose in diabetic patients following myocardial infarction. In the DIGAMI study, 'diabetes' was defined as either a previous diagnosis of diabetes or a blood glucose on admission above 11 mmol/l. This latter group will include patients with previously undiagnosed diabetes and patients with stress hyperglycaemia. The publication of a feasibility study in *Diabetes Care* showed that use of a high-dose insulin infusion regimen in patients with suspected myocardial infarction was associated with a lower blood glucose at 24 hours compared to conventional control.[46] There was a slight but significant decrease in potassium in both intervention and control groups, and this was greater in the infusion group. The initial insulin infusion rate was around 5 units/hour, and the infusion rate was

Table 4.4   Protocol used by coronary care unit nurses for insulin–glucose infusions in the original DIGAMI study[47]

Infusion: 500 ml 5% glucose with 80 IU of soluble insulin (~1 IU/6 ml).

- Start with 30 ml/h. Check blood glucose after 1 h. Adjust infusion rate according to the protocol and aim for a blood glucose level of 7 to 10 mmol/l.
- Blood glucose should be checked after 1 h if infusion rate has been changed, otherwise every 2 h.
- If the initial decrease in blood glucose exceeds 30%, the infusion rate should be left unchanged if blood glucose is >11 mmol/l and reduced by 6 ml/h if blood glucose is within the targeted range of 7 to 10.9 mmol/l.
- If blood glucose is stable and < 10.9 mmol/l after 10 PM, reduce infusion rate by 50% during night.

Blood glucose: > 15 mmol/l: Give 8 IU of insulin as an intravenous bolus injection and increase infusion rate by 6 ml/h.

11 to 14.9 mmol/l: Increase infusion rate by 3 ml/h

7 to 10.9 mmol/l: Leave infusion rate unchanged

4 to 6.9 mmol/l: Decrease infusion rate by 6 ml/h

<4 mmol/l: Stop infusion for 15 min. Then test blood glucose and continue testing every 15 min until blood glucose is ≥ 7 mmol/l. In the presence of symptoms of hypoglycaemia, administer 20 ml of 30% glucose intravenously. The infusion is restarted with an infusion rate decreased by 6 ml/h when blood glucose is ≥ 7 mmol/l.

subsequently altered every 1 to 2 hours depending on the blood glucose concentration, which was performed using a reflectance meter (Table 4.4). Seventeen per cent of the insulin-infusion group had an episode of hypoglycaemia within the first 24 hours, but this was not associated with any adverse effects.

Of the 1240 patients eligible for inclusion in the completed study, only 620 (50%) were randomized, and the commonest reasons for exclusion were unwillingness or inability to follow the study protocol. Patients in the insulin–glucose group (n = 306) received standard coronary care unit therapy, the insulin–glucose infusion, then subcutaneous insulin four times daily for at least 3 months. Control patients (n = 314) were treated according to standard coronary care practice and did not receive insulin unless it was clinically indicated. There was substantial overlap in the treatments received by the two groups of patients, with the majority of subjects in the control group receiving at least one injection of insulin during their admission and many being treated with insulin at the time of discharge from hospital. During the hospital stay 55% of the control patients received at least one injection of soluble insulin and 43% of the control group were receiving insulin treatment at the time of hospital discharge, compared to 87% in the insulin–glucose group.

The results of the completed study demonstrated a statistically significant reduction in mortality in patients who had received the insulin–glucose infusion followed by a multi-dose insulin regimen compared with a control group who received conventional therapy.[47] There was a non-significant reduction in mortality at the time of discharge from hospital, and at 3 months. After 1 year of follow-up the mortality in the control group was 26% and in the insulin-infusion group 19%, a relative reduction in mortality of one-third. The reduction in mortality was particularly evident for patients who had a low cardiovascular risk profile and no previous insulin treatment.[47]

When specific causes of death were analysed there was a trend towards fewer cardiovascular deaths of all kinds, and specifically for sudden death in the insulin–glucose group compared to the control group, but this was not statistically significant.[48] This may be due to the small number of deaths from specific causes in each group. The most common cause of death in all patients was congestive heart failure.

Similar mortality results were seen when longer follow-up data were published.[49] With a mean follow-up of 3.4 years the mortality in the insulin–glucose group was 33% compared with 44% in the control group, a relative risk reduction of 28% (Fig. 4.4). A detailed analysis of patients in prespecified subgroups showed that it was only in patients who were identified as being at low risk and who were not previously receiving insulin therapy that benefit was obtained. There was no statistically significant benefit in patients at high risk who were not previously on insulin, and no benefit was obtained in patients who were previously treated with insulin therapy regardless of risk stratification.

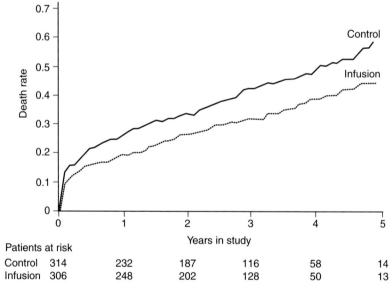

Figure 4.4 Actuarial mortality curves from the DIGAMI study during long term follow up in patients receiving insulin–glucose infusion and the control group. The mean follow-up was 3.4 years (range 1.6–5.6 years). The absolute reduction in risk was 11%; relative risk = 0.72 (0.55 to 0.92), p = 0.011. (Based on data published in reference 49.)

This interesting study has provoked much intense debate. The authors were aware of the limitations of the study, including the fact that there was a considerably lower than predicted overall mortality rate. They concluded that 'the long-term overall mortality in diabetic patients with acute myocardial infarction *could* be further reduced by the administration of insulin–glucose infusion followed by multi-dose subcutaneous insulin'. Possible mechanisms which they suggested for the reduced mortality in the insulin–glucose group included:

- effects on free fatty acids, which may potentiate ischaemic injury through several mechanisms;
- an effect similar to the use of insulin–glucose–potassium infusion on intracellular potassium in the ischaemic zone, preserving myocardium and causing less extensive myocardial damage; and
- possible effects of extended insulin treatment in improving metabolism in the non-infarcted areas, reducing the gradual remodelling of the left ventricular myocardium.

The authors also commented that the institution of insulin therapy might have been paralleled by a general improvement in the care of the patient, contributing to the beneficial outcome.[46]

Other possible explanations are:

- the inclusion in the control group of a larger number of patients with stress hyperglycaemia and previously undiagnosed diabetes,
- the withdrawal of therapy with sulphonylureas which may cause harm by having effects on potassium channels in the heart,[50,51] and affecting ischaemic preconditioning.[51]

Glucose–insulin–potassium (GIK) has also been advocated for the treatment of non-diabetic patients following myocardial infarction. A recent meta-analysis of this therapy including nine suitable studies, but not including the DIGAMI study, has demonstrated that mortality was reduced from 21% in the placebo group to 16.1% in the GIK group.[52] The authors suggested that the value of this therapy in the era of thrombolysis and acute revascularization by primary angioplasty can only be fully resolved by conducting large, randomized trials. In one small-scale randomized trial GIK seemed to be of particular benefit when combined with reperfusion strategies, principally thrombolysis,[53] and confirmation is required from large-scale studies.

Implementation of the DIGAMI results

From the results of DIGAMI it is not possible to determine whether the improvement in mortality was because of improved metabolic control with the intravenous insulin at the time of infarction, the improved control with subcutaneous insulin after discharge, the withdrawal of sulphonylurea therapy, or a combination of all three. If the intravenous insulin was important, how tight should glycaemic control be and could the same benefit be obtained without the risk of hypoglycaemia? If chronic treatment was important, do these patients need multiple injections or would more limited insulin treatment regimens suffice? It is hoped that some of the questions raised by the first DIGAMI study will be answered following the completion of DIGAMI 2. This compares a group who will receive insulin–glucose infusion followed by multi-dose, subcutaneous insulin, a second group who will receive the same initial treatment followed by conventional treatment, and a third group who will continue pre-existing therapy for diabetes. Concomitant pharmacological therapy is strictly defined, as are treatments for the complications of myocardial infarction.

Secondary prevention of myocardial infarction

Beta-blockers

It is 20 years since the Norwegian timolol multi-centre study first showed that treatment with beta-blockers reduced mortality following myocardial infarction.[54] In the non-diabetic patients overall mortality was reduced from 16% to 10% by timolol, and in the diabetic subgroup timolol reduced overall mortality from 30% to 11%.[55] Meta-analysis from nearly 50 trials of beta-blockers given during or after acute myocardial infarction has confirmed the general benefit of beta-blockers. Only six of these studies, including the Norwegian timolol study, reported results stratified for diabetes. Analysis has confirmed an improved survival in diabetic patients, both when beta-blockers are given at the time of the infarction and when they are given on long-term follow up.[56] There is some suggestion that beneficial effects of beta-blockers in diabetic patients following myocardial infarction may be greater than in non-diabetic subjects. Despite clinical evidence of efficacy in routine clinical practice outside the study situation,[57] the use of beta-blockers in routine clinical practice following myocardial infarction in people with diabetes has been surprisingly limited,[57] possibly because of erroneous fears of obscuring the symptoms of hypoglycaemia.

In the era of evidence based medicine it is remarkable that myths about the possible adverse effects of beta-blockers on hypoglycaemia persist. Firstly, it has been suggested that diabetic patients may be less suitable for beta-blockers because of diminished awareness and warning of impending hypoglycaemia. Secondly, it has been suggested that beta-blockers may diminish the recovery from hypoglycaemia. To avoid these potential problems it has been suggested that selective beta-blockers should be used, implying that there is some credibility in the fears concerning the use of non-selective beta-blockade. A detailed description of the effects of beta-blockers on hypoglycaemia is beyond the scope of this chapter, and has been previously reviewed in detail.[58] In summary, beta-blockers do modify some of the physiological and hormonal responses to hypoglycaemia, but the perception of a low blood glucose and cognitive function are not adversely affected. Conflicting results have been obtained in studies which have directly examined the effect of beta-blockade on glucose recovery.

Other aspects on the use of beta-blockers in patients with diabetes are considered in Chapter 7.

ACE inhibitors

A relatively small amount of evidence is currently available for the beneficial effects of ACE inhibitors following myocardial infarction in diabetic patients.[56] Trials of ACE inhibitors in myocardial infarction can be divided into studies that started therapy during or shortly after myocardial infarction (acute trials) and studies that started therapy after myocardial infarction, in subjects with either clinical congestive cardiac failure or with echoradiographic evidence of left ventricular dysfunction. In the Gruppo Italiano per lo Studio della Sopravvivenza nell'Infarto miocardico (GISSI-3) study lisinopril was started within the first 24 hours following myocardial infarction and continued at doses between 2.5 and 10 mg for 6 weeks. Subgroup data for people with diabetes showed that lisinopril reduced the mortality at 6 weeks in patients with type 2 diabetes,[59] and the effect was substantially better than in non-diabetic subjects. Treatment with lisinopril was associated with a decreased 6-week mortality in diabetic patients, falling from 12.4% in the placebo group to 8.7% in the group who received lisinopril. This benefit was still seen at 6 months despite withdrawal of treatment at 6 weeks, and at 6 months the mortality was 16.1% in the placebo group and 12.9% in the treatment group.

Other studies, including substantial numbers of diabetic patients, have demonstrated the benefit of long-term therapy in patients with left ventricular dysfunction following myocardial infarction, but limited subgroup analysis of the diabetic cohorts has not been published. Data from the Studies of Left Ventricular Dysfunction (SOLVD) trials and registry showed that enalapril reduced mortality in diabetic patients and non-diabetic subjects to a similar extent.[60] On the basis of these studies ACI inhibitors have been recommended for use in diabetic patients who have suffered a myocardial infarction and who have either congestive cardiac failure or systolic dysfunction, defined as a left ventricular ejection fraction of less than 40%.[56]

The results of the Heart Outcomes Prevention Evaluation (HOPE) study have now extended these indications to include any patient following myocardial infarction regardless of left ventricular function[61] (see Chapter 7).

Treatment of hyperlipidaemia

A detailed examination of hyperlipidaemia and diabetes is provided in Chapter 6. Evidence for the efficacy of cholesterol lowering with statins in diabetic patients following myocardial infarction comes from post-hoc subgroup analysis of three published studies, and there are no published studies exclusively in diabetic patients. The Scandinavian Simvastatin Survival Study (4S) was the first lipid lowering study to show a reduction in overall mortality.[62] This study included patients with previous myocardial infarction or angina pectoris who had a serum cholesterol of 5.5–8.0 mmol/l, and triglycerides < 2.5 mmol/l. Treatment with simvastatin 20 mg reduced the incidence of major coronary heart disease (CHD) events, with a reduced CHD mortality and a reduced all cause mortality compared to the placebo control group. Within the study there were 202 patients with diabetes, and subgroup analysis showed that the absolute clinical benefit in diabetic subjects was, if anything, greater than in non-diabetic subjects, with a 55% reduction in any CHD event including myocardial infarction and a 43% reduction in total mortality.[62] The benefit from simvastatin was independent of any benefit from aspirin or beta-blockers.

Similar findings were found in the Cholesterol And Recurrent Events (CARE) trial[63] and the Long-term Intervention with Pravastatin in Ischaemic Disease (LIPID) study.[64] It is not certain whether these drugs have a specific action or whether this represents a class effect for all statins. It is also not clear whether the benefit is directly related to the reduction in serum cholesterol or whether these drugs have other effects such as stabilizing the atheromatous plaques. It is advisable, therefore, to treat patients with diabetes and myocardial infarction with either simvastatin or pravastatin, increasing the dose until the serum cholesterol is at least less than 5.0 mmol/l.

The VA-HIT study has shown that treatment with gemfibrozil is of benefit in patients who have relatively normal cholesterol concentrations following myocardial infarction, but low HDL cholesterol levels.[65] Other aspects of the treatment of dyslipidaemia in patients with diabetes are described in Chapter 6.

Other acute coronary syndromes

The acute coronary syndromes comprise two groups:

- ST segment elevation myocardial infarction as described above and
- unstable angina and non-Q wave myocardial infarction.

Unstable angina can be defined as chest pain that is more frequent, severe or prolonged than the patient's usual angina symptoms, occurs at rest or minimal exertion or is difficult to control with drugs.[66] Non-Q wave myocardial infarction presents with similar symptoms to unstable angina, but is accompanied by a rise in cardiac enzyme concentration, including troponin concentrations, without new Q waves on the electrocardiogram. The pathophysiology of these syndromes is thought to be initiated by rupture of the fibrous plaque of an athersclerotic plaque, leading to intracoronary thrombosis. There may also be a role for acute inflammatory markers. Transient obstruction by a platelet-rich white clot is considered causal in most episodes of unstable angina, whereas fibrin-rich red clot is associated with total coronary occlusion and infarction with ST segment elevation.

Several clinical studies have demonstrated that thrombolytic therapy should be avoided in patients with unstable angina, as the use of thrombolytic therapy in unstable angina or non-Q wave myocardial infarction is of no benefit and may actually increase the rates of death, myocardial infarction or bleeding. The current treatment strategy consists of the risk stratification of patients, early and aggressive medical therapy and an expedited invasive assessment of patients who fail to respond, or who are at ongoing high risk, with a view to intervention with either percutaneous transluminal coronary angioplasty or coronary artery bypass grafting. The recent Clopidogrel in Unstable angina to prevent Recurrent Events (CURE) study showed that aspirin combined with clopidogrel gave better results than aspirin alone, and this study included a substantial number of patients with diabetes.[67]

In a study of patients admitted to the emergency department because of acute chest pain or other symptoms raising the suspicion of myocardial infarction, but in whom the diagnosis was not confirmed, 14% had a history of diabetes.[68] The mortality in the diabetic patients was approximately twice that of the non-diabetic patients.[68] Two small comparative studies have demonstrated that the prognosis is worse for diabetic patients compared to non-diabetic patients with unstable angina[69] and non-Q myocardial infarction[38] respectively, and patients with diabetes are usually initially allocated to intermediate or high risk groups. These risk groups should be treated with aspirin and low-molecular weight heparin, and should be considered for early treatment with glycoprotein IIb/IIIa inhibitors.

Summary and future prospects

The mortality from the acute coronary syndromes is increased in people with diabetes. Multiple pharmaceutical and interventional strategies are of benefit, but there are still a significant number of patients with diabetes who do not receive these treatments. The role of insulin in the management of myocardial infarction is unclear, both in the patient with diabetes and in the non-diabetic patient. Interestingly, a recent study of patients in the high dependency unit has shown marked benefit from intravenous insulin in reducing mortality.[70] The majority of these patients were admitted to the high dependency unit following cardiac surgery, and studies are ongoing to determine whether similar benefit is obtained for patients who are admitted to the high dependency unit with other conditions. It is possible that in the future all patients who are admitted to hospital with serious medical and surgical conditions will be given intravenous insulin, and that patients with diabetes will need particular considerations because of the greater upset to glucose metabolism.

References

1. Haffner SM, Lehto S, Ronnemaa T et al. Mortality from coronary heart disease in subjects with type 2 diabetes and in nondiabetic subjects with and without prior myocardial infarction. N Engl J Med 1998;339:229–34.
2. Nesto RW, Zarich S. Acute myocardial infarction in diabetes mellitus: lessons learned from ACE inhibition. Circulation 1998;97:12–15.
3. Herlitz J, Malmberg K. How to improve the cardiac prognosis for diabetes. Diabetes Care 1999;22(Suppl 2):B89–96.
4. Simmons D, Bhoopatkar M. Diabetes and hyperglycaemia among patients with myocardial infarction in a multiethnic population. Aust NZ J Med 1998;28:207–209.
5. Herlitz J, Malmberg K, Karlson BW et al. Mortality and morbidity during a five-year follow-up of diabetics with myocardial infarction. Acta Med Scand 1988;224:31–8.
6. Herlitz J, Bang A, Karlson BW. Mortality, place and mode of death and reinfarction during a period of 5 years after acute myocardial infarction in diabetic and non-diabetic patients. Cardiology 1996;87:423–8.
7. Aronson D, Rayfield E, Cheseboro JH. Mechanisms determining course and outcome of diabetic patients who have had acute myocardial infarction. Ann Intern Med 1997;126:296–306.
8. Granger CB, Califf RM, Young S et al and the Thrombolysis and Angioplasty in Myocardial Infarction (TAMI) study group. Outcome of patients with diabetes mellitus and acute myocardial infarction treated with thrombolytic agents. J Am Coll Cardiol 1993;21:920–5.
9. Lehto S, Pyorala K, Miettinen H et al. Myocardial infarct size and mortality in patients with non-insulin-dependent diabetes mellitus. J Intern Med 1994;236:291–7.
10. Bradley RF, Schonfeld A. Diminished pain in diabetic patients with acute myocardial infarction. Geriatrics 1962;17:322–6.
11. Zammit Maempel JV. Effect of diabetes on the course of acute myocardial infarction in Malta. Israel J Med Sci 1978;14:424–31.
12. Day JJ, Bayer AJ, Chadha JS, Pathy MSJ. Myocardial infarction in old people. The influence of diabetes mellitus. J Am Geriatr Soc 1988;36:791–4.
13. Airaksinen KE. Silent coronary artery disease in diabetes – a feature of autonomic neuropathy or accelerated atherosclerosis? Diabetologia 2001;44:259–66.
14. Faerman I, Faccio E, Milie J et al. Autonomic neuropathy and painless myocardial infarction in diabetic patients. Histological evidence of their relationship. Diabetes 1977;26;1147–58.
15. Toyry JP, Niskaneen LK, Mantysaari MJ et al. Occurrence, predictors, and clinical significance of autonomic neuropathy in NIDDM. Ten-year follow-up from the diagnosis. Diabetes 1996;45:308–15.

16. Bhatnagar SK, Al-Yusuf AR, Al-Asfoor AR. Abnormal autonomic function in diabetic and nondiabetic patients after first acute myocardial infarction. Chest 1987;92:849–52.

17. Fisher BM, Frier BM. Evidence for a specific heart disease of diabetes in humans. Diabet Med 1990;7:478–89.

18. Bell DSH. Diabetic cardiomyopathy. A unique entity or a complication of coronary artery disease? Diabetes Care 1995;18:708–14.

19. Brown HB, Waugh NR, Jennings PE. Microangiopathy as a prognostic indicator in diabetic patients suffering from acute myocardial infarction. Scot Med J 1992;37:44–6.

20. Fava S, Azzopardi J, Muscat HA, Fenech FF. Factors that influence outcome in diabetic subjects with myocardial infarction. Diabetes Care 1993;16:1615–18.

21. ISIS-2 (Second International Study of Infarct Survival) collaborative group. Randomised trial of intravenous streptokinase, oral aspirin, both, or neither among 17,187 cases of suspected acute myocardial infarction: ISIS-2. Lancet 1988;ii:349–60.

22. Antiplatelet Trialists' Collaboration. Collaborative overview of randomised trials of antiplatelet therapy-I: prevention of death, myocardial infarction, and stroke by prolonged antiplatelet therapy in various categories of patients. Br Med J 1994;308:81–106.

23. Harpaz D, Gottlieb S, Graff E et al. Effects of aspirin treatment on survival in non-insulin-dependent diabetic patients with coronary artery disease. Israeli Bezafibrate Infarction Prevention Study Group. Am J Med 1998;105:494–9.

24. Yudkin JS. Which diabetic patients should be taking aspirin? Br Med J 1995;311;641–2.

25. Hansson L, Zanchetti A, Carruthers SG et al for the HOT study group. Effects of intensive blood-pressure lowering and low-dose aspirin in patients with hypertension: principal results of the Hypertension Optimal Treatment (HOT) randomised trial. Lancet 1998;351:1755–62.

26. Fibrinolytic Therapy Trialists' (FTT) collaborative group. Indications for fibrinolytic therapy in suspected acute myocardial infarction: collaborative overview of early mortality and major morbidity results from all randomised trials of more than 1000 patients. Lancet 1994;343:311–22.

27. Gray RP, Yudkin JS, Patterson DL. Enzymatic evidence of impaired reperfusion in diabetic patients after thrombolytic therapy for acute myocardial infarction: a role for plasminogen activator inhibitor? Br Heart J 1993;70:530–6.

28. Mak KH, Moliterno DJ, Granger CB et al for the GUSTO-I investigators. Influence of diabetes mellitus on clinical outcome in the thrombolytic era of acute myocardial infarction. J Am Coll Cardiol 1997;30:171–9.

29. Woodfield SL, Lundergan CF, Reiner JS et al for the GUSTO-I angiographic investigators. Angiographic findings and outcome in diabetic

patients treated with thrombolytic therapy for acute myocardial infarction: the GUSTO-I experience. J Am Coll Cardiol 1996;28:1661–9.

30. Barbash GI, White HD, Modan M, Van de Werf F for the investigators of the International Tissue Plasminogen Activator/Streptokinase Mortality Trial. Significance of diabetes mellitus in patients with acute myocardial infarction receiving thrombolytic therapy. J Am Coll Cardiol 1993;22:707–13.

31. Jelesoff NE, Feinglos M, Granger CB, Califf RM. Outcomes of diabetic patients following acute myocardial infarction: a review of the major thrombolytic trials. Coron Art Dis 1996;7:732–43.

32. Ward H, Yudkin JS. Thrombolysis in patients with diabetes. Br Med J 1995;310:3–4.

33. Yudkin JS. Managing the diabetic patient with acute myocardial infarction. Diabet Med 1998;15:276–81.

34. Hansen H-HT, Kjaergaard SC, Bulow I et al. Thrombolytic therapy in diabetic patients with acute myocardial infarction. Diabetes Care 1996;19:1135–7.

35. Weaver WD, Simes RJ, Betriu A et al. Comparison of primary coronary angioplasty and intravenous thrombolytic therapy for acute myocardial infarction: a quantitative review. J Am Med Assoc 1997;278:2093–8.

36. Thomas K, Ottervanger JP, de Boer M-J et al. Primary angioplasty compared with thrombolysis in acute myocardial infarction in diabetic patients. Diabetes Care 1999;22:647–9.

37. Waldecker B, Waas W, Haberosch W et al. Type 2 diabetes and acute myocardial infarction. Angiographic findings and results of an invasive therapeutic approach in type 2 versus nondiabetic patients. Diabetes Care 1999;22:1832–8.

38. Gowda MS, Vacek JL, Hallas D. One-year outcomes of diabetic versus nondiabetic patients with non-Q-wave acute myocardial infarction treated with percutaneous transluminal coronary angioplasty. Am J Cardiol 1998;81:1067–71.

39. Schomig A, Kastrati A, Dirschinger J et al for the Stent versus Thrombolysis for Occluded Coronary Arteries in Patients with Acute Myocardial Infarction study investigators. Coronary stenting plus platelet glycoprotein IIb/IIIa blockade compared with tissue plasminogen activator in acute myocardial infarction. N Engl J Med 2000;343:385–91.

40. Tiefenbrunn AJ, Chandra NC, French WJ et al. Clinical experience with primary percutaneous transluminal coronary angioplasty compared with alteplase (recombinant tissue-type plasminogen activator) in patients with acute myocardial infarction: a report from the Second National Registry of Myocardial Infarction (NRMI-2). J Am Coll Cardiol 1998;31:1240–5.

41. Danchin N, Vaur L, Genes N et al. Management of acute myocardial infarction in intensive care units in 1995:a nationwide French survey of practice and early hospital results. J Am Coll Cardiol 1997;30:1598–1605.

42. Gwilt DJ, Nattrass M, Pentecost BL. Use of low-dose insulin infusions in diabetics after myocardial infarction. Br Med J 1982;285:1402–404.

43. Gwilt DJ, Petri M, Lamb P et al. Effect of intravenous insulin infusion on mortality among diabetic patients after myocardial infarction. Br Heart J 1984;51:626–30.

44. Clark RS, English M, McNeill GP, Newton RW. Effect of intravenous infusion of insulin in diabetics with acute myocardial infarction. Br Med J 1985;291:303–305.

45. Davies RR, Newton RW, McNeill GP et al. Metabolic control in diabetic subjects following myocardial infarction: difficulties in improving blood glucose levels by intravenous insulin infusion. Scot Med J 1991;36:74–6.

46. Malmberg KA, Efendic S, Ryden LE for the Multicenter Study Group. Feasibility of insulin–glucose infusion in diabetic patients with acute myocardial infarction. A report from the multicenter trial: DIGAMI. Diabetes Care 1994;17:1007–14.

47. Malmberg K, Ryden L, Efendic S et al on behalf of the DIGAMI study group. Randomized trial of insulin–glucose infusion followed by subcutaneous insulin treatment in diabetic patients with acute myocardial infarction (DIGAMI study): effects on mortality at 1 year. J Am Coll Cardiol 1995;26:57–65.

48. Malmberg K, Ryden L, Hamsten A et al. on behalf of the DIGAMI study group. Effects of insulin treatment on cause-specific one-year mortality and morbidity in diabetic patients with acute myocardial infarction. Eur Heart J 1996;17:1337–44.

49. Malmberg K for the DIGAMI (Diabetes Mellitus, Insulin Glucose Infusion in Acute Myocardial Infarction) study group. Prospective randomised study of intensive insulin treatment on long term survival after acute myocardial infarction in patients with diabetes mellitus. Br Med J 1997;314:1512–15.

50. Muhlhauser I, Sawicki PT, Berger M. Possible risk of sulphonylureas in the treatment of non-insulin-dependent diabetes mellitus and coronary artery disease. Diabetologia 1997;40:1492–3.

51. Smits P. Cardiovascular effects of sulphonylurea derivatives. Diabetologia 1997;40:S160–S161.

52. Fath-Ordoubadi F, Beatt KJ. Glucose–insulin–potassium therapy for treatment of acute myocardial infarction: an overview of randomized placebo-controlled trials. Circulation 1997;96:1152–6.

53. Diaz R, Paolasso EA Piegas LS et al, on behalf of the ECLA (Estudios Cardiologicos Latinoamerica) collaborative group. Metabolic modulation of acute myocardial infarction. Circulation 1998;98:2227–34.

54. The Norwegian Multicentre Study Group. Timolol-induced reduction in mortality and reinfarction in patients surviving acute myocardial infarction. N Engl J Med 1981;304:801–807.

55. Gundersen T, Kjekshus J. Timolol treatment after myocardial infarction in diabetic patients. Diabetes Care 1983;6:285–90.

56. MacDonald TM, Butler R, Newton RW, Morris AD for the DARTS/MEMO collaboration. Which drugs benefit diabetic patients for secondary prevention of myocardial infarction? Diabet Med 1998;15:282–9.

57. Gottlieb SS, McCarter RJ, Vogel RA. Effect of beta-blockade on mortality among high-risk and low-risk patients after myocardial infarction. N Engl J Med 1998;339:489–97.

58. Kerr D. Drugs and alcohol. In: Frier B, Fisher BM, eds. Hypoglycaemia and Diabetes. Clinical and Physiological Aspects. London: Edward Arnold, 1993:328–36

59. Zuanetti G, Latini R, Maggioni AP et al for the GISSI-3 investigators. Effect of the ACE inhibitor lisinopril on mortality in diabetic patients with acute myocardial infarction. Circulation 1997;94:4239–45.

60. Shindler DM, Kostis JB, Yusuf S et al for the SOLVD investigators. Diabetes mellitus, a predictor of morbidity and mortality in the Studies of Left Ventricular Dysfunction (SOLVD) trials and registry. Am J Cardiol 1996;77:1017–20.

61. Heart Outcomes Prevention Evaluation (HOPE) study investigators. Effects of ramipril on cardiovascular and microvascular outcomes in people with diabetes mellitus: results of the HOPE study and MICRO-HOPE substudy. Lancet 2000;355:253–9.

62. Pyorala K, Pedersen TR, Kjekshus J et al, the Scandinavian Simvastatin Survival Study (4S) group. Cholesterol lowering with simvastatin improves prognosis of diabetic patients with coronary heart disease. A subgroup analysis of the Scandinavian Simvastatin Survival Study (4S). Diabetes Care 1997;20:614–20.

63. Goldberg RB, Mellies MJ, Sacks FM et al for the CARE investigators. Cardiovascular events and their reduction with pravastatin in diabetic and glucose-intolerant myocardial infarction survivors with average cholesterol levels: subgroup analyses in the Cholesterol And Recurrent Events (CARE) trial. Circulation 1998;98:2513–19.

64. The Long-Term Intervention with Pravastatin in Ischaemic Disease (LIPID) study group. Prevention of cardiovascular events and death with pravastatin in patients with coronary heart disease and a broad range of initial cholesterol levels. N Engl J Med 1998;339:1349–57.

65. Rubins HB, Robins SJ, Collins D et al for the Veterans Affairs High-Density Lipoprotein Cholesterol Intervention Trial study group. Gemfibrozil for the secondary prevention of coronary heart disease in men with low levels of high-density lipoprotein in cholesterol.. N Engl J Med 1999;341:410–18.

66. Maynard SJ, Scott GO, Riddell JW, Adgey AAJ. Management of acute coronary syndromes. Br Med J 2000;321:220–3.

67. The Clopidogrel in Unstable Angina to prevent Recurrent Events trial investigators. Effects of clopidogrel in addition to aspirin in patients with acute coronary syndromes without ST-segment elevation. Lancet 2001;345:494–502.

68. Karlson BW, Strombom U, Ekvall H-E, Herlitz J. Prognosis in diabetics in whom the initial suspicion of acute myocardial infarction was not confirmed. Clin Cardiol 1993;16:559–64.

69. Fava S, Azzopardi J, Agius-Muscat H. Outcome of unstable angina in patients with diabetes mellitus. Diabet Med 1997;14:209–13.

70. Van den Berghe G, Wouters P, Weekers F et al. Intensive insulin therapy in critically ill patients. N Engl J Med 2001;345:1359–67.

chapter 5

Effects of treatment of hyperglycaemia and hypertension on cardiovascular outcomes in diabetes

Peter H Winocour

Introduction

The management of hyperglycaemia and hypertension in diabetes has been facilitated by the results from recent intervention studies. However, limitations inherent to clinical research need to be taken account of in the application of research findings to day-to-day individual clinical practice. There has understandably been a great deal of hyperbole from both protagonists and critics accompanying these reports. In this chapter the impact of the management of hypertension and hyperglycaemia in diabetes on cardiovascular outcomes is critically assessed. The evidence base for, and the practical feasibility of applying recent national and international guidelines are examined.

Epidemiology

There is an independent relationship between coronary heart disease (CHD) and diabetes, with an additive impact of co-existent hypertension on CHD outcome in people with diabetes. It is worth taking a closer look at the separate and combined impact of these factors in both type 1 and type 2 diabetes before examining the impact of treatment of hyperglycaemia and hypertension on cardiovascular outcomes.

The literature in this area is not totally consistent, and there may be some difficulties inherent in this area of epidemiology:

■ There is a tendency to equate CHD with cardiovascular disease (CVD), whereas in terms of risk factor associations these may not be synonymous. This is particularly evident when discriminating CHD from cerebrovascular disease.

■ The definition of CHD itself is not always as clear as might first appear, and is often defined in qualitative terms as 'possible' or 'definite', based on symptoms and electrocardiographic abnormalities, as opposed to the harder endpoints of definite myocardial infarction or mortality.

■ The impact of risk markers on morbidity and on mortality may differ.

■ Finally, and particularly pertinent to diabetes, there is the frequent co-existence and confounding impact of non-atherosclerotic cardiac disease, due to underlying diabetic cardiomyopathy and hypertensive and autonomic neuropathic influences on cardiac structure and function (see Chapter 2).

The evidence that type 2 diabetes (and more subtle disturbances of glucose intolerance) is associated with a 2- to 4-fold excess risk of CVD events and mortality is indisputable.[1] This has been demonstrated both in men and women (the latter in particular at greatest relative risk), and in many different ethnic groups, including populations at high and low CVD risk.[2-9] The situation is much less clear when examining the relationship between the *degree* of hypergly-caemia and CHD and CVD outcome.[2-6]

There are sound pathophysiological bases whereby increasing hyperglycaemia could aggravate CVD. Increased oxidative stress, thrombogenicity, glycation and oxidative modification of lipoproteins, endothelial damage and the frequent clustering of traditional and putative CVD risk markers (often in insulin-resistant subjects) have previously been correlated with poor blood glucose control.

Type 2 diabetes

It is important to examine the studies which have actually examined the relationship. One of the largest prospective studies involved over 1000 Finnish men and women with type 2 diabetes over 7 years.[9] Whereas univariate analyses confirmed that increasing tertiles of fasting blood glucose and HbA1 predicted CHD mortality, low HDL cholesterol and triglycerides were more powerful predictors after adjustment for other independent factors. Perhaps more importantly, the relationship for all CHD events was not evident for HbA1, and the cutoffs selected for discrimination of risk were fasting glucose levels > 13.4 mmol/l and HbA1 > 10.7%. This suggests that the relationship between glycaemia and CHD might operate in a trimodial distribution, with a doubling of risk with minor glucose intolerance, and a further 50–100% risk magnification, not at the point of diabetes diagnosis where the microvascular (retinopathy) risk is measurable, but where blood glucose control is considered extremely poor by most standards.

By contrast, the United Kingdom Prospective Diabetes Study (UKPDS) (see below) suggested a graded relationship with HbA1c,[6] which was independent of other CVD risk factors.[3]

To put the relationship between degree of glycaemia and outcome further into perspective, in most populations the relative excess CVD risk of minimal microalbuminuria (> 10 μg/minute overnight) is equivalent to that of poor glucose control,[10] and the impact of clini-cal Albustix proteinuria further magnifies the risk 3.5-fold.[11] Interest-ingly, there is a possibility that where there is a low incidence of

CHD, such as in Japan, there is no appreciable impact of microalbuminuria on diabetic CHD.[12]

Type 1 diabetes

In type 1 diabetes the situation is quite different, not least because of the younger age of the study population and the very low background age-matched rates of CHD. This needs to be borne in mind when considering the much greater impact of diabetes-related factors on relative as opposed to absolute risk. Several studies confirm that the unusual occurrence of mortality in type 1 diabetic subjects under 50 years of age is due to CHD and other types of CVD in 30–40% of cases, in contrast to less than 5% of cases in the non-diabetic population.[13–15] Cases of CHD seem to be confined virtually exclusively to those with established diabetic nephropathy.[16,17]

The impact of glycaemic control on CVD and all-cause mortality in type 1 diabetes has been examined in two reasonably sized studies over 10 years. In the Wisconsin epidemiological study of 1210 subjects with type 1 diabetes, the impact of other factors, notably age, smoking, hypertension and proteinuria (and to a lesser extent microalbuminuria), remained significant predictors in multiple regression analysis.[8] By contrast, the impact of glycaemic control (assessed by glycated haemoglobin measurements) was less consistent. The hazard ratio for CHD death for a 1% increase in HbA1c was 1.18 (confidence intervals (CI) 1.00 to 1.40), with similar hazard ratios for all-cause and stroke mortality.[8]

In a study of 939 cases from the Steno hospital in Denmark, HbA1c was an independent significant predictor of all cause mortality (relative risk 1.11 (CI 1.03 to 1.20), but not of cardiovascular mortality.[13] The Pittsburgh Epidemiology of Complications study put the impact of glycaemia into clinical perspective. It retrospectively confirms that those who escaped cardiovascular (and other) complications had lower levels of HbA1c and blood pressure, and improved lipid profiles.[18]

This could suggest that complication reduction in diabetes may be a consequence of multiple risk factor control, a central feature of some of the intervention studies to be discussed later in this chapter.

The impression gained is that the presence of hyperglycaemia confers a state of increased risk of CHD in both type 1 and type 2 diabetes, but that the degree of hyperglycaemia itself exerts only a modest impact, unless extremely high. In assessing the impact of improved blood glucose control on cardiovascular disease in diabetes, trial design would need to take account of background incidence of events in conventionally treated diabetic subjects, and the anticipated benefit with better glycaemic control over a suitable period of follow-up.

Based on the information to be presented, it can be estimated that the minimum event rate would be 3% per annum, in a study lasting 15 years, involving over 4000 subjects, with an anticipated CVD risk reduction of at least 30%. In prefacing the data in both type 1 and type 2 diabetes it will be appreciated that such a study has not been and probably never will be carried out.

Impact of treatment of hyperglycaemia on CHD

Type 1 diabetes

Strictly speaking it is not possible to reject the null hypothesis, given the lack of appropriate studies investigating this issue. There is a vague suggestion that 'early atherosclerosis is retarded by improved long term blood glucose control in type 1 diabetes' from an offshoot of the Stockholm Diabetes Intervention Study.[19] This was conceived and initiated in the 1980s. After 10–12 years, 31 subjects on intensive insulin therapy were compared with 28 who received standard insulin therapy. This led to a mean HbA1c of 7.1% and 8.2%, respectively, and the standard therapy group were noted to have increased 'stiffness' and intimal-medial thickness of the common carotid artery. There was no formal assessment of cardiac function, and in vivo assessment of endothelial-derived and non-endothelial-dependent brachial artery vasodilation was not different between the groups. There were, respectively, one and two macrovascular events in the intensive and standard treatment groups!

The Diabetes Control and Complications Trial (DCCT) was a landmark in our understanding of the impact of tight glycaemic control on the initiation and progression of microvascular disease.[20] It is not surprising that the effect on macrovascular disease was (much) more modest. 'Only' 1441 subjects were studied, half each in the primary and secondary prevention cohorts. The mean age at trial entry was 27 years (as you would expect in type 1 diabetes); 'hypertension, hypercholesterolaemia, and severe diabetic complications' were exclusion criteria, and the mean follow-up was only 6.5 years, so there were very few cardiovascular events. The difference in HbA1c (intensive 7.1% versus conventional 9%) was associated with a significant reduction in LDL-cholesterol and a non-significant 41% reduction in the incidence of 'all major cardiovascular and peripheral vascular events'. This superficially impressive statistic belies the low event rate (presented as 0.5 versus 0.8 events per 100 patient years) and the consequent wide confidence intervals (−10% to +68%).

In summary, there is no current evidence that improving glycaemic control reduces CHD events in type 1 diabetes in a clinically important fashion.

Type 2 diabetes

Type 2 diabetes is more relevant than type 1 diabetes in investigating the impact of improved glycaemia on CHD; first given that this is a more appropriate older constituency with a much higher background incidence of CHD, and second because we now have an opportunity to review the data with a historical perspective.

University Group Diabetes Program (UGDP)

Views may have been coloured by more senior physicians who remember the University Group Diabetes Program (UGDP) debacle.[21,22] The headlines from this North American study published in 1976–78 suggested that tolbutamide and fixed doses of lente insulin treatment were associated with an upward trend in cardiovascular deaths after 3.5 years of the study. This has been refuted with the results of the UKPDS (see below), but at the time the UGDP generated considerable controversy, and concern that sulphonylureas could be cardiotoxic and insulin potentially atherogenic.

With hindsight, it can be seen that there were serious flaws in the study design:

- only 823 subjects
- a higher baseline CVD risk in the tolbutamide group, and
- somewhat doubtful attainment of better glycaemic control.

Since UGDP, three studies have examined the impact of intensified control on vascular complications in type 2 diabetes. As with type 1 diabetes, the data on reducing microvascular complications is irrefutable, and the data on macrovascular complications, and CHD in particular, are much more flimsy.

Kumamoto study

The Kumamoto study of 110 Japanese diabetic subjects with type 2 diabetes used intensive or conventional insulin therapy (and attained an average HbA1c over 6 years of 7.1% versus 9.4%, respectively), with important reductions in the development and progression of retinopathy and nephropathy.[23] Baseline ECG examination was normal in all subjects at study initiation. Of interest, the mean body mass index of this Japanese type 2 diabetic cohort was 19–23, in contrast to 27–31 in the European studies to be discussed. Thus there may exist marked differences in the degree of insulin insensitivity between these two populations.

In contrast to the DCCT study, lipid levels did not alter in the Kumamoto study. The authors presented data (0.6 versus 1.3 total CVD events per 100 patient years, non-significant difference) which they interpreted as 'intensive glycaemic control seems to have a beneficial effect on the progression of macrovascular complications'. In fact, the number of 'hard' macrovascular endpoints was two with intensive treatment (one with claudication, one sudden death from presumed myocardial infarction), in comparison to four endpoints with conventional treatment (one death from cerebral infarction, two patients with claudication and one patient who developed angina). Thus, in this small study of short duration in a population at low background CHD risk, CHD was not demonstrably affected by this degree of improved glycaemic control.

Steno study

The Danish 'Steno type 2 randomized study' employed multifactorial intervention in 160 type 2 diabetic subjects with microalbuminuria followed up for just under 4 years. Half were randomized to stepwise intensive treatment (behaviour modification and pharmacological therapy—tight glucose control (HbA1c target 6.5%), and use of antihypertensive and lipid lowering agents, as well as aspirin). The study was primarily designed to examine the impact on microvascular disease.[24]

As an open trial of small numbers, any conclusions from such a study must be viewed as tentative at best, but it does reflect the likely clinical impact of what we might currently consider 'best practice'. The target blood pressure was < 140/85 mm Hg, and metabolic targets were HbA1c < 6.5%, total cholesterol < 5.0 mmol/l, triglycerides < 1.7 mmol/l and HDL cholesterol > 1.1 mmol/l. All subjects received an ACE inhibitor irrespective of blood pressure, and aspirin was given to all those with CHD or peripheral vascular disease. At trial entry, roughly 25% already had ECG evidence of CHD.

Relevant cardiovascular endpoints and all-cause mortality were graded by severity into three categories:

- Total mortality, with two deaths with standard treatment and four deaths with intensive treatment.
- The incidence of non-fatal strokes, myocardial infarctions, or coronary or peripheral vascular surgery was 14 cases versus 10 cases in the standard and intensive groups, respectively.
- In the final category of developing ischaemia on ECG or ankle:brachial pressure index there were 34 events versus 17 events in the standard and intensive groups, respectively. However, over 75% of the events in this latter category related to peripheral vascular measures.

As a result, pooling *all macrovascular* events in three categories led to a significant ($p = 0.03$) reduction with the intensive approach. If cardiac as opposed to cerebrovascular and peripheral vascular outcomes are examined, then 23 versus 18 events were recorded, the difference mainly made up from changes in resting or stress electro-cardiograms. As with the UKPDS, the benefits of reducing the primary microvascular endpoints were much more impressive.

United Kingdom Prospective Diabetes Study (UKPDS)

The United Kingdom Prospective Diabetes Study (UKPDS) deserves the cliché 'landmark study', given its scope, duration, sample size and positive findings. In some respects, the questions that remain are a legacy of the complexity of the study design and, with regard to CHD, the absence of any concurrent effort to treat dyslipidaemia. The issue of antihypertensive therapy in UKPDS is discussed later in the chapter, and by necessity the UKPDS was, like the Steno study, partly multi-factorial, in that 50% of the cohort were enrolled in the hypertension intervention wing of the study. Pragmatically we need to accept that the benefits probably reflect the 'package' of both glycaemic and blood pressure control in a sizeable proportion at highest absolute risk.

In respect of the impact of glycaemic control, almost 4000 newly diagnosed middle aged (mean age 54 years) type 2 diabetic subjects were studied, and followed up for 10 years.[25] There was initial random allocation to standard treatment with diet or intensive treat-ment with one of three sulphonylureas, or insulin. However, with time the progressive decline in beta cell function meant that additional therapy was required in around 20% of cases in all subgroups. In addition, metformin treatment was a further add on in 10% of cases overall.

Three aggregate endpoints were used to examine the benefit of intensive treatment (target fasting glucose < 6 mmol/l): any of 21 prespecified diabetes-related endpoints, diabetes-related death or all-cause mortality.

Although there were several macrovascular exclusion criteria (myocardial infarction in the previous year, current angina or heart failure, 'more than one major vascular event'), at least 10% (and up to 25% of women) had previous myocardial infarction or possible/probable ischaemia on baseline electrocardiograms at entry into the study.

The three major aggregated cardiovascular endpoints were:

■ myocardial infarction
■ stroke
■ amputation/death from peripheral vascular disease (PVD).

Data were derived from cumulating the following single endpoints: fatal and non-fatal myocardial infarction, sudden death, heart failure, angina, fatal and non-fatal stroke, and the PVD endpoints.

Intensive treatment led to a mean HbA1c of 7% over 10 years (compared to 7.9% with 'conventional' therapy). While this is a testimony to the rigorous care patients received, it may have somewhat diminished the impact of the study in that in routine practice clinic HbA1c levels are usually on average 8.5–9%.

The results are very clear in one respect—neither sulphonylurea nor insulin therapy is associated with an excess of CVD events. This effectively consigns the fears that arose from the UGDP study to oblivion.

The incidence of myocardial infarction overall was 27% over the 10-year study. There was no difference between intensive and conventional treatment groups in the proportion of patients who had a silent myocardial infarction, cardiomegaly/heart failure, angina, stroke or peripheral vascular disease endpoints. The major benefit was the significant reduction in microvascular endpoints, particularly retinopathy.

However, intensive treatment led to a relative risk reduction (RR = 0.84) for 'all myocardial infarction' which was of borderline significance (p = 0.052). The raw data reveal that this was through a reduction in sudden death and non-fatal myocardial infarction, but not in fatal myocardial infarction. This can also be presented as demonstrating that over 150 subjects would require intensive treatment for

10 years in order to prevent one myocardial infarction. There was no suggestion that the CHD incidence was altered by the type of intensive treatment, although in the embedded study of metformin in obese subjects, overall mortality was lowered by metformin.[26]

Overall, it is reasonable to conclude that tight blood glucose control has no more than a marginal impact on cardiovascular disease in general, and on coronary heart disease in particular, regardless of the type of diabetes.

Hypertension

Epidemiology in type 1 and type 2 diabetes

The nature, prevalence and impact of hypertension is different in type 1 and type 2 diabetes. A great deal of early research did not make this distinction, which may have led to invalid assumptions. Hypertension in type 1 diabetes has been linked to alterations in the renin–angiotensin system, altered vascular reactivity to pressor agents, altered cation transport mechanisms and increased exchangeable sodium, endothelial and glomerular dysfunction. Whereas all these factors can operate in type 2 diabetes, central obesity, renal atherosclerotic disease and insulin insensitivity/hyperinsulinaemia are the predominant factors accounting for the link[27] (see Chapter 1).

This is supported by the 10–20% evolution of type 2 diabetes in individuals with essential hypertension over a 10–12 year period.[28,29] The metabolic impact of antihypertensive medication has also received attention, and important data from Uppsala and Gothenburg in Sweden have demonstrated that thiazides and beta-blockers in particular (and especially in combination) independently increase the incidence of diabetes. This is particularly apparent in obese individuals. The increased insulin insensitivity demonstrated with such therapy during euglycaemic clamp studies has been considered an important contribution to such an outcome, by compounding insulin resistance in individuals with a genetic predisposition to type 2 diabetes.[28–30]

Type I diabetes

In type 1 diabetes, the prevalence of hypertension varies between 10 and 30%.[27,31,32] The most basic issue in this population is how to define hypertension, and there is now consensus that this should be established on age- and gender-matched norms. Thus levels above 130/85 mm Hg may be identified as hypertensive in individuals aged < 30 years of age. Based on epidemiological associations and outcome studies to be discussed later, there is an acceptance that values > 140/90 mm Hg should be considered for treatment in diabetes in general.

Hypertension is intimately linked with the evolution of diabetic nephropathy in type 1 diabetes, and is present in 30% with microalbuminuria and over 60% with macroalbuminuria.[31,32] There is an additional increase in hypertension associated with ageing.

Given these caveats the relationship between hypertension and macrovascular disease has been clearly established in type 1 diabetes, but most notably for CHD where there is coexistent nephropathy, and for peripheral vascular disease, particularly among smokers. The less clear relationship between blood pressure and cerebrovascular disease in type 1 diabetes reflects the relative rarity of this complication.

It can be argued that at a clinical level sophisticated epidemiological analyses to tease out the independent impact of hypertension from other variables are artificial in that intensive clinical efforts will concentrate on hypertensive type 1 patients who are older, albuminuric and have additional vascular risk factors or established vascular disease.

A 10-year follow-up of over 900 Danish subjects with type 1 diabetes has given a useful perspective on the relative risk of cardiovascular mortality from hypertension,[13] defined as > 160/95 mm Hg or prevailing antihypertensive treatment. The relative risk was 2.35 on multiple regression analyses, roughly equivalent to the impact of smoking, but statistically less important than age or overt nephropathy (proteinuria). Cardiovascular death attributed to microalbuminuria was less clearly linked in this study.

A 15-year follow-up of over 5000 Finnish type 1 diabetic subjects confirmed that diabetic nephropathy was associated with a 10-fold relative risk of both CHD and stroke.[17]

Type 2 diabetes

In type 2 diabetes the prevalence of hypertension is over 50%,[27] partly reflecting the impact of obesity and insulin resistance. The relationship with microalbuminuria and nephropathy is not as intimate as in type 1 diabetes, which may reflect the non-specific nature of microalbuminuria in this population, not least from the frequent coexistence of clinical or subclinical atherosclerosis, which may itself be implicated in glomerular leakage of albumin. More than 60% of hypertensive type 2 diabetic subjects have microalbuminuria and an equivalent proportion of microalbuminuric type 2 diabetic subjects are hypertensive. As in type 1 diabetes, hypertension is virtually endemic when proteinuria supervenes.[33,34]

The Framingham and Whitehall studies confirmed the important relationship between hypertension and macrovascular disease in diabetes, although the Multiple Risk Factor Intervention Trial (MRFIT) and UKPDS studies were able to demonstrate in much larger cohorts the synergistic impact of additional risk factors.[27]

In UKPDS 35% of males and 46% of females had hypertension at inception to the study with newly diagnosed type 2 diabetes.[35] The original cohort comprised over 3600 individuals and hypertension was defined as mean blood pressure ≥ 160 mm Hg systolic and ≥ 90 mm Hg diastolic 2 and 9 months after diagnosis of diabetes, or taking antihypertensive therapy. Given the current concepts and guidelines to be discussed, it will be appreciated that this prevalence of hypertension is likely to be an underestimate.

In respect of the relationship between blood pressure and prevalent and evolving cardiovascular disease it should be appreciated that there were important vascular exclusion criteria:

- myocardial infarction in the previous year
- current angina or heart failure

- more than one 'major vascular episode'
- accelerated hypertension
- serum creatinine levels > 175 μmol/l.

These are common considerations in the majority of intervention trials that will be discussed.

Notwithstanding these facts, patients with hypertension had up to 3-fold greater prevalence of a previous cerebrovascular and/or cardiac vascular event, in comparison to normotensive subjects. This was particularly notable among men.[35] Such a history confirms that diabetes does not simply lead to macrovascular damage but that the close and complex relationship may reflect a common combination of antecedent aetiological factors for both conditions.

Inevitably, those with hypertension had a much greater prevalence (21–27% versus 11–18%) of electrocardiographic features of possible/probable CHD at trial entry. During a median follow-up of almost 8 years in over 2600 subjects with complete data, stepwise regression analysis revealed that the evolution of CHD (aggregate measures of angina, fatal and non-fatal myocardial infarction) was associated with blood pressure, especially systolic. The hazard ratio between the upper and lower tertiles was 1.8 (CI 1.3 to 2.5), but importantly CHD outcome was also predicted by raised LDL cholesterol and glucose, reduced HDL cholesterol and smoking.[3] The practical importance is the frequent clustering of hypertension with these metabolic variables in the UKPDS, and the recognition that the impact on cardiovascular prognosis is additive/synergistic.

Data on the evolution of stroke, cardiac failure and amputation/peripheral vascular disease in UKPDS also show a relationship with baseline hypertension. More recently, an observational study from the UKPDS demonstrated a continuous relationship between systolic blood pressure and the evolution of cardiovascular mortality and specific events (stroke, myocardial infarction, cardiac failure and lower extremity amputation/deaths from peripheral vascular disease).[36]

The observed reduction in cardiac failure and stroke following the treatment of hypertension was greater than expected from the observational findings on the prognostic impact of systolic blood pressure, although the non-significant reduction in myocardial infarction and peripheral vascular disease was consistent with the observational findings. This raised the possibility of additional benefits of the primary agents (beta-blockers and ACE inhibitors), and will be discussed later in more detail.

The synergistic impact of multiple risk factors had already been clearly demonstrated in the Multiple Risk Factor Intervention Trial (MRFIT). Among over 5000 men receiving treatment for diabetes there was > 20% overall mortality (> 10% cardiovscular mortality), at least three times greater than for non-diabetic subjects. Systolic blood pressure significantly predicted CHD and stroke mortality, especially among smokers and where total cholesterol exceeded 6.5 mmol/l.[1]

The relationship between hypertension, diabetes and macrovascular outcome is best defined in Caucasian populations, yet there are data suggesting that hypertension is at least as prevalent, if not more so, among the Afro-Caribbean population in the UK, and among African Americans.[37–39] The importance lies in the suggested greater incidence of cerebrovascular disease among these populations, potential therapeutic issues (see below), and the exaggerated impact of blood pressure on renal failure, also evident amongst the Indo-Asian population in the UK.[40]

As with type 1 diabetes, the common but not inevitable co-occurrence of hypertension with albuminuria-proteinuria is important in greatly magnifying the prevalence of CHD and the mortality from CVD.[10,11,41,42]

Clustering of risk factors operates to magnify the CVD risk from diabetes and hypertension, and cardiovascular morbidity and mortality has been clearly linked to adverse socio-economic status in diabetes in the UK.[43,44] This appeared predominantly a consequence of the excess of hypertension and smoking, and may partly explain why a similar phenomenon was not seen in a larger survey of the entire Finnish population, where there appeared much smaller social class differences in smoking and hypertension.[45]

Direct and indirect impact of treatment of hypertension on atherothrombosis

A detailed discussion of the pathophysiology of atherosclerosisis and thrombosis is beyond the scope of this chapter, but it is important to reflect on the mechanisms whereby hypertension and the various antihypertensive agents can affect these processes.

In broad terms they may interact with the function and structure of the endothelium, the myocytes and fibroblasts, circulating factors such as lipoproteins, platelets and clotting factors, and overall arteriolar, arterial and cardiac structure and function. Thus, hypertension may accelerate coronary atherosclerosis, leading to a higher proportion of cases with triple vessel disease.[46] Hypertension will also adversely affect coronary haemodynamics and could thereby accelerate atherosclerotic plaque rupture and thrombosis.

From a practical point of view, hypertension and increased peripheral resistance can lead to left ventricular hypertrophy, itself an independent important predictor of cardiovascular events.

The issue of additional selective antihypertensive class effects on CVD will be discussed later in more detail, but there is potential for the various types of hypotensive agents to exert other beneficial (and potentially adverse) effects on atheroscerosis and CVD.

A large body of such work rests on animal models, which are beyond the scope of this chapter. Human angiographic studies have focused on whether specific drug classes affect the progression or regression of atherosclerosis, particularly with respect to restenosis following angioplasty.

Small studies with calcium antagonists in the late 1980s and mid-1990s produced conflicting reports of benefit in established atherosclerosis, with any favourable effect limited to minimizing development of early lesions.[47] Similarly, the impact of ACE inhibitors on coronary atherosclerosis has been disappointing, without any detectable impact on post-angiographic restenosis.[48] The HOPE study (see below) has raised the question as to other beneficial non-hypotensive modes of action whereby ACE inhibitors may reduce cardiovascular disease.

Data on carotid doppler estimates of atherosclerosis following treatment with calcium antagonists, alpha-blockers and ACE inhibitors is generally more positive, but has not yet been translated into a specific advantage in cerebrovascular outcomes, and in general carotid atheroma is not an ideal surrogate for coronary heart disease.

There are, of course, a large number of real and theoretical class specific benefits which may impact on CVD outcomes:

- Specific cardioprotection by beta-blockers and certain calcium antagonists may operate by reducing myocardial oxygen consumption and workload, as well as minimizing arrhythmogenicity.
- ACE inhibitors (and possibly AII receptor antagonists) may have unique effects on endothelial function and, along with thiazide diuretics, may improve left ventricular dysfunction and cardiac failure.

The independent benefits of specific classes on left ventricular hypertrophy have been examined in large meta-analyses, with ACE inhibitors apparently more effective than beta-blockers, alpha-blockers, calcium antagonists and thiazide diuretics in this respect.[49–51]

Finally there is clearly documented variation in the impact of drug classes on lipids, lipoproteins, measures of free radical and anti-oxidant activity, and circulating clotting factors and endothelial constituents such as PAI-1, von Willebrand factor, ACE and growth factors. Modulation of the renin–angiotensin–aldosterone system at both a paracrine and endocrine level may affect vascular disease.

Most of these differences are of hypothetical importance, with the exception of the metabolic effects on lipid and glucose metabolism.

Treatment of hypertension and the prevention of cardiovascular disease

The history of this subject extends over four decades and looks likely to run for many more given the inherent difficulties of even the best designed studies, data manipulation by meta-analyses, and perhaps new pressures resulting from studies being precipitately curtailed, or from findings of other studies being overplayed.

In this section, studies of essential hypertension will be reviewed before discussing the key issue of antihypertensive therapy in diabetes. This is important since several of the later studies incorporated diabetic subjects and such information needs to be put in the context of the overall study; and second because some of the critical debates still raging require us to be acquainted with the facts.

The key issues are:

1. Does blood pressure lowering improve all cardiovascular outcomes?
2. Are there differences in cardiovascular outcome between men and women, elderly and younger populations, and between Caucasian and other ethnic groups?
3. What is the impact of smoking on antihypertensive therapy?
4. How low should blood pressure be reduced?
5. Are all classes of antihypertensive therapy equivalent in their impact on CVD?
6. How important are adverse metabolic and other effects of antihypertensive agents?
7. How applicable are trial data to routine clinical practice e.g. in subjects routinely excluded from trial entry, such as a recent major CVD event?

Modern antihypertensive drug trials effectively started with the publication of the Veterans' Administration Study of moderate hypertension (diastolic $105 \leq 115$ mm Hg) in 1970.[52] Drug therapy reduced strokes, cardiac failure and major renal endpoints, but not myocardial infarction.

This study first identified the issue of greater absolute benefit in the elderly patients at highest absolute CVD risk, and also noted the limited power to evaluate the impact on myocardial infarction. This latter point is of some interest, as all subsequent studies have chosen composite CVD endpoints as the primary outcome measure, with meta-analysis confirming that antihypertensive treatment reduces the incidence of coronary heart disease.

The benefits of antihypertensive therapy for mild to moderate diastolic hypertension on stroke and coronary heart disease are summarized in Figs 5.1 and 5.2.[53] These studies were published in the mid- and late 1980s and confirmed that modest reduction in diastolic pressure (mean reduction 6–8 mm Hg) reduced the incidence of stokes by 35–50% in comparison to placebo. The MRC study in particular evaluated over 17 000 men and women aged 35 to 64 years, and the key benefits were most apparent for those treated with thiazide diuretics.[54] Women and men both derived clinical benefit. Much has been made of the subgroup analyses in respect of the lesser impact of propanolol on strokes, particularly among smokers, and the possible contrasting reduction in all CHD morbidity among non-smokers treated with propanolol. These were not prespecified endpoints and must be treated with caution.

The Metoprolot Atherosclerosis Prevention in Hypertensives (MAPHY) study in far fewer subjects failed to confirm any coronary benefit among non-smokers treated with beta-blockers.[55]

Other important practical issues emerged which have been replicated in later studies. Most importantly, the 'small print' in the study design allowed for additional antihypertensive therapy to enable target blood pressure attainment, particularly with thiazide use in 25–33% of cases. The 20% drop out rate in a study population raises issues of compliance in a wider context, highlighted by the commoner side effect profile of beta-blockers.

Studies of the elderly population

The results of drug treatment in elderly hypertensive subjects are generally consistent with those in younger subjects. However, as the absolute risks of heart failure and stroke are greater, so the absolute benefits are greatest in the higher risk elderly population. The six main studies are summarized in Table 5.1. In 1985 the first trial of diuretic therapy (EWPHE) involved only 840 individuals,[56] a far cry from later studies of 4500 to 6500 elderly men and women.[57,58]

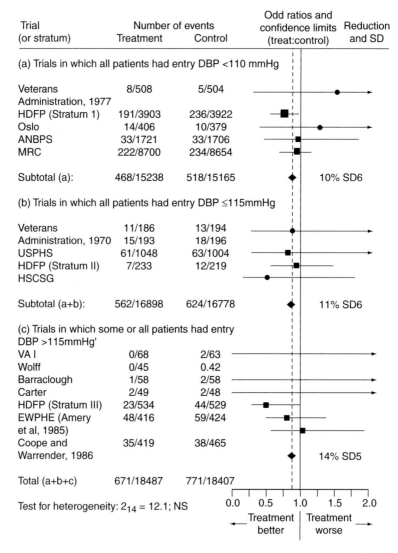

Trial (or stratum)	Number of events Treatment	Control	Odd ratios and confidence limits (treat:control)	Reduction and SD
(a) Trials in which all patients had entry DBP <110 mmHg				
Veterans Administration, 1977	8/508	5/504		
HDFP (Stratum 1)	191/3903	236/3922		
Oslo	14/406	10/379		
ANBPS	33/1721	33/1706		
MRC	222/8700	234/8654		
Subtotal (a):	468/15238	518/15165		10% SD6
(b) Trials in which all patients had entry DBP ≤115mmHg				
Veterans Administration, 1970	11/186	13/194		
	15/193	18/196		
USPHS	61/1048	63/1004		
HDFP (Stratum II)	7/233	12/219		
HSCSG				
Subtotal (a+b):	562/16898	624/16778		11% SD6
(c) Trials in which some or all patients had entry DBP >115mmHg'				
VA I	0/68	2/63		
Wolff	0/45	0.42		
Barraclough	1/58	2/58		
Carter	2/49	2/48		
HDFP (Stratum III)	23/534	44/529		
EWPHE (Amery et al, 1985)	48/416	59/424		
Coope and Warrender, 1986	35/419	38/465		14% SD5
Total (a+b+c)	671/18487	771/18407		

Test for heterogeneity: $2_{14} = 12.1$; NS

0.0   0.5   1.0   1.5   2.0

← Treatment better | Treatment worse →

Figure 5.1 *Reductions in coronary heart disease in antihypertensive trials.*[53]

The headline results of EWPHE[56] were significant reductions in cardiac and overall cardiovascular mortality. Interesting findings were a significant 43% reduction in mortality from myocardial infarction, an insignificant

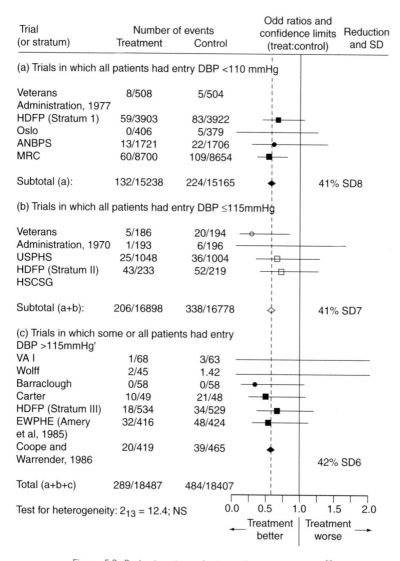

Trial (or stratum)	Number of events		Odd ratios and confidence limits (treat:control)	Reduction and SD
	Treatment	Control		
(a) Trials in which all patients had entry DBP <110 mmHg				
Veterans Administration, 1977	8/508	5/504		
HDFP (Stratum 1)	59/3903	83/3922		
Oslo	0/406	5/379		
ANBPS	13/1721	22/1706		
MRC	60/8700	109/8654		
Subtotal (a):	132/15238	224/15165		41% SD8
(b) Trials in which all patients had entry DBP ≤115mmHg				
Veterans Administration, 1970	5/186	20/194		
USPHS	1/193	6/196		
HDFP (Stratum II)	25/1048	36/1004		
HSCSG	43/233	52/219		
Subtotal (a+b):	206/16898	338/16778		41% SD7
(c) Trials in which some or all patients had entry DBP >115mmHg'				
VA I	1/68	3/63		
Wolff	2/45	1.42		
Barraclough	0/58	0/58		
Carter	10/49	21/48		
HDFP (Stratum III)	18/534	34/529		
EWPHE (Amery et al, 1985)	32/416	48/424		
Coope and Warrender, 1986	20/419	39/465		42% SD6
Total (a+b+c)	289/18487	484/18407		

Test for heterogeneity: 2_{13} = 12.4; NS

0.0   0.5   1.0   1.5   2.0

← Treatment better | Treatment worse →

Figure 5.2 *Reductions in stroke in antihypertensive trials.*[53]

reduction in stroke mortality, and demonstration of a J-shaped curve, with attained blood pressure and mortality, which should remain an important practical clinical issue in this particular population.

Table 5.1 Percentage reduction in stroke and CHD events in antihypertensive drug studies in the elderly

	EWPHE[56]	STOP[57]	SHEP[58]	MRC in elderly[59]	SYSTEUR[65]	STOP-2[66 a]
Total cardiovascular mortality	27%*↓	43%***↓	20%*↓	29%**↓	27% ns↓	1%↓ns
CHD mortality	38%*↓		20%*↓		27% ns↓	
MI mortality	43%*↓	25%**↓	43%**↓		56% ns↓	
Stroke mortality	32% ns↓	73%**↓	29%**↓		27% ns↓	
Non-fatal MI	+3% ns↑		33%**↓		20% ns↓	
Non-fatal CVA	52%*↓		37%**↓		44%**↓	
All MI (fatal and non-fatal)		13%**↓	27%***↓	19%↓	30% ns↓	4%↑ns
All CVA (fatal and non-fatal)		47%***↓	—	25%↓	42%**↓	11%↓ns

*p < 0.05; **p < 0.01; ***p < 0.001.
All studies placebo controlled except a newer versus conventional treatments.

The larger STOP study was able to demonstrate the expected reduction in stroke morbidity and mortality, and a reduction in fatal and non-fatal myocardial events.[57]

The next issue to be addressed in the elderly was whether treatment of isolated systolic (as opposed to diastolic) hypertension reduced morbidity and mortality from stroke. The SHEP study was a well-designed study including both men and women, treated with thiazides initially, with beta-blockers added as necessary.[58] Fourteen per cent of the subjects were Afro-American, and 10% had non-insulin-treated diabetes. There was a clear cut reduction (risk reduction (RR) 0.64) in total strokes, and a significant reduction (RR 0.73) in the combined secondary endpoint of non-fatal myocardial infarction and fatal CHD.

The benefits observed in the SHEP study seemed to be confined to thiazide treatment. There was no evidence that addition of atenolol conferred additional benefit. This was also the broad conclusion of the MRC study in the elderly, which also included mild diastolic hypertension, excluded diabetic subjects, and compared diuretic, beta-blocker or placebo.[59] Both stroke *and* coronary events were reduced with diuretics, especially in non-smokers (only stroke incidence was reduced when active treatment overall was compared to placebo). Furthermore, there was a higher rate of side effects and drop-outs with atenolol.

These studies together suggest that blood pressure reduction is important in that it reduces strokes and probably cardiac events in the elderly, and that this is best achieved with thiazide diuretics as the first line drug. There seems *no* support for the idea that beta-blockers might have any advantageous cardioprotective role in hypertensive subjects of any age without evidence of major CHD. There also remains an issue of the benefits of hypotensive therapy possibly being more limited amongst smokers.

Studies of 'newer' antihypertensive agents and 'tight blood pressure control' (Table 5.2)

The last few years have seen publication in the general and elderly populations of several major studies examining the impact of calcium

Table 5.2 Antihypertensive studies involving subjects with and without type 2 diabetes

Study name	Subjects in trial	Diabetic subjects in trial (no (%))	Outcomes (relative risk) in DM	Comments
SHEP[58]	4 736	583 (10%)	Major CVD 0.66* CVA 0.78 ns MI/CHD 0.46*	Placebo controlled
HOT[60]	18 790	1650 (8%)	Major CVD 0.49**	Comparison of tight control (diastolic BP 80 vs 90 mm Hg)
CAPP[61]	10 985	572 (5%)	Major CVD 0.59* Stroke 1.02 ns All MI 0.34*	Comparison of captopril vs conventional drugs
STOP2[66]	6 614	721 (10.9%)	Equivalent prevention of cardiovascular mortality or major CHD/CVA event	Comparison of ACE inhibitors/calcium, antagonists vs conventional drugs

Table 5.2 continued

NORDIL[63]	10 881	727 (6.5%)	Equivalent reduction of major CVD, CVA, MI	Comparison of diltiazem vs conventional drugs
INSIGHT[64]	6 321	1302 (20.6%)	Equivalent reduction of CVD events	Comparison of nifedipine vs conventional drugs
Syst-Eur[65]	4 695	492 (10%)	Greater reduction in overall mortality, CVD mortality, CVD events	Nitrendipine vs placebo
ALLHAT[62]	24 335	8300 (35.5%)	Increased risk of combined CVD 1.24*** and heart failure 2.14***	Comparison of doxazosin vs thiazide
HOPE[79]	9 297	3577 (38.4%)	Major CVD event or mortality 0.75*** All MI 0.78** All CVA 0.67**	Ramipril vs placebo added to other CVD drugs

$*p < 0.05$; $**p < 0.01$; $***p < 0.001$.

antagonists, ACE inhibitors and alpha-blockers, and the issue of how low to reduce blood pressure. The design of these more recent studies has been to include much larger numbers of subjects, often more broadly representative of a wider hypertensive constituency, and in particular often including a significant proportion of men and women with diabetes. In addition, these were not placebo controlled trials, an appropriate ethical modification.

HOT

The Hypertension Optimal Treatment (HOT) study evaluated almost 19 000 subjects with moderate diastolic hypertension (100–115 mm Hg) aged up to 80 years, followed for a mean period of 3.8 years. There was an 8% prevalence of diabetes in each of the three target diastolic blood pressure categories ($\leq$ 90, $\leq$ 85, $\leq$ 80 mm Hg) . The study objectives were to elucidate the optimum target diastolic blood pressure and the benefit of additional aspirin in reducing major cardiovascular events.[60]

The specific hypotensive agent evaluated was the calcium antagonist felopidine, with the addition of ACE inhibitors, beta-blockers and diuretics through a five-step regimen. This is an important aspect of this study, in that effectively the issue of benefits of one drug class over another were relegated below the issue of reducing blood pressure by whatever means required, the practical approach necessary in routine clinical practice.

Diastolic blood pressure was reduced by 20–24 mm Hg, and the lowest risk of cardiovascular events occurred at achieved levels of 83–87 mm Hg. With the important exception of the diabetic subgroup, the majority of the major primary endpoints were not significantly altered by more intensive blood pressure lowering. The addition of aspirin to 50% of subjects significantly reduced all major cardiovascular events by 15%, and 'all myocardial infarction' was reduced by a more impressive 36%.

Important points emerge from careful reading of the report. First, it was well conducted, with only 2.6% of subjects lost to follow up. The full five-step regimen was required in 20% of cases, i.e. ACE inhibitors or beta-blockers added with titration to top dosage, and the addition of a diuretic. Only 50% in the most intensive (≤ 80 mm Hg) group reached the target, and the benefits were likely to be evident if 140/90 mm Hg was attained, and no J-shaped curve was seen. The event rate in this study was lower than in other studies and control populations, most likely reflecting the impact of effective blood pressure control.

CAPP

The Catopril Project (CAPP) study followed shortly afterwards.[61] Captopril was compared to conventional thiazide or beta-blocker in 11 000 younger men and women (up to 66 years) with diastolic blood pressure > 100 mm Hg, followed for 5 years. Target pressure was <90 mm Hg, and the drop-out rate was minimal. Roughly 5% in each group had diabetes. As in the HOT study, this was not a strict comparison of drug classes. Diuretics and calcium antagonists were added to either group, and thiazides and beta-blockers could be combined, but the frequency of these variations is not stated.

There were no important differences between the 'captopril' and 'conventional' groups in achieved blood pressure, nor in the composite primary CVD endpoint. As with any study the subgroup evaluations should be treated with caution, although they are likely to be more meaningful where they bear out recurring themes from other studies. Stroke incidence was greater in the 'captopril' group (relative risk 1.25), but this is attributed to the higher baseline blood pressure prerandomization. There was no difference in cardiac failure overall, a finding to be contrasted with the later Antihypertensive and Lipid-Lowering Treatment to Prevent Heart Attack Trial (ALLHAT) study (v.i.).[62]

In respect of diabetes, captopril treatment led to significantly fewer cardiac events (especially myocardial infarction) in the 572 subjects with baseline diabetes, and importantly was associated with a significant 14% reduction in the incidence of newly diagnosed diabetes. This concurs with the findings with another ACE inhibitor (ramipril) in the HOPE study (see below), but in CAPP may more realistically just as likely reflect the established support for finding an adverse metabolic effect of thiazide and beta-blocker use (particularly in combination).

Studies with calcium antagonists

The story of calcium antagonists in hypertension (and diabetic hypertension in particular) is controversial. It is evident that hype has overridden substance in this debate, and that calcium antagonists are integral to effective hypertension control in a substantial proportion of patients. Two recent studies provide useful information to illuminate the debate.

NORDIL

The Nordic Diltiazem Study (NORDIL) study of almost 11 000 men and women aged less than 75 compared diltiazem with diuretics and/or beta-blockers over a 4.5 year period.[63] Diabetes was present in 6.5–6.9% of cases in the randomized groups. The target diastolic pressure was 90 mm Hg, and as in the previously mentioned recent studies, other drug classes were added in 50% of cases, including the use of ACE inhibitors. Such a strategy led to reductions of blood pressure of 20–23/19 mm Hg, with no difference in the combined primary endpoint of all cardiovascular events or the secondary endpoints of cardiac failure or myocardial infarction, in either the total study population or the diabetic subgroup. The incidence of fatal/non-fatal stroke was significantly reduced by 20% in the diltiazem group, and there was no difference in the evolution of new diabetes between the two study groups.

An important issue focussed on in this particular study was the development of side-effects. As expected, headaches were more common in the diltiazem group, whereas fatigue and dyspnoea were more evident in the diuretic–beta-blocker group. These factors are perhaps relevant to the important drop-out from active treatment of 23% and 7% in the two groups, respectively.

INSIGHT

Nifedipine (and by implication other dihydropyridine calcium channel blockers) had previously received a 'bad press' on the back of the clinical effects of the standard short lived preparation. The Intervention as a Goal in Hypertension Treatment (INSIGHT) study is important that it also restores a degree of credibility to this class of drugs, using the sustained action (GITS) preparation.[64]

This study involved over 6000 men and women aged 55–80 years with either systolic blood pressure ≥ 160 or diastolic blood pressure $\geq 95\,\text{mm Hg}$ and one of many additional cardiovascular risk factors (20.6% had diabetes) for a period of 51 months. Nifedipine GITS was compared with co-amilozide, with the option of add-on atenolol or enalapril, and the primary outcome was the composite of cardiovascular death, myocardial infarction, cardiac failure or stroke. Blood pressure fell by $33/17\,\text{mm Hg}$ and there was no difference between the groups for the composite or individual primary end points.

The drop-out rate in this study was $> 30\%$, and it has been argued that as analysis was on an intention to treat basis, then a high early drop-out rate might have masked differences between the groups. From a practical point of view it highlights the considerable effort in maintaining compliance outside the setting of a research study. The difficulty with fluid retention was particularly evident with nifedipine, whereas 'serious adverse events' (life threatening, disabling or requiring hospital admission) were more prevalent with co-amilozide. The diabetic subgroup required additional hypotensive therapy more frequently, a statistic not commented on in the other studies.

INSIGHT achieved identical blood pressure lowering to that seen in the HOT study, and nifedipine was not associated with any excess total mortality or cancer incidence.

Other studies with calcium antagonists

The issue regarding different class effects was also examined in the elderly in the Syst-Eur (mean age 70) and the STOP-2 (76 years) studies. Syst-Eur was placebo-controlled and evaluated the impact of nitrendipine with optional add-on ACE inhibitor and thiazide in isolated systolic hypertension over 2 years.[65] Over 4600 men and women were entered; 10% of the subjects had diabetes. The primary endpoint was stroke, and a highly significant 42% reduction in this outcome was achieved with an average $23\,\text{mm Hg}$ reduction in blood pressure. An additional 26% reduction in fatal/non-fatal cardiac endpoints was noted, but only a trend toward reduction in the incidence of cardiac failure. As with the later studies of calcium antagonists in a younger population, there was no difference in overall mortality or cancer incidence.

STOP-2 was designed to compare 'conventional' and 'newer' antihypertensive agents in the elderly (aged 70–84) with moderate hypertension (systolic ≥ 180 mm Hg and/or diastolic ≥ 105 mm Hg), and there was no placebo arm.[66] Over 6500 subjects were randomized to a thiazide, beta-blocker, ACE inhibitor or calcium antagonist. The study lasted 54 months and included 11% with diabetes. The study design allowed for dose titration and addition of another drug class (required in 46%) aiming at a target of 160/95 mm Hg. Although the authors stated that no patient was lost to follow up or refused to continue with the study, 34–39% of subjects withdrew from their original treatment regimens.

The combined primary endpoint mortality from stroke, myocardial infarction or CVD was equivalent with 'old' and 'new' agents in the total study group and among the diabetic subgroup. Morbidity in the form of all myocardial infarctions and cardiac failure was reduced by 22–23% with ACE inhibitors in comparison to calcium antagonists, although all events were comparable between the calcium antagonist and conventional groups. Interestingly (and in contrast to HOPE and CAPP), ACE inhibitor use was not associated with a reduced incidence of new diabetes.

Broadly equivalent benefit with dihydropyridines has been suggested in elderly Chinese hypertensive subjects, most notably the Shanghai Trial of Nifedipine in the Elderly (STONE) study, where stroke incidence and total mortality were reduced, but there was no impact on the incidence of fatal/non-fatal myocardial infarction or cancer.[67]

ALLHAT
Two other well-publicized, large-scale trials of anti-hypertensive agents have recently been published. The ALLHAT study includes over 24 000 hypertensive white, Hispanic and Afro-American men and women. One component was published early.[62] Subjects have mild hypertension (> 140/90 mm Hg) and at least one additional risk factor for CHD (35% with diabetes). The study design comprises initial dose

titration (of thiazide, calcium antagonist, ACE inhibitor or alpha-blocker) followed by two additional steps adding beta-blockers and other agents in 25–33% of cases.

Although the main part of the study is on-going, one component was published early.[62] The primary composite endpoint of fatal CHD and non-fatal myocardial infarction was comparable between the main thiazide and alpha-blocker (doxazosin) group. The doxazosin arm of the trial was discontinued at the request of the safety monitoring board because of a doubling of the relative risk of cardiac failure and a less dramatic 1.25 relative risk of combined cardiovascular disease (including angina and stroke) compared to the thiazide arm. An excess of adverse outcomes with doxazosin was also noted in the diabetic subgroup, and also amongst Afro-Americans and those over the age of 65. Given that the 'new' drug performed less well than the standard comparator drug, termination of this study component was justified. From a practical point of view this does not establish a definite risk with doxazosin, simply an advantage for the use of a thiazide as *first-line* treatment of hypertension in most clinical situations, unless there are clear contra-indications.

The practice of early trial termination when the primary endpoints have not been reached and circumstances develop that were not prespecified for trial termination has been carried out under more dubious circumstances in several other studies, raising concern about the validity of any conclusions drawn from these studies.

HOPE

The Heart Outcomes Prevention Evaluation (HOPE) study in many respects is the most challenging study yet of antihypertensive agents,[68,69] although it was not constructed as a hypotensive study. Its findings were more dramatic than any other study to date, and suggested that the treatment of 1000 patients at high cardiovascular risk with the ACE inhibitor ramipril for 4 years prevented about 150 CVD events in 70 patients. In particular, the study claimed that the benefits were observed in almost 5000 cases without hypertension, and only a small part of the benefit was derived from a hypotensive action given the modest 3/2 mm Hg reduction in blood pressure.

In HOPE, over 9000 men and women with established coronary, cerebrovascular or peripheral arterial disease, *or* diabetes plus at least one additional CVD risk factor (38% of the total trial sample), were randomized to placebo or ramipril, with a composite primary endpoint of myocardial infarction, stroke or CVD death. At trial entry over 75% were on antiplatelet agents, 39% were on beta-blockers, 28.5% on lipid lowering agents, 15% on diuretics and over 46% were on calcium antagonists.

Roughly 47% had hypertension (> 160/90 mm Hg, or were on antihypertensive therapy), but presumably the prevalence with mild hypertension (> 140/90 mm Hg) was greater. Patients were excluded if they had cardiac failure, were known to have a left ventricular ejection fraction reduced to less than 0.40 or had experienced a stroke or myocardial infarction in the preceding month.[68]

From a practical point of view, almost 10% of the original eligible patients were excluded from randomization (including elevations of potassium or creatinine) and during the study treatment was permanently discontinued in 29% on ramipril (27% on placebo). This high drop-out rate for both treatment arms is also troubling. In particular the details of 1101 individuals who withdrew for 'other' reasons are important. This constituted the vast majority of withdrawals, and it would be important to know if the specific reasons for withdrawals differed from those 'other' reasons behind 1074 cases withdrawing from placebo treatment. The incidence of hyperkalaemia–renal impairment is of importance given the 42% prevalence of peripheral vascular disease, and the possibility that this would have been associated with subclinical renal vascular disease, which may be present in up to 15% of type 2 diabetes cases.

The trial was stopped 6 months early when the major endpoint was clearly achieved.[69] Compared to placebo, ramipril produced highly significant benefits:

- a 22% reduction in the primary endpoint
- a 20% reduction in myocardial infarction
- a 15–16% reduction in all cause mortality and revascularization procedures

- a 23% reduction in cardiac failure
- a 34% reduction in new diagnoses of diabetes.

This impact on reducing the development of diabetes seems to be a class effect of ACE inhibitors different to that observed with thiazides and beta-blockers, where the trend may be towards a greater incidence of diabetes. The benefits were considered independent of gender, age, concomitant therapy or the presence of microalbumuria and were statistically significant after 2 years of treatment.

While the clinical outcomes undoubtedly improved, the mechanism of the benefit is unclear. Improved left ventricular function is one likely explanation whether or not a small minority had reduced left ventricular ejection fraction. What of the impact on blood pressure? Amongst the 'hypertensive' group, an ACE inhibitor would be a logical addition to the other antihypertensive agents. It is not clear what hypotensive impact it had on this subgroup—if, as is likely, this was more than 3/2 mm Hg, such a reduction might have explained the benefit in this group, but what about those without hypertension? First some would have had mild hypertension and may have derived benefit from a hypotensive effect. A lack of blood pressure response in normotensive subjects in ACE inhibitors is well recognized, especially in the context of diabetes, and this may have diminished the average blood pressure achieved for the total study population. However, reduction of microalbuminuria in the diabetic subgroup might have additional specific benefits. Other mechanisms such as the impact on the endothelium and the renin–angiotensin system are speculative.

The benefits observed are also difficult to disentangle from the fact that a high proportion of the study group were on other agents acting on the cardiovascular system. Thus it is unclear whether a synergistic effect was observed and whether the impact of ramipril on CVD outcome would be less marked in the absence of these other treatments, particularly aspirin.

Another question remaining to be answered is whether this outcome is a class effect likely with other ACE inhibitors? The results of ongoing similar studies of ACE inhibitors (PEACE, EUROPA) will be vital if they confirm the findings of HOPE. As with beta-blockers, aspirin and statins, the HOPE study suggests a role for ramipril in secondary prevention of CHD and strokes, with 80% at trial entry having established CHD.

Summary of studies of hypotensive therapy in non-diabetic subjects

1. It would appear that all cardiovascular outcomes can be improved assuming there is a substantial reduction in blood pressure.
2. Antihypertensive therapy is effective regardless of gender, age and ethnic background, but in absolute terms delivers most where there is greatest risk (e.g. the elderly).
3. The question of the effect of smoking on the outcome of blood pressure lowering is still not resolved, and may possibly attenuate the benefit derived from beta-blockers.
4. The target blood pressure should ideally be 140/90 in younger individuals, with recognition that this may only be achievable by using a combination of at least three drug classes, and in less than 90% of cases.
5. The big question of whether a specific drug class has a preferential effect on CVD may be an academic one. Blood pressure control by whatever means is required. In practice this should be thiazides initially, with addition of other agents clinically tailored to the individual. Thus ACE inhibitors would be preferable to beta-blockers in managing a hypertensive individual with obstructive airways disease and cor pulmonale.
6. The real adverse metabolic effects of thiazides and beta-blockers have been shown to be subordinate to their impact on CVD in trials. However, in clinical practice tailoring of hypotensive drug selection will rightly affect selection; for example there may be reservations using beta-blockers in individuals with hypertriglyceridaemia who are at risk of pancreatitis. Furthermore there was an appreciable 2–6% incidence of hyponatraemia, hypokalaemia, hyperuricaemia and impaired renal function with diuretics, and

over 25% of subjects on nifedipine in the INSIGHT study had side-effects from fluid retention.[64] These side-effects will often lead to poor compliance or curtailment of therapy.

7. The major trials can serve as a guide to routine clinical practice, and clinicians should resist efforts to constrain a correct individualized approach to patient care. A good example would be blood pressure control 3 months after a stroke, subjects previously routinely excluded from the trials.

Treatment of hypertension in diabetes

Before discussing the impact of hypertension on cardiovascular disease in type 1 and type 2 diabetes, the impact on microvascular disease requires consideration. In both types of diabetes antihypertensive therapy has led to important improvements both in retinopathy and also in evolution and progression of microalbuminuria, at least over periods of up to 5 years. It is outside the scope of this chapter to focus in great detail on this issue, but worth noticing that the data on microalbuminuria–nephropathy with antihypertensive therapy, and ACE inhibitors in particular, is not evident after 10 years in UKPDS,[70] in contrast to more encouraging findings from HOPE and other studies,[71,72] which did not extend beyond 5 years' follow-up.

Impact of treatment of hypertension on CVD in type 1 diabetes

The close relationship between nephropathy and hypertension in type 1 diabetes extends to studies which establish the benefits of antihypertensive therapy and ACE inhibitors, in particular in delaying the progression of nephropathy at all stages. In addition there is increasing evidence that retinopathy likewise benefits from effective blood pressure lowering. In contrast, there are no published studies evaluating the impact of hypotensive therapy on CVD in type 1 diabetes in subjects without diabetic complications.

Collaborative study group

Studies that have examined the impact of different antihypertensive agents on CVD have not had a large enough sample size or event rate to examine the issue definitively. One placebo-controlled study of captopril lasted 3 years and examined 409 type 1 diabetic subjects with established nephropathy, of whom 75% were already hypertensive. Appreciable reductions in renal endpoints were demonstrated with captopril, including a 50% reduction in the combined endpoint of death, dialysis or renal transplantation that was independent of any disparity in attained blood pressure.[73]

As the endpoint was a doubling of serum creatinine the impact on CVD was difficult to ascertain, but over 3% experienced non-fatal CVD events which required study withdrawal. There are no data provided to inform us whether these events were more common in the placebo group.

Impact of treatment of hypertension on CVD in type 2 diabetes

In 1998 the Fosinopril versus Amlodipine Cardiovascular Events randomised Trial (FACET)[74] and Appropriate Blood Pressure Control in Diabetes (ABCD)[75] studies in hypertensive type 2 diabetic subjects were published and caused a controversy. It is important to recognize that they were studies of short duration, small sample size and with totally different primary endpoints from those that were focused on. They partly supported the earlier findings from the MIDAS study,[76] all of which suggested that in contrast to alternative antihypertensive agents (thiazides and ACE inhibitors), three different dihydropyridine calcium antagonists (isradipine, nisodipine and amolodipine) were particularly associated with an excess of fatal and non-fatal CVD events among diabetic subjects.

ABCD

The ABCD study[75] was designed to examine whether intensive as opposed to moderate blood pressure control would prevent or slow the progression of nephropathy, a concept similar to that in the HOT study.

In addition, a secondary hypothesis was to establish comparative benefit from a calcium antagonist and an ACE inhibitor. Blood pressure control was equivalent between the groups and, if anything, those who received the ACE inhibitor had a higher baseline CVD risk. Although over 50% in each group discontinued study medication, the study was terminated after 67 months when a 5.5-fold excess of fatal/non-fatal myocardial infarction was observed in the group assigned nisoldipine as opposed to enalapril. The incidence of stroke was also increased (relative risk 1.6).

FACET

FACET was an open-labelled trial of up to 3.5 years in duration that examined the metabolic effects of fosinopril and amlodipine in hypertensive type 2 diabetes.[74] Both treatments effectively lowered blood pressure, with equivalent metabolic effects on glycaemia and lipids, and there was a low drop-out rate of roughly 10% in each group. Fosinopril treatment led to a significantly lower risk (RR 0.49) of the composite secondary endpoint of acute myocardial infarction, stroke or hospitalized angina.

MIDAS

The Multicenter Isradipine Diuretic Atherosclerosis Study (MIDAS) study compared isradipine and a thiazide and was designed to examine their impact on carotid artery intimal medial thickness assessed by ultrasound in non-diabetic hypertensive subjects over 3 years.[76,77] In this respect there was no difference between the two treatments. Systolic (but not diastolic) blood pressure was reduced more effectively with thiazide treatment, which may be important as this group also had fewer major vascular events, especially among those who had evidence of deteriorating glucose tolerance during follow-up.

Later studies involved more than three times the number of hypertensive diabetic subjects treated with these drugs.[60,63,64] They showed reductions in CVD events with calcium antagonists comparable to conventional therapy, and focused attention more on the importance of the degree of blood pressure lowering than on the agents that achieved the reduction.

Hypertension in Diabetes Study (HDS)

The UKPDS differs from other studies of the impact of antihypertensive therapy in several respects. First, it evaluated the impact of *both* intensive blood glucose and blood pressure control. As yet, analyses which could separate out the independent benefits of each have not been published, and despite statistical correction, it should be conceded that the combined package delivered a large proportion of the improvements. This is in some ways similar to the benefits of adding ramipril to established treatments for cardiovascular disease in the HOPE study,[69] or the result from intensified multifactorial intervention in a report from the Steno group.[24]

Second, the UKPDS studied newly diagnosed type 2 diabetic subjects and was able to follow them up for over 8 years, so it is likely that the natural history of the evolution of CVD would differ from studies where CVD was more evident at trial entry. Indeed, this is supported by, for example, the 'raw data' of CVD events in comparison to the HOPE study,[69] the incidence being greater in the latter study.

There were two hypertension studies nested within the UKPDS. First an evaluation of the benefits of 'tight' blood pressure control, similar to the HOT study,[70] and second a comparison of the relative impact of beta-blockers and ACE Inhibitors.[78] However, as with so many studies which superficially evaluate the benefit of one drug class, stepwise addition of other agents in 29% of cases was necessary to attain target blood pressure levels.

The major outcomes of 'tight' blood pressure control (144/82 compared to 154/87 mm Hg after 8.4 years) were significant reductions in diabetes-related mortality (32%, mainly CVD), strokes (44%), cardiac failure (56%) and retinopathy treatment (35%). A non-significant 21% reduction in myocardial infarction and similar modest reductions (with wide confidence intervals) in amputation rates and progression of nephropathy were noted. Overall, it was estimated that the number needing treatment (NNT) for 10 years was 6.1 to prevent one vascular event or 15 to prevent one death.

In the comparison of beta-blockers and ACE inhibitors, there was an equivalent hypotensive response and requirement for at least two additional classes of hypotensive agent. Withdrawal/non-compliance was recorded for 22% receiving captopril and 35% receiving the beta-blocker, and as expected there was a greater incidence of weight gain and fatigue with atenolol and more cough with the ACE inhibitor. There was no significant difference in rates of diabetes-related mortality, strokes, myocardial infarction, cardiac failure or peripheral vascular disease.

MICRO-HOPE study

Within the HOPE study 3577 diabetic subjects were studied, of whom 60% had established CHD and 50% had documented hypertension. Rampiril or placebo was added to other treatments for CVD (55% on aspirin, 44% on calcium channel blockers, 20% on diuretics, 23% on hypolipidaemic agents and 28% on beta-blockers).[79]

As with the major study, ramipril treatment was associated with significant 25% reductions in the combined primary outcome of myocardial infarction (22%), stroke (33%) or death from CVD (37%). The NNT to prevent one event was 15. There was a 33% drop-out from ramipril, and the majority were for reasons not defined in detail. Reassuringly there was no difference in serum creatinine levels between the groups among those who completed the study. Despite a marginal 2/1 mm Hg change in blood pressure, a reduction in CVD events comparable to that of UKPDS was noted.

Steno study

As mentioned earlier, the Steno study implemented stepwise intensive therapy targeting hyperglycaemia, hypertension, dyslipidaemia and microalbuminuria in 80 type 2 diabetic subjects. The primary endpoint was the development of clinical nephropathy (albuminuria > 300 mg/l). As a consequence, almost half were converted to insulin, 71 received antihypertensive therapy, 70 ACE inhibitors, 31 aspirin, 35 hypolipidaemic agents and two received HRT. A composite CVD endpoint (fatal and non-fatal) was observed in significantly fewer (26 versus 42) who received this intensive approach.[24]

Thus the benefits of antihypertensive therapy in diabetes would seem to be most apparent when combined with other strategies to improve the metabolic and vascular state. The lack of major outcome studies where all such aspects (including hypolipidaemic agents) are evaluated will be rectified with the ALLHAT study.

Practical aspects of the management of hypertension in diabetes

There are many guidelines for the management of hypertension which have been developed in response to the bewildering intervention studies and their interpretation. Some of these are summarized in Table 5.3 and demonstrate that intervention thresholds range between 130 and 160 mm Hg systolic and between 85 and 95 mm Hg diastolic pressure.[80–83] More interestingly (and perhaps even more unfeasable) are the target blood pressures of < 125–140/ 75–85 mm Hg. This is not therapeutic nihilism but a recognition of the findings of the intervention studies, and observations from routine clinical practice. For example, in the UKPDS there were major investments of time and effort, involving 3–4 monthly visits over a period of 8.4 years.

Despite this intensive treatment (with at least three agents in 29% of cases), only 56% of cases attained a blood pressure of < 150/85 mm Hg. Interestingly, one case in 25 continued with moderate hypertension (≥ 180/105) despite this strategy. Treatment of hypertension in type 1 diabetes poses similar challenges in meeting targets,[32] and there is documentation that among hypertensive diabetic patients in England one-third were untreated and more than 50% had suboptimal control on therapy.[84] There are earlier reports that talk of the 'rule of halves', whereby blood pressure detection and effective management is only achieved in 50% of cases.[85] It seems that, optimistically, the targets of the august bodies producing guidelines can also only be achieved in 50% of cases at best. In this respect they are unrealistic, as are the targets chosen for elderly diabetics without careful consideration.

When it comes to the question of the class of antihypertensive agents to be used there would seem merit in advocating that thiazide

Table 5.3 Guidelines on management of hypertension in diabetes

	Intervention threshold		Target blood pressure	
	Systolic BP	Diastolic BP	Systolic BP	Diastolic BP
British Hypertension Society[80]	140	90	< 140	< 80
St Vincent Declaration[82]				
age < 40 or end organ damage	140	90	≤ 140	≤ 85
age ≥ 40 and no end organ damage	160	95	≤ 140	≤ 85
American Diabetes Association[83]	140	90	≤ 130	≤ 85
Joint National Committee VI[81]	130	85	≤ 130	≤ 85
with proteinuria (> 1 g/24 h)	130	85	≤ 125	≤ 75

diuretics are the most appropriate first-line agents for use in diabetes. Thereafter a strong case could be made for the use of ACE inhibitors in as maximal a dose as possible. These treatments would not be appropriate where there was established or evolving hyponatramia/hyperkalaemia, respectively, and individuals with concurrent angina might be better suited to beta-blockers or diltiazem. Addition of other drug classes will then be necessary in at least 30% of cases.

Individual tailoring of drug classes might also be required for the demonstrable metabolic benefits of alpha-blockers and ACE inhibitors in dyslipidaemic hypertriglyceridaemic states, in contrast to beta-blockers.[28-30] The presence of impotence or chronic obstructive pulmonary disease similarly might favour alpha-blockers over beta-blockers.[86,87]

Given the high likelihood of the need for multiple hypotensive agent therapy, some of the strict criteria for one class over another are somewhat academic. Thus in clinical practice the arguments over the lack of benefits of calcium antagonists in FACET, ABCD and MIDAS are difficult to reconcile with the findings from HOT, NORDIL and INSIGHT, and the ALLHAT concern about doxazosin may also prove impractical.

This is supported by the fact that calcium antagonists in particular are frequently used in addition to the other drug classes where superior efficacy is claimed. Thus in UKPDS, 27% and 36% of the captopril and atenolol groups, respectively received calcium antagonists,[78] and the figure was 44% in the MICRO-HOPE study.[79] Of the many subgroup analyses that have been reported one important subgroup analysis that is presently lacking is to compare outcome of those who did or did not receive calcium antagonists in addition to the main drug under study.

In routine clinical practice perhaps the most important limiting factor will be compliance (see Chapter 10). The drop-out rate from the large studies on the grounds of unsuitability or side-effects is sizeable. An important database in Scotland had put the issue of drug compliance in diabetes into sharp focus, with over 50% of patients apparently non-compliant with their oral hypoglycaemic therapy.[88]

Given that antihypertensive agents (often three in number) will be required in addition to two or three oral hypoglycaemic agents, aspirin and hypolipidaemic therapy (also possibly dual statin–fibrate combination therapy), polypharmacy and adherence to it is probably the next great challenge for the effective prevention of diabetic cardiovascular disease.

The future approach to this may be able to effectively channel findings from pharmacogenetic studies whereby those most amenable to, for example, ACE inhibitors would receive them, based on ACE gene polymorphism.[89]

The financial aspects of this area also merit discussion. Whereas cost-effective analyses have shown that effective blood pressure control is achievable at reasonable cost,[90,91] it would be hoped that efforts to widen the constituency who could benefit will be undertaken by the pharmaceutical agency. In particular, in addition to evaluation of new classes of antihypertensive agents that improve efficacy, introduction of treatments containing active constituents of different antihypertensive drug classes and conceivably also hypoglycaemic and hypolipidaemic and antiplatelet agents presents the most immediate challenge in the pharmacological fight against macrovascular disease. Those lifestyle changes of diet and exercise subject to individual willpower are no less important, but perhaps even less achievable in sedentary overprovided Westernized societies (see Chapter 9).

References

1. Stamler J, Vaccaro O, Neaton JD, Wentworth D. Diabetes, other risk factors, and 12-year cardiovascular mortality for men screened in the Multiple Risk Factor Intervention Trial. Diabetes Care 1993;16:434 –44.
2. Coutinho M, Wang Y, Gerstein H, Yusuf S. The relationship between glucose and incident cardiovascular events. Diabetes Care 1999;22:233–40.
3. Turner RC, Millns H, Neil HAW et al. Risk factors for coronary heart disease in non-insulin dependent diabetes mellitus: United Kingdom Prospective Diabetes Study (UKPDS 23). BMJ 1998;316:823–8.

4. Andersson DKG, Svardsudd K. Long-term glycaemic control relates to mortality in type 2 diabetes. Diabetes Care 1995;18:1534–43.
5. Kuusisto J, Mykkanen L, Pyorala K, Laakso M. NIDDM and its metabolic control predicts coronary heart disease in elderly subjects. Diabetes 1994;43:960–7.
6. Stratton IM, Adler AI, Neil HAW et al. Association of glycaemia with macrovascular and microvascular complications of type 2 diabetes (UKPDS 35): prospective observational study. BMJ 2000;321:405–12.
7. Lowe LP, Liu K, Greenland P et al. Diabetes, asymptomatic hyperglycaemia and 22-year mortality in black and white men: the Chicago Heart Association Detection Project in Industry Study. Diabetes Care 1997;20:163–9.
8. Moss SE, Klein R, Klein BEK, Meur SM. The association of glycaemia and cause specific mortality in a diabetic population. Arch Intern Med 1994;154:2473–9.
9. Lehto S, Ronnemaa T, Haffner SM et al. Dyslipidaemia and hyperglycaemia predict coronary heat disease events in middle-aged patients with NIDDM. Diabetes 1997;46:1354–9.
10. Macleod JM, Lutale J, Marshall SM. Albumin excretion and vascular deaths in NIDDM. Diabetologia 1995;38:610–16.
11. Nelson RG, Pettitt DJ, Carraher MJ et al. Effect of proteinuria on mortality in NIDDM. Diabetes 1988;37:1499–504.
12. Araki S, Haneda M, Togawa T et al. Microalbuminuria is not associated with cardiovascular death in Japanese NIDDM. Diabetes Res Clin Pract 1997;35:35–40.
13. Rossing P, Hougaard P, Borch-Johnsen K, Parving HH. Predictors of mortality in insulin dependent diabetes: 10 year observational follow up study. BMJ 1996;313:779–84.
14. Krowlewski AS, Kosinski EJ, Warram JH et al. Magnitude and determinants of coronary heart disease in juvenile-onset insulin-dependent diabetes mellitus. Am J Cardiol 1987;59:750–5.
15. Laing SP, Swerdlow AJ, Slater SD et al. The British Diabetic Association Cohort Study, II: cause-specific mortality in patients with insulin-treated diabetes mellitus. Diabet Med 1999;16:466–71.
16. Borch-Johnsen K, Andersen PK, Deckert T. The effect of proteinuria on relative mortality in Type 1 (insulin dependent) diabetes mellitus. Diabetologia 1985;28:590–6.
17. Tuomilehto J, Borch-Johnsen K, Molarius A et al. Incidence of cardiovascular disease in Type 1 (insulin-dependent) diabetic subjects with and without diabetic nephropathy in Finland. Diabetologia 1998;41:784–90.
18. Orchard TJ, Dorman JS, Maser RE, Becker DJ et al. Factors asociated with avoidance of severe complications after 25 yr of IDDM. Pittsburgh Epidemiology of Diabetes Complications Study 1. Diabetes Care 1990;13:741–7.

19. Jensen-Urstad KJ, Reichard PG, Rosfors JS et al. Early atherosclerosis is retarded by improved long-term blood glucose control in patients with IDDM. Diabetes 1996;45:1253–8.
20. The Diabetes Control and Complications Trial Research Group. The effect of intensive treatment of diabetes on the development and progression of long-term complications in insulin-dependent diabetes mellitus. N Engl J Med 1993;329:977–86.
21. University Group Diabetes Program. A study of the effects of hypogly-caemic agents on vascular complications in patients with adult-onset diabetes. VI. Supplementary report on non-fatal events in patients treated with tolbutamide. Diabetes 1976;25:1129–53.
22. Knatterud GL, Klimt CR, Levin ME et al for the University Group diabetes Program. Effects of hypoglycaemic agents on vascular complications in patients with adult-onset diabetes. VII. Mortality and selected non-fatal events with insulin treatment. JAMA 1978;240:37–42.
23. Ohkubo Y, Kishikawa H, Araki E et al. Intensive insulin therapy prevents the progression of diabetic microvascular complications in Japanese patients with non-insulin-dependent diabetes mellitus: a randomised prospective 6-year study. Diabetes Res Clin Pract 1995;28:103–17.
24. Gaede P, Vedel P, Parving HH, Pedersen O. Intensified multifactor-ial intervention in patients with type 2 diabetes mellitus and microal-buminuria: the Steno type 2 randomised study. Lancet 1999;353:617–622.
25. The UK Prospective Diabetes Study (UKPDS) Group. Intensive blood-glucose control with sulphonylureas or insulin compared with conven-tional treatment and risk of complications in patients with Type 2 diabetes (UKPDS 33). Lancet 1998;352:837–53.
26. UK Prospective Diabetes Study (UKPDS) Group. Effect of intensive blood glucose control with metformin on complications in overweight patients with Type 2 diabetes (UKPDS 34). Lancet 1998;352:854–65.
27. Williams B. Diabetes and Hypertension. A Fatal Attraction Explained. Publishing Initiative Books, 1997.
28. Skarfors ET, Selinus KI, Lithell HO. Risk factors for developing non-insulin dependent diabetes: a 10 year follow up of men in Sweden. BMJ 1991;3030:755–60.
29. Skarfors ET, Lithell HO, Selinus I, Aberg H. Do antihypertensive drugs precipitate diabetes in predisposed men? BMJ 1989;298:1147–52.
30. Bengtsson C, Blohme G, Lapidus L, Lundgren H. Diabetes in hyperten-sive women: an effect of antihypertensive drugs or the antihypertensive state per se? Diabet Med 1988;5:261–4.
31. Norgaard K, Feldt-Rasmussen B, Borch-Johnsen K et al. Prevalence of hypertension in Type 1 (insulin-dependent) diabetes mellitus. Diabetolo-gia 1990;33:407–10.

32. Collado-Mesa F, Colhoun HM, Stevens LK et al. Prevalence and management of hypertension in Type 1 diabetes mellitus in Europe:the EURODIAB IDDM complications study. Diabet Med 1999;16:41–8.
33. Gall MA, Rossing P, Damsbo P et al. Prevalence of micro- and macroalbuminuria, arterial hypertension, retinopathy and large vessel disease in European Type 2 (non-insulin-dependent) diabetic patients. Diabetologia 1991;34:655–61.
34. Winocour PH, Marshall SM. Microalbuminuria. Biochemistry, epidemiology and clinical practice. Cambridge University Press, 1998.
35. The Hypertension in Diabetes Study Group. Hypertension in Diabetes Study (HDS): 1. Prevalence of hypertension in newly presenting Type 2 diabetic patients and the association with risk factors for both cardiovascular and diabetic complications. J Hypertens 1993;11:309–17.
36. Adler AI, Stratton IM, Neil HAW et al. Association of systolic blood pressure with macrovascular and microvascular complications of type 2 diabetes (UKPDS 36): prospective observational study. BMJ 2000;321:412–19.
37. UK Prospective Diabetes Study Group. UK Prospective Diabetes Study XII: Differences between Asian, Afro-Caribbean and White Caucasian Type 2 Diabetic patients at diagnosis of diabetes. Diabet Med 1994;11:670–7.
38. Pacy PJ, Dodson PM, Beevers M et al. Prevalence of hypertension in white, black and Asian diabetics in a district hospital diabetic clinic. Diabet Med 1985;2:125–30.
39. Douglas JG. Hypertension and diabetes in blacks. Diabetes Care 1990;13 (Suppl 4):1191–5.
40. Raleigh VS. Diabetes and hypertension in Britain's ethnic minorities: implications for the future of renal services. BMJ 1997;314:209–13.
41. Schmitz A, Vaeth M. Microalbuminuria: a major risk factor in non-insulin-dependent diabetes . A 10-year follow-up study of 503 patients. Diabet Med 1988;5:126–34.
42. Foley RN, Culleton BE, Parfrey PS et al. Cardiac disease in diabetic end-stage renal disease. Diabetologia 1997;40:1307–12.
43. Chaturvedi N, Jarrett J, Shipley MJ, Fuller JH. Socio-economic gradient in morbidity and mortality in people with diabetes: cohort study findings from the Whitehall study and the WHO multinational study of vascular disease in diabetes. BMJ 1998;316:100–106.
44. Kelly WF, Mahmood R, Kelly MJ et al. Infuence of social deprivation on illness in diabetic patients . BMJ 1993;307:1115–16.
45. Koskinen SVP, Martelin TP, Valkonen T. Socio-economic differences in mortality among diabetic people in Finland: five year follow up. BMJ 1996;313:975–8.
46. De Cesare N, Polese A, Cozzi S et al. Coronary angiographic patterns in hypertensive compared to normotensive patients. Am Heart J 1991;121:1101–106.

47. Leonetti G, Cuspidi G. Hypertension and coronary heart disease. In: Kaplan NM, ed. Metabolic Aspects of Hypertension. Science Press 1994: 5.1–5.24.
48. MERCATOR study group. Does the new angiotensin inhibitor cilazipril prevent restenosis after percutaneous transluminal coronary angioplasty? The results of the MERCATOR-study: a multi-center randomized double-blind placebo-controlled trial. Circulation 1992;86:100–10.
49. Schmieder RE, Martus P, Klingbeil A. Reversal of left ventricular hypertrophy: a meta-analysis of randomised double-blind studies. JAMA 1996;275:1507–13.
50. Gottdiener JS, Reda DJ, Massie BM et al. Effect of single drug therapy on reduction of left ventricular mass in mild to moderate hypertension. Circulation 1997;95:2007–14.
51. Dahlof B, Pennert K, Hansson L. Reversal of left ventricular hypertrophy in hypertensive patients. A meta-analysis of 109 treatment studies. Am J Hypertens 1992;5:95–110.
52. Veterans' Administration Cooperative Study Group on Antihypertensive Agents. Effects of treatment on morbidity in hypertension: II. Results in patients with diastolic pressures averaging 90 through 114 mm Hg. JAMA 1970;213:1143–92.
53. Collins R, Peto R, MacMahon S et al. Blood pressure, stroke and coronary heart disease. Part 2. Short term reductions in blood pressure: overview of randomised drug trials in their epidemiological context. Lancet 1990;335:827–38.
54. Medical Research Council Working Party. MRC trial of treatment of mild hypertension: principal results. BMJ 1985;291:97–104.
55. Wikstrand J, Warnold I, Olsson G et al. Primary prevention with metoprolol in patients with hypertension. Mortality results from the MAPHY Study. JAMA 1988;259:1976–82.
56. Amery A, Birkenhager W, Brixxo P et al. Mortality and morbidity results from the European Working Party on High Blood Pressure in the Elderly Trial. Lancet 1985;I:1351–4.
57. Dahlof B, Lindholm LH, Hansson L et al. Morbidity and mortality in the Swedish Trial in Old Patients with Hypertension (STOP-Hypertension). Lancet 1991;338:1281–5.
58. SHEP Cooperative Research Group. Prevention of stroke by antihypertensive drug treatment in older persons with isolated systolic hypertension. Final Results of the Systolic Hypertension in Elderly Program (SHEP). JAMA 1991;265:3255–64.
59. MRC Working Party. Medical Research Council Trial of treatment of hypertension in older adults: principal results. BMJ 1992;304:405–12.
60. Elmfeldt D, Julius S, Menard J et al for the HOT study group. Effects of intensive blood-pressure lowering and low dose aspirin in patients with hypertension: principal results of the Hypertension Optimal Treatment (HOT) randomised trial. Lancet 1998;351:1755–62.

61. Hansson L, Lindholm LH, Niskanen L et al for the Captopril Project (CAPP) study group. Lancet 1999;353:611–16.

62. ALLHAT Collaborative Research Group. Major cardiovascular events in hypertensive patients randomized to doxazosin vs chlorthalidone. The Antihypertensive and Lipid-Lowering Treatment to Prevent Heart Attack Trial (ALLHAT). JAMA 2000;283:1967–75.

63. Hansson L, Hedner T, Lund-Johansen P et al. Randomised trial of effects of calcium antagonists compared with diuretics and β-blockers on cardiovascular morbidity and mortality in hypertension: the Nordic Diltiazem (NORDIL) study. Lancet 2000;356:359–65.

64. Brown MJ, Palmer CR, Castaigne A et al. Morbidity and mortality in patients randomised to double-blind treatment with a long-acting calcium-channel blocker or diuretic in the International Nifedipine GITS study: Intervention as a Goal in Hypertension Treatment (INSIGHT). Lancet 2000;356:366–72.

65. Tuomilehto J, Rastenyte D, Birkenhanger WH et al for the Systolic Hypertension in Europe Trial Investigators (Syst-Eur). Effects of calcium-channel blockade in older patients with diabetes and systolic hypertension. N Engl J Med 1999;340:677–84.

66. Hansson L, Lindholm LH, Ekbom T et al. Randomised trial of old and new antihypertensive drugs in elderly patients: cardiovascular mortality and morbidity in the Swedish Trial in Old Patients with Hypertension-2 study. Lancet 1999;354:1751–6.

67. Gong L, Zhang W, Zhu Y et al. Shanghai trial of nifedipine in the elderly (STONE). J Hypertens 1996;14:1237–45.

68. The HOPE Study Investigators. The HOPE (Heart Outcomes Prevention Evaluation) Study: The design of a large simple randomised trial of an angiotensin-converting enzyme inhibitor (ramipril) and vitamin E in patients at high risk of cardiovascular events. Can J Cardiol 1996;12:127–37.

69. The Heart Outcomes Prevention Evaluation Study Investigators. Effect of an angiotensin-converting-enzyme inhibitior, ramipril, on cardiovascular events in high risk patients. N Engl J Med 2000;342:145–53.

70. UK Prospective Diabetes Study Group. Tight blood pressure control and risk of macrovascular and microvascular complications in Type 2 diabetes: UKPDS 38. BMJ 1998;317:705–13.

71. Ravid M, Savin H, Jutrin I et al. Long-term stabilising effect of angiotensin-converting enzyme inhibition on plasma creatinine and proteinuria in normotensive Type 2 diabetic patients. Ann Intern Med 1993;118:577–81.

72. The Microalbuminuria Captopril Study Group. Captopril reduces the risk of nephropathy in IDDM patients with microalbuminuria. Diabetologia 1996;39:587–93.

73. Lewis EJ, Hunsicker LG, Bain RP, Rohde RD. The effect of angiotensin-converting-enzyme inhibition on diabetic nephropathy. N Engl J Med 1993;329:1456–62.

74. Tatti P, Guarisco R, Pahor M et al. Outcome results of the Fosinopril versus Amlodipine cardiovascular events randomized trial (FACET) in patients with hypertension and NIDDM. Diabetes Care 1998;21:597–603.

75. Estacio RO, Jeffers BW, Hiatt WR et al. The effect of Nisoldipine as compared with Enalapril on cardiovascular outcomes in patients with non-insulin-dependent diabetes and hypertension. N Engl J Med 1998;338:645–52.

76. Borhani NO, Mercuri M, Borhani PA et al. Final outcome results of the multicenter Isradipine diuretic atherosclerosis study (MIDAS). JAMA 1996;276:785–91.

77. Byington RP, Craven TE, Furberg CD, Pahor M. Isradipine, raised glyco- sylated haemoglobin, and risk of cardiovascular events. Lancet 1997;350:1075–6.

78. UK Prospective Diabetes Study Group. Efficacy of atenolol and capto- pril in reducing risk of macrovascular and microvascular complications in Type 2 diabetes: UKPDS 39. BMJ 1998;317:713–20.

79. HOPE study investigators. Effects of ramipril on cardiovascular and microvascular outcomes in people with diabetes mellitus: results of the HOPE study and the MICRO-HOPE study. Lancet 2000;355:253–9.

80. Ramsay LE, Williams B, Johnson GD et al. Guidelines for management of hypertension: report of the third working party of the British Hyper- tension Society. J Human Hypertens 1999;13:569–92.

81. The Joint National Committee on prevention, detection, evaluation and treatment of high blood pressure. The sixth report of the Joint National Committee on prevention, detection, evaluation and treatment of high blood pressure. Arch Intern Med 1997;157:2413–46.

82. Krans HMJ, Porta M, Keen H, Staehr Johansen K eds. Diabetes care and research in Europe: The St Vincent Declaration Action Programme. Implementation document, 2nd edn. Guidelines on cardiovascular disease and stroke. 1995.

83. ADA Consensus panel. treatment of hypertension in diabetes. Diabetes Care 1993;16:1394–401.

84. Colhoun HM, Dong W, Barakat MT et al. The scope for cardiovascular disease risk factor intervention among people with diabetes mellitus in England: a population-based analysis from the Health Surveys for England 1991–1994. Diabet Med 1999;16:35–40.

85. Smith WCS, Lee AJ, Crombie IK, Tunstall-Pedoe H. Control of blood pressure in Scotland: the rule of halves. BMJ 1990;300:981–3.

86. Giordano M, Matsuda M, Sanders L et al. Effects of angiotensin-convert- ing enzyme inhibitors, Ca^{2+} channel antagonists, and α-adrenergic block- ers on glucose and lipid metabolism in NIDDM patients with hypertension. Diabetes 1995;44:665–71.

87. Zemel P. Sexual dysfunction in the diabetic patient with hypertension. Am J Cardiol 1988;61:27H–33H.

88. Donnan PT, MacDonald TM, Morris AD, for the DARTS/MEMO Collaboration. Adherence to prescribed oral hypoglycaemic medication in a population of patients with type 2 diabetes: a retrospectve cohort study. Diabetic Med 2002;19:279–84.

89. Keavney BD, Dudley CRK, Stratton IM et al. UK Prospective Diabetes Study (UKPDS) 14: association of angiotensin-converting enzyme insertion/deletion polymorphism with myocardial infarction in NIDDM. Diabetologia 1995;38:948–52.

90. UK Prospective Diabetes Study Group. Cost effectiveness analysis of improved blood pressure control in hypertensive patients with Type 2 diabetes: UKPDS 40. BMJ 1998;317:720–6.

91. Golan L, Birkmeyer JD, Welch HG. The cost-effectiveness of treating all patients with angiotensin-converting enzyme inhibitors. Ann Intern Med 1999;131:660–7.

chapter 6

Lipids and diabetes

John Hinnie

Introduction

The contribution of lipids to cardiovascular disease and the possible therapeutic options to counteract their effect have been the subject of much research interest in recent years, and will no doubt continue to be so for some time to come. To date many of the available data on this topic have been obtained from non-diabetic patients. Although current knowledge can be extrapolated to diabetic patients, there is very little data available for diabetic subjects specifically.

It is widely accepted that diabetes mellitus can be accompanied by an unfavourable plasma lipid profile and that this is a major risk factor for cardiovascular disease, contributing to the 2–6-fold increase in risk of myocardial infarction seen in people with diabetes compared to the general population.[1-3] This may be because of the association of diabetic dyslipidaemia with the insulin resistance syndrome, which itself contributes to cardiovascular risk (see Chapter 1), or because this type of dyslipidaemia is in itself atherogenic.

In the future, further research data will become available for both diabetic and non diabetic patients, and indeed there are several large multi-centre studies ongoing which contain large numbers of subjects with diabetes. This chapter presents what is currently known about lipid abnormalities in diabetes in relation to cardiovascular disease, as well as possible treatment options. It has been written in a way that will allow the reader to integrate any future advances in knowledge into their clinical practice with ease.

The plasma lipids

Cholesterol (some of which is bound to fatty acid to form cholesterol esters), triglyceride and phospholipid are the lipids present in plasma. They are not very soluble in water and are not therefore found free in the plasma. In order that they may be transported through plasma, they bind with various more water soluble proteins to form lipoproteins (these can be thought of as detergents, which make lipids more soluble in plasma). It is therefore more correct to refer to them as plasma lipoproteins rather than plasma lipids, and the terms are often used interchangeably. The plasma lipoproteins may be divided into four classes, each containing different amounts of the various types of lipids along with proteins. The four classes have different physical and chemical properties and they can therefore be separated in the laboratory and quantified. The most widely used separation technique is centrifugation, where the lipoproteins are separated

Table 6.1 Terms used for the plasma lipoproteins

Term	Centrifugation density	Electrophoresis position
Chylomicrons	< 0.95	Origin of electrophoresis strip
VLDL or pre-beta-lipoprotein	0.95–1.006	Pre-beta region
LDL or beta-lipoprotein	1.006–1.063	Beta region
HDL or alpha-lipoprotein	1.063–1.210	Alpha region

according to their density. This gives rise to familiar terms such as high and low density lipoprotein (HDL and LDL). They can also be separated according to their electrical charge by electrophoresis. This gives rise to terms such as alpha- and beta-lipoprotein. Alpha and beta simply refer to the band on the electrophoresis strip where the lipoproteins are present. Alpha is band 1 and beta band 2, etc. Lipoprotein classifications based on separation by these techniques are fortunately more or less interchangeable (Table 6.1).

Chylomicrons

These are the least dense of the lipoproteins. They comprise mainly triglyceride (> 90%) derived from dietary fat, while cholesterol content is low. Chylomicrons can be separated in the centrifuge at densities < 0.95 and remain at the origin on electrophoresis. They appear in plasma following the ingestion of a fat, reaching the bloodstream via the thoracic duct.

Very low density lipoprotein or pre-beta-lipoprotein

The main triglyceride-containing lipoprotein in plasma in the fasting state, very low density lipoprotein (VLDL), comprises about 60% triclyceride and 15% cholesterol. VLDL can be separated on the centrifuge at densities between 0.95 and 1.006 and is also known as pre-beta-lipoprotein because of its electrophoretic behaviour.

Low density lipoprotein or beta-lipoprotein

Whereas the chief lipid component of chylomicrons and VLDL is triglyceride, cholesterol is the main lipid of LDL. About 45% of LDL is cholesterol, while the triglyceride content is low (10%). LDL can be separated on the centrifuge at densities between 1.006 and 1.063 and is also known as beta-lipoprotein because of its electrophoretic behaviour.

High density lipoprotein or alpha-lipoprotein

Unlike the other lipoproteins which comprise mainly lipid, HDL consists of a roughly equal proportion of protein and lipid. The chief lipid is not triglyceride or cholesterol but phospholipid. Only about

20% of HDL is cholesterol, while the triglyceride content is less than 5%. HDL can be separated on the centrifuge at densities between 1.063 and 1.210 and is also known as alpha-lipoprotein because of its electrophoretic behaviour.

Lipids and cardiovascular risk

It has been shown in numerous studies (many of which are discussed in this chapter) that it is not simply total cholesterol levels which determine the proportion of cardiovascular risk attributable to plasma lipids. High levels of low density lipoprotein cholesterol (LDL-C) increase the risk of cardiovascular events, while low levels of high density lipoprotein cholesterol (HDL-C) have a similar effect, especially in the presence of high triglyceride levels. The two common classes of drugs used to treat hyperlipidaemia (the statins and the fibrates), not surprisingly, tend to increase HDL-C and lower LDL-C and triglyceride levels.

Lipid abnormalities in diabetes

The dyslipidaemias seen in type 1 and type 2 diabetes tend to differ, although they both contribute to the increased cardiovascular risk seen in people with diabetes. It is convenient to talk of these dyslipidaemias as if they are two distinct entities, but in clinical practice this is not the case and a spectrum of lipid abnormalities is seen in diabetic patients. Why should this be so? When the disorders of plasma lipoprotein metabolism in diabetes are classified according to whether the patient has type 1 or type 2 diabetes it is essential to remember that an attempt is being made to classify the nature of the lipoproteins in the plasma on the basis of one element (i.e. type 1 or type 2 diabetes) which can contribute to deranged lipoprotein metabolism. Diet, exercise, obesity, alcohol consumption and inherited abnormalities of lipid metabolism will all also determine the exact plasma lipid profile seen in a specific individual.

Type 1 diabetes

The typical dyslipidaemia seen in type 1 diabetics differs from that seen in type 2. In type 1 diabetes there is more likely to be elevation of total cholesterol with a rise in LDL-C, decreased HDL-C and increased triglyceride (in the form of increased VLDL and chylomicrons). The relative decrease in HDL-C in type 1 diabetes is less marked than in type 2 diabetes. The main determinants of hyperlipidaemia in type 1 diabetes are poor glycaemic control along with age, obesity and nephropathy.

Type 2 diabetes
Lipid abnormalities occur more commonly in type 2 diabetes than they do in type 1, and can be found even in patients with type 2 who have reasonable glycaemic control. The characteristic pattern of lipids seen in type 2 diabetes differs from that found in type 1 diabetes and is often referred to as 'diabetic dyslipidaemia'. This comprises elevated serum triglyceride (mainly in the form of VLDL), decreased HDL-C with a less marked rise in total and LDL-C concentrations than is seen in type 1 diabetes. Although total LDL-C is relatively normal, the distribution of LDL subfractions is altered so that small dense LDL particles predominate. Such dyslipidaemia is also present in patients with impaired glucose tolerance as opposed to frank diabetes and is accepted as one of the components of the insulin resistance syndrome sometimes called syndrome X or alternatively Reaven's syndrome.[4] This consists of central (truncal) obesity, hypertension, insulin resistance, diabetic dyslipidaemia and premature atherosclerosis (see Chapter 1).

Evidence for benefit from intervention

In the following discussion the generally accepted principles of what constitutes a significant result are adhered to. Therefore percentages quoted for differences between treatment and control groups are all statistically significant (i.e. $p = 0.05$ or less) unless otherwise designated not significant (ns).

There is no evidence from large randomized, double-blind, placebo-controlled trials conducted solely on people with diabetes to shows reduction in morbidity and mortality in people with diabetes successfully treated with lipid modifying agentst. However, a few large scale trials of lipid lowering have included some patients with type 2 diabetes and data from these trials will be discussed later.

First let us consider the evidence that lipid lowering is worthwhile in the general population. Compelling evidence that cholesterol lowering is beneficial in the prevention of coronary heart disease is available from several large randomized controlled trials. These studies did not look at people with diabetes alone but rather at a more general population. It would seem reasonable, however, to extrapolate these results to the diabetic population. It is useful to consider these trials under the headings of primary and secondary prevention, i.e. where the population studied either does (secondary prevention) or does not (primary prevention) have pre-existing coronary heart disease. However, it is worth bearing in mind that many people with diabetes have silent myocardial ischaemia, so that the distinction between primary and secondary prevention in diabetic subjects may be somewhat artificial.

Primary prevention studies (Table 6.2)

A recent meta-analysis of four such primary prevention trials showed that drug treatment reduced the odds of coronary heart disease events by 30% and of coronary heart disease mortality by 29%.[5] The four trials concerned used:

- colestyramine for 7 years (the LRC or Lipid Research Clinic trial[6])
- gemfibrozil for 5 years (the HHS or Helsinki Heart Study[7])
- pravastatin for 5 years (WOSCOPS or West of Scotland Coronary Prevention Study[8])
- lovastatin for 5 years (AFCAPS/TexCAPS or Air Force/Texas Coronary Prevention Study[9]).

Further details of these trials are shown in Table 6.2. Looking at these four studies individually, the respective reductions in coronary heart disease events and coronary heart disease mortality were as follows: LRC, 19% (ns) and 22% (ns); HHS, 35% and 27% (ns), WOSCOPS, 32% and 32%; AFCAPS/TexCAPS, 42% and 32% (ns).

Table 6.2 Details of primary prevention trials of lipid lowering

Trial	LRC	HHS	WOSCOPS	AFCAPS/TexCAPS
Total no. of patients	3806	4081	6595	6605
Percentage of females	0	0	0	15
Average initial cholesterol (mmol/l)	7.5	7.4	7.0	5.7
Drug regime	24 g/day	600 mg twice/day	40 mg/day	20–40 mg/day
Average fall in cholesterol (%)	8.5	10	20	18

Secondary prevention studies (Table 6.3)

Large randomized, controlled secondary prevention studies also provide conclusive evidence that lipid lowering is worthwhile. In the Scandinavian Simvastatin Survival Study (4S), patients with a myocardial infarction in the previous 6 months or angina with a positive exercise ECG were treated for 5.4 years with simvastatin.[10] Combined coronary heart disease (CHD) morbidity and mortality fell by 33%, while there was a 42% decrease in CHD deaths. Similarly there was a 37% reduction in the need for coronary artery surgery or angioplasty. A second trial, using pravastatin for 5 years in patients with a myocardial infarction diagnosed 3 to 20 months previously (the Cholesterol And Recurrent Events or CARE trial[11]), showed a 24% fall in CHD events while CHD mortality fell by 20%. The need for coronary artery surgery or angioplasty was reduced by 27%. The Long

Table 6.3 Details of secondary prevention trials of lipid lowering

Trial	4S	CARE	LIPID	VA-HIT
Total no. of patients	4444	4159	9014	2531
Percentage of females	18	14	17	0
Initial cholesterol (mmol/l)	5.5–8.0[a]	5.4[b]	5.6[c]	HDL-C ≤ 1.0[d] LDL-C ≤ 3.6
Drug regime	20 mg/day[a]	40 mg/day	40 mg/day	600 mg twice/day
Average fall in cholesterol	3.0–5.2%[a]	20%	18%	4%[d] (triglycerides fell by 31%)

[a]In 4S, initial total cholesterol levels were in the range 5.5–8.0 mmol/l. The initial dose of simvastatin was 20 mg/day, and the aim was to decrease total cholesterol to between 3.0 and 5.2 mmol/l. In two patients the dose was reduced to 10 mg/day while in 37% it was increased to 40 mg/day.
[b]In CARE, the average initial total cholesterol was 5.4 mmol/l.
[c]In LIPID, the median total cholesterol was 5.6 mmol/l.
[d]In VA-HIT entry criteria for lipids were HDL-C ≤ 1.0 and LDL-C ≤ 3.6. Total cholesterol fell by 4% and triglycerides by 31% in the treatment group.

term Intervention with Pravastatin in Ischaemic Disease (LIPID) study looked at patients with a myocardial infarction or unstable angina 3 to 36 months previously and followed them for 6.1 years.[12] In this study total CHD morbidity and mortality decreased by 24%, while there was also a 24% decrease in CHD deaths. Similarly there was a 20% reduction in the need for coronary artery surgery or angioplasty. One interesting finding from the LIPID trial was a 19% fall in the predefined endpoint of stroke.

In the Veterens' Affairs Cooperative Study Programme High Density Cholesterol Intervention Trial (VA-HIT)[13] patients with coronary heart disease were treated for 5.1 years with gemfibrozil, resulting in a 23% fall in non-total myocardial infarction and a 22% fall in coronary heart disease deaths (ns).

Statins in people with diabetes

Although there have been no trials of lipid lowering therapy in diabetic patients published to date, subgroup analyses on diabetic patients are available from the WOSCOPS primary prevention study and the 4S, CARE and LIPID secondary prevention studies.

In WOSCOPS,[8] pravastatin reduced both CHD morbidity and mortality by 32% in the whole study population. Approximately 1% of the 6595 participants in this trial had diabetes and subgroup analysis on them showed a similar reduction in CHD morbidity and mortality.

There were 202 diabetic patients in 4S.[14] Simvastatin reduced coronary heart disease incidence by 55% over 5 years in these diabetic subjects, suggesting at least as great a benefit as in the non-diabetic participants. In CARE there were 586 patients with diabetes[11] and their CHD incidence declined by 25% with pravastatin, again suggesting that patients with diabetes gained as much benefit as non-diabetics. Only 164 patients with diabetes took part in LIPID,[12] and although CHD incidence fell by 19%, the result did not reach levels of significance.

Although the number of people with diabetes in these trials was small, it seems that the effect of statin treatment is similar among people with and without diabetes. Indeed, since cardiovascular risk is greater in patients with diabetes than in the general population, the effect of statin treatment represents a larger absolute risk reduction in people with diabetes, compared to the general population.

Fibrates in people with diabetes

The evidence that fibrates reduce cardiovascular events in people with diabetes is less compelling than that available for statins. As with the statins, subgroup analysis of trials in the general population does suggest that fibrates are beneficial. In the Veterans Affairs High Density Lipoprotein Cholesterol Intervention Trial (VA-HIT, a randomized, controlled secondary prevention trial), a 25% reduction in the risk of vascular events was seen in diabetic patients treated with gemfibrozil for 5.1 years.[13] This result compared favourably with the 22% reduction in vascular events seen in the trial as a whole.

The recently published Diabetes Atherosclerosis Intervention Study (DAIS) showed that treatment with micronized fenofibrate (200 mg/day) for at least 3 years reduced progression of coronary artery stenosis in type 2 diabetics (27% were women) who had at least one visible coronary lesion on angiography.[15] Not all of the patients had clinical coronary heart disease so that DAIS could be said to have looked at both primary and secondary prevention. The increase in percentage diameter stenosis was 2.11% versus 3.65%, and the decrease in minimum lumen diameter was 0.06 mm versus 0.10 mm in treatment and control groups respectively, showing that treatment with fenofibrate had a significant effect on the progression of coronary artery stenosis. DAIS was not designed to look at clinical endpoints, but there was a 24% (ns) reduction in the total number of deaths, myocardial infarction, angioplasty and coronary bypass in the intervention group.

Should we treat dyslipidaemia in people with diabetes?

It has to be conceded that there is a relative lack of evidence that treating lipid abnormalities in people with diabetics per se is worthwhile. However, as we have seen, there is irrefutable evidence from large randomized controlled trials that shows treatment of non-diabetic patients with statins or fibrates reduces the relative risk of cardiovascular events. Bearing in mind that subgroup analysis of diabetic subjects in these large trials suggests that they enjoy similar benefits from treatment, it would seem reasonable to extrapolate these results to the diabetic population.

Assessment of lipid abnormalities in people with diabetes

When considering cardiovascular disease prevention in diabetes, lipids are not the only risk factor to be considered. The risk of cardiovascular disease is also influenced by factors such as age, sex, obesity, smoking, blood pressure and glycaemic control (see Chapter 2). It should also be remembered that good glycaemic control will decrease serum cholesterol and triglyceride, as well as decreasing overall risk independently of any effect on lipids. The United Kingdom Prospective Diabetes Study (UKPDS) provides evidence that control of blood glucose and blood pressure reduces cardiovascular risk. This study, which looked at type 2 diabetics, but the diabetes control and complications trial suggested that tight glucose control also reduces cardiovascular risk in type 1 diabetic subjects.[18] Lipid levels cannot be considered in isolation therefore and an assessment of the patient's overall cardiovascular risk should be made, especially if hypolipidaemic agents are being considered.

At the first consultation, diabetic patients should be fully assessed to exclude secondary causes of hyperlipidaemia (see Table 6.4) and to establish the patient's overall cardiovascular risk profile. It is particularly important to identify excessive alcohol intake, cigarette smoking, obesity, sedentary lifestyle, hypertension and pre-existing myocardial ischaemia. An underlying primary hyperlipidaemia may

Table 6.4 Secondary causes of hyperlipidaemia (excluding diabetes mellitus)

Hypothyroidism
Excessive alcohol intake
Chronic renal failure
Nephrotic syndrome
Obstructive liver disease

also be present in addition to the abnormalities secondary to diabetes, so that severe hyperlipidaemia in diabetic patients can be due to an underlying primary disorder exacerbated by poor glycaemic control.

Plasma lipid samples should be taken after a 12 hour overnight fast. Cholesterol levels are unaffected by fasting, but triglyceride levels rise after a meal mainly due to an increase in chylomicrons. If the samples show hyperlipidaemia, a second fasting sample should be taken about 2 weeks later to confirm the diagnosis. If the two consecutive samples show persistent abnormalities, intervention should be considered.

It should be remembered that in patients with acute myocardial infarction, serum cholesterol will fall soon after the onset of pain. This effect generally lasts for 6 weeks at most if no complications ensue from the infarction. However, it is still worthwhile measuring lipids in the first 24 hours following an infarct since the finding of a raised cholesterol may give the patient some impetus for risk factor modification in the early stages following the acute event. It is imperative, however, that lipids are measured at 6 weeks or so.

Total cholesterol, HDL-C and triglyceride should be measured, along with LDL-C where available. If direct measurement of LDL-C is not available, it can be calculated from the Freidwald equation[19]:

$$LDL\text{-}C = \text{total cholesterol} - \left[HDL\text{-}C + \frac{\text{total triglyceride}}{2.2}\right]$$

where all concentrations are in mmol/l. Note, however, that this equation does not give an accurate estimate of LDL-C when (as can be the case in poorly controlled diabetic patients) triglyceride levels are greater than 4.5 mmol/l. The fasting triglyceride level should be established before initiating drug therapy, as abnormalities can influence which hypolipidaemic drug is chosen. For example, resins may cause a rise in plasma triglyceride levels.

Estimation of cardiovascular risk

The estimation of an individual's cardiovascular risk simply by clinical judgement is not adequate. Estimating risk can be carried out more satisfactorily with a thorough consultation and the measurement of relevant parameters. Once this has been achieved then the information obtained can be used in one of the available models for the calculation of the individual's overall cardiovascular risk. Many such models exist, some more sophisticated than others, some even requiring a computer to carry out the calculations. However, from a practical point of view the Coronary Risk Prediction Chart produced as part of the Joint British Recommendations on Prevention of Coronary Heart Disease in Clinical Practice[20] is adequate. These charts are now widely available, having been recently incorporated into the British National Formulary. The information required is the patient's age, sex, smoking habit, systolic blood pressure, serum total cholesterol to HDL-C ratio and whether the patient has diabetes.

From the coronary risk chart, the individual's risk of a non-fatal myocardial infarction or coronary death over the next 10 years can be obtained. Although the charts compute risk using decade of life rather than an individual's age in years, a more precise estimate of risk is possible. For example, bearing in mind that risk increases exponentially with age, in the 5th decade risk will be closer to that of a 50 year old in the first 6 years of the decade (i.e. 50 to 55 years), but closer to that of a 60 year old in the last 4 years of the decade (i.e. 56 to 59 years). One important risk factor not employed in the calculation is a positive family history of premature coronary heart disease. By this is meant under 55 years in men and under 65 years in women in a first degree relative. Such a finding would increase an individual's risk by a factor of 1.5.

Blood pressure and lipids should be measured on more than one occasion to give a more accurate estimate of their true value. Annual diabetic hospital review is insufficient for the frequent monitoring necessary for introducing lipid lowering or antihypertensive medication. Therefore, agreed management protocols between hospital and general practice, which include hypertension and hyperlipidaemia, are required (see Chapter 10). While there are separate charts for diabetic and non-diabetic patients, one weakness in the calculation of risk using these charts is that the dyslipidaemias seen in type 1 and type 2 diabetic patients differ. In type 1 diabetes HDL-C tends to be relatively high and does not have the protective effect that it appears to have in non-diabetics. This point is conceded in the Joint British Recommendations, and they suggest that the total cholesterol in mmol/l is used rather than the total cholesterol/HDL-C ratio to compute the risk in a person with type 1 diabetes. It should be borne in mind that risk will be underestimated by using blood pressure and lipid values recorded after the commencement of treatment (including dietary intervention). This is because long term levels of these values are more relevant than those obtained following treatment. Similarly, an individual who has only recently given up cigarettes should not be classified as a non-smoker. One final point to bear in mind is that the charts cannot be used to predict risk for patients who already have pre-existing cardiovascular disease, familial hypercholesterolaemia or significant renal dysfunction. Patients with pre-existing cardiovascular disease should be considered under the heading of secondary prevention, and we will return to this later.

When to introduce lipid lowering drugs

At what level of risk is the introduction of hypolipidaemic drugs justified for primary prevention in diabetics? The Joint British Recommendations on Prevention of Coronary Heart Disease in Clinical Practice[20] suggest that evidence from clinical trials shows that all individuals with a calculated risk of 15% or more will benefit from lipid lowering. They also concede that the effort involved in identifying these individuals and the cost of treating them is probably prohibitive. However, diabetic patients should be considered separately in this context. They are at increased risk compared to non-diabetic subjects and no extra effort is required to identify them. If we accept that it is possible to apply the evidence from primary and secondary prevention trials to diabetic patients (as we have seen subgroup analysis would suggest this is a reasonable thing to do) then those with a risk of 15% or more for non-fatal myocardial infarction or coronary death in the next 10 years should be treated.

The decision to use hypolipidaemic agents in patients with diabetes for secondary prevention (i.e. in patients with established coronary heart disease) is more straightforward. Consideration of the data available from trials of secondary prevention has led the Joint British Recommendations on Prevention of Coronary Heart Disease in Clinical Practice[20] to suggest commencing a statin if serum cholesterol exceeds 5.0 mmol/l and triglycerides are less than 5.0 mmol/l despite diet.

Since, as we have seen, there are no CHD prevention trials of lipid lowering therapy in diabetic patients alone, the most appropriate lipid lowering drug in this group of patients when hypertriglyceridaemia is present is less certain. Diabetic patients with high triglycerides may well benefit from a fibrate drug, or the combination of a statin and a fibrate, but the situation is unclear at present.

The presence of microalbuminuria is a strong predictor of coronary risk in diabetics and where this is present, then the patient should considered in the category of secondary prevention.[21]

Treatment of hyperlipidaemia in diabetes

As with non-diabetic patients, the initial step in the treatment of hyperlipidaemia in diabetes involves lifestyle modification. Dietary advice should be given as part of the early input that all newly diagnosed diabetics should receive from the diabetes care team, and should be aimed at improving glycaemic control and optimizing body mass index as well as lowering serum lipid levels. Lifestyle measures, such as stopping smoking and modifying alcohol intake where applicable, as well as regular exercise, should also be instituted (see Chapter 9). These measures (if complied with) often produce an improved lipid profile in type 1 diabetes, but may be insufficient to correct the dyslipidaemia of type 2 diabetes.

If hyperlipidaemia persists after these measures, lipid-lowering drugs should be considered. It is important to stress that lifestyle modifications should be continued while a patient is taking a hypolipidaemic agent. This should be mentioned when the drug is started, and reinforced at subsequent visits. Patients should also be made aware that therapy will probably be lifelong. They should be counselled on possible side-effects, and instructed to return if they experience any problems. They should be told to consult immediately if they have muscle pains or weakness while taking a statin or fibrate, as both these drugs can cause myositis. Women of child-bearing age should be counselled about contraception. Patients should be told to avoid taking other drugs at the same time as a resin, as the resin can reduce their absorption. Other drugs should be taken either 1 hour before or 4 to 6 hours after the resin.

Hypolipidaemic agents

The statins and fibrates are widely prescribed today, even by practitioners who are not experts in the field of lipids. The resins were widely prescribed prior to the advent of the statins and fibrates but have been superceded by these drugs now. Nevertheless, I think it is worthwhile retaining them in the armoury of even the non-expert since they are effective and relatively free of side-effects even though they are more inconvenient to take than the more modern options. They may therefore be of use in the occasional patient where statins and fibrates cannot be used. The more exotic hypolipidaemic agents such as nicotinic acid derivatives, omega-3-marine triglycerides and probucol are best reserved for patients who have not responded to other drugs. In my experience, these patients should be fully assessed at a specialist lipid or cardiovascular risk factor clinic before starting further such medications.

The statins

Statins inhibit the enzyme hydroxymethylglutaryl co-enzyme A (HMG-Co A) reductase, an early step in cholesterol synthesis. They reduce cholesterol synthesis, causing an upregulation of LDL receptor synthesis which in turn promotes cholesterol removal from the blood. The statins have a potent effect on cholesterol levels, and can lower total cholesterol by up to 30%. LDL-C falls by up to 40%, while HDL-C rises by up to 10%. In addition, they can lower triglycerides by up to 15% at higher doses.

The fibrates

The fibrate group of drugs works partly by stimulating the enzyme lipoprotein lipase which breaks down triglyceride-rich lipoprotein. These drugs reduce both total cholesterol (by up to 25%) and triglyceride (by up to 50%), while elevating HDL-C by up to 30% and lowering LDL-C by 25% to 30%.

The resins

These drugs work by binding bile acids in the gut and preventing their reabsorption. This causes an increase in the synthesis of bile acids from cholesterol in the liver and consequently a fall in plasma cholesterol. Resins lower both total cholesterol (by up to 20%) and LDL-C (by up to 30%). They can cause triglycerides and HDL-C to rise by up to 5%. They may still be useful when statins or fibrates cannot be used.

Pregnancy and lactation

The safety of hypolipidaemic agents has not been fully assessed in pregnant or lactating females. Consequently their use is not recommended, although the resins are not absorbed from the gut and therefore are probably safe. Women of child-bearing age should be advised to use a reliable form of contraception while taking hypolipidaemic agents. In those taking a resin, folate levels should be checked and supplements given if necessary. It is recommended that statins and fibrates are stopped 1 month prior to a planned conception. Although probucol should only be prescribed in the setting of a specialist clinic, it is worth pointing out that it persists in adipose tissue for some time and should therefore be stopped 6 months before a planned conception.

Prescribing statins

Atorvostatin (Lipotor, 10 mg, 20 mg or 40 mg tablets) should be taken once daily. It is best to start with 10 mg and increase at monthly intervals according to the response. The maximum daily dose is 80 mg.

Fluvastatin (Lescol, 2 mg or 40 mg capsules) should be taken once daily. It is best to start with 20 mg and increase to 40 mg after one month according to the response. The maximum daily dose is 80 mg.

Pravastatin (Lipostat, 10 mg, 20 mg or 40 mg tablets) should be taken once daily. It is best to start with 10 mg and increase the dose at monthly intervals, according to the response. The maximum daily dose is 40 mg.

Simvastatin (Zocor, 10 mg, 20 mg, 40 mg or 80 mg tablets) should be taken once daily. It is best to start with 10 mg and increase at monthly intervals according to the response. The maximum daily dose is 80 mg. A maximum of 10 mg daily should be given when a fibrate, nicotinic acid or cyclosporin are also being prescribed.

Prescribing fibrates

There is little to choose between the various fibrates. It is probably best to stick with one or two fibrates, and gain experience with them. The once daily preparations of bezafibrate (Bezalip-Mono), ciprofibrate (Modalim), fenofibrate (Lipantil Micro 200 and Lipantil Micro 267) have obvious advantages.

Bezafibrate (non-proprietary bezafibrate (200 mg tablets), Bezalip (200 mg tablets), Bezalip-Mono (400 mg tablets)). Bezalip-Mono is taken once daily, while non proprietary bezafibrate or Bezalip should be taken as a single tablet three times daily, after meals.

Ciprofibrate (Modalim, 100 mg tablet) should be taken as a single 100 mg daily dose after a meal—the evening is usually most convenient.

Fenofibrate (Lipantil Micro, 67 mg, 200 mg or 267 mg capsules of 'micronized' fenofibrate, Supralip 160). Lipantil micro can be taken as one 67 mg capsule three times daily or one 200 mg capsule once daily. In resistant cases the dose can be increased to one 267 mg capsule daily.

Gemfibrozil (non-proprietary gemfibrozil, Lopid. Both come as 300 mg capsules or 600 mg tablets) This should be taken in two divided doses. The recommended dose is 0.9–1.5 g per day divided into two doses. The dose of Supralip 160 is one tablet daily.

Prescribing resins

Colestyramine (non-proprietary colestyramine, Questran, Questran light. All come in powder form and are supplied in 4 g sachets). It is best to start with two sachets per day. The dose can be increased, at monthly intervals, up to nine sachets a day in divided doses. Although a maximum of nine sachets can be given, few patients can tolerate this amount. These preparations should not be taken as a powder, but can be mixed with water, fruit juice, etc.

Colestipol (Colestid granules, Colestid Orange. Both come in granule form and are supplied in 5 g sachets). It is best to start with one to two sachets per day in divided doses. This can be increased at monthly intervals to a maximum of six sachets a day in a single or divided doses. As with colestyramine, colestipol should not be taken in its dry form.

Drug interactions

Statins
Co-administration of a statin and a fibrate may predispose to myositis. This important interaction was part of the reason for the withdrawal of cerivastatin from the market, as several severe cases of myositis were seen when this drug was co-prescribed with gemfibrozil. In normal volunteers, simvastatin has a mild potentiating effect on warfarin and digoxin levels and doses may need to be adjusted accordingly.

Fibrates

Fibrates potentiate the effect of oral anticoagulants, so it is often necessary to adjust warfarin doses. They also improve glucose utilization, which can potentiate antidiabetic medication—insulin and oral hypoglycaemic doses may need to be adjusted.

Co-administration of fibrates with monamine oxidase inhibitors with hepatotoxic potential is not recommended. The hypolipidaemic properties of fibrates are reduced by oestrogen-containing drugs. Co-administration of a fibrate and a statin may predispose to myositis-type problems and should be used with caution.

Resins

Resins can reduce or delay the absorption of some drugs. It is important to monitor concomitant medications, such as digoxin, propranolol, thyroxine, warfarin and tetracycline, and adjust the dose where necessary. A resin should be taken at least 1 hour before or 4–6 hours after other drugs.

Adverse effects

Statins

Minor rises in transaminases can occur soon after starting a statin, but do not require withdrawal of therapy in my experience. However, the statin should be discontinued if the transaminases rise to more than three times the upper limit of normal.

Transient minor rises in creatine kinase can be seen in patients on a statin, but do not merit withdrawal of the drug. However a few (< 0.1%) patients will develop a myopathy, with marked rise in creatine kinase. If this occurs the statin should be discontinued immediately.

The incidence of myopathy is increased by concomitant use of cyclosporin, fibrate or nicotinic acid. Liver function tests and creatine kinase should be checked after 1 month, 3 months and then at 6-monthly intervals. As mentioned above, major problems with myotoxicity were encountered with cerivastatin when it was combined with gemfibrozil.

Fibrates

Anorexia, nausea and abdominal discomfort are the most common side-effects of fibrates, but are usually only transient. Headache, urticaria, pruritus and impotence are less common side-effects. A myositis-like syndrome, with or without a rise in creatine kinase has very rarely been reported. Clofibrate, one of the earliest fibrates which is no longer used, was associated with an increased incidence of gallstones, and this should be borne in mind when prescribing a fibrate.

Haematological abnormalities, including a fall in haemoglobin, leukocytes or platelets, have been seen with fibrate therapy, but are an extremely rare occurrence. A rise in transaminases is also rare. Full blood count, liver function tests and creatine kinase should be checked after 1 month, 3 months and then at 6-monthly intervals.

Rhabdomyolysis has occurred in patients with renal disease. Fibrates should therefore be used at reduced dose in mild renal impairment, but should not be used in severe renal disease.

Resins

Resins have gastrointestinal side-effects, including nausea, vomiting, heartburn, abdominal discomfort, constipation, diarrhoea and flatulence. Hypoprothrombinaemia (with increased bleeding times) has occurred on prolonged therapy, but is extremely rare. It can be treated with parenteral vitamin K, in the acute phase, followed by oral vitamin K supplements. In the rare event of treating a child with a resin, I would routinely prescribe supplements of fat-soluble vitamins.

Follow-up of hyperlipidaemia in diabetes

Patients starting hypolipidaemic therapy need regular follow-up. They should be questioned about possible side-effects and should be tested for any haematological or biochemical abnormalities. They should also be encouraged to maintain any lifestyle changes.

Response to lipid-lowering drugs is not predictable, so plasma lipid levels should be measured to ensure the response is adequate.

Patients taking a statin, fibrate or resin should have their lipid levels checked at monthly intervals and the dose and/or drug should be adjusted until an adequate response is obtained.

Subsequently, lipid levels should then be checked every 6–12 months. If one fibrate is ineffective then another should be tried. The response to statins is more predictable and most patients respond. Failure to respond to a resin indicates poor compliance which is relatively common with these drugs.

Conclusions

Dyslipidaemia is common in people with diabetes, and contributes to the risk of cardiovascular disease. The evidence for a reduction in cardiovascular risk with lipid lowering in people with diabetes is based on small numbers of subjects. Some evidence is available from Primary[8] and secondary prevention[11,12,14] studies to show a benefit with statin treatment in diabetic patients. There is also some evidence that fibrates reduce cardiovascular risk in the context of secondary prevention in people with diabetes.[13]. The recently completed Heart Protection Study[22] contained a large number of patients with diabetes in both primary and secondary prevention categories (simvastatin) benefit from statin therapy. Detailed analysis of this and other studies are ongoing. Results presented to date suggest that both categories will help clarify the role of lipid-lowering in reducing cardiovascular risk in people with diabetes.

References

1. Stamler J, Dyer AR, Shekelle RB. Relationship of baseline major risk factors to coronary and all-cause mortality, and longevity: findings from long-term follow-up of Chicago cohorts. Cardiology 1993;82:191–222.
2. Abbott RD, Donahue RP, MacMahon SW. Diabetes and the risk of stroke: the Honolulu Heart Project. JAMA 1987;257:949–52.
3. Arnow W, Ahn C. Incidence of heart failure in 2,737 older persons with and without diabetes mellitus. Chest 1999;115:867–8

4. Reaven GM. Insulin resistance and human disease: a short history. J Basic Clin Physiol 1998;9(2–4):387–406.

5. Pigone M, Phillips C, Murlow C. Use of lipid lowering drugs for primary prevention in coronary heart disease: meta-analysis of randomised trials. BMJ 2000;231:983–6.

6. Lipid research clinics coronary primary prevention trial results. II: The relationship of reduction in incidence of coronary heart disease to cholesterol lowering. JAMA 1984;251:365–74.

7. Frick M, Elo O, Haapa K et al. Helsinki heart study: primary prevention trial with gemfibroszil in middle aged men with dyslipidemia. Safety of treatment changes in risk factors, and incidence of coronary heart disease, N Engl J Med 1987;317:1237–45.

8. Shepherd J, Cobbe SM, Ford I et al. Prevention of coronary heart disease with pravastatin in men with hypercholesterolemia: West of Scotland Coronary Prevention Study Group. N Engl J Med 1995;333:1301–7.

9. Downs JR, Clearfield M, Weis S et al. Primary prevention of acute coronary events with lovastatin in men and women with average cholesterol levels: results of AFCAPS/TexCAPS, Air Force/Texas coronary atherosclerosis prevention study. JAMA 1998;79:1615–22.

10. Scandinavian Simvastatin Survival Study Group. Randomised trial of cholesterol lowering in 4444 patients with coronary heart disease: the Scandinavian simvastatin survival study. Lancet 1994;344:1383–9.

11. Sacks FM, Pfeffer MA, Moye LA et al. The effect of pravastatin on coronary events after myocardial infarction in patients with average cholesterol levels. N Engl J Med 1996;335:1001–9.

12. The Long Term Intervention with Pravastatin in Ischaemic Disease (LIPID) Study Group. Prevention of cardiovascular events and death with pravastatin in patients with coronary disease and a broad range of initial cholesterol levels. N Engl J Med 1998;339:1349–57.

13. Rubins HB, Robins SJ, Collins D et al. Gemfibrozil for the secondary prevention of coronary heart disease in men with low levels of high density lipoprotein cholesterol.Veterans Affairs High Density Lipoprotein Cholesterol Intervention Trial Study Group. N Engl J Med 1999;341:410–18.

14. Pyorala K, Pederson TJ, Kjerkshus J et al and the Scandinavian Simvastatin Survival Study (4S) Group. Cholesterol lowering with simvastatin improves prognosis of diabetic patients with coronary heart disease. Diabetes Care 1997;20:614–20.

15. Diabetes Atherosclerosis Intervention Study Investigators. Effect of fenofibrate on progression of coronary-artery disease in type 2 diabetes: Diabetes Atherosclerosis Intervention Study, a randomised study. Lancet 2001;357:905–10.

16. UK Prospective Diabetes Study (UKPDS) Group. Intensive blood glucose control with sulphonylureas or insulin compared with conventional

treatment and risk of complications in patients with type 2 diabetes (UKPDS 33). Lancet 1998;352:837–53.

17. UK Prospective Diabetes Study (UKPDS) Group. Tight blood pressure control and risk of macrovascular and microvascular complications in type 2 diabetes UKPDS 38. BMJ 1998;317:703–13.

18. Diabetes Control and Complications Trial Research Group. Effect of intensive diabetes management on macrovascular event and risk factors in the diabetes control and complications trial (DCCT). Am J Cardiol 1995;75:894–903.

19. Friedwald WT, Levy RI, Fredrickson DS. Estimation of the concentration of low density lipoprotein cholesterol in plasma without the use of the preparative ultracentrifuge. Clin Chem 1972;18:499–502.

20. Joint British Recommendations on Prevention of Coronary Heart Disease in Clinical Practice. British Cardiac Society, British Hyperlipidaemia Association, British Hypertension Society, endorsed by British Diabetic Association. Heart 1998;80(Suppl 2):S1–S29.

21. Durrington PN. Serum high density lipoprotein in diabetes mellitus: an analysis of factors which influence its concentration. Clin Chem Acta 1980;104:11–23.

22. Heart Protection Study Collaborative Group. MRC/BHF Heart Protection Study of cholesterol lowering with simvastartin in 20,536 high risk individuals: a randomised, placebo-controlled trial. Lancet 2002;360:7–22.

chapter 7

Coronary heart disease in patients with diabetes – pharmacological treatment

Geraldine M Brennan and Andrew D Morris

Introduction

Patients with diabetes have a significantly increased absolute risk of developing coronary heart disease (CHD).[1,2] In diabetic individuals who have no preceding history of coronary disease, the risk of developing an acute myocardial infarction is equivalent to that in a non-diabetic individual with a previous event.[3] Following myocardial infarction, diabetic patients are more likely to develop cardiac failure and cardiogenic shock, resulting in a greater short- and long-term mortality.[4] The primary and secondary prevention of CHD in patients with diabetes is therefore a key component of diabetes management. The St Vincent Declaration[5] set a 5-year target to reduce morbidity and mortality from coronary heart disease in diabetes by 'a vigorous programme of risk factor reduction'. Over the past decade, the effectiveness of pharmacological interventions for the treatment of CHD has been addressed by many well-designed randomized controlled trials. However, none of these has focused specifically on individuals with diabetes and, at best, evidence has been limited to subgroup analysis. This chapter will focus on the pharmacological aspects of CHD risk factor management in people with diabetes, based on current evidence, where this is available. It will highlight some of the real and perceived adverse effects of cardiovascular drugs in people with diabetes and the issue of effective uptake of these interventions, particularly of secondary prevention strategies, in the diabetic population. We will therefore discuss:

1. The pharmacological treatment of established coronary vascular disease and risk reduction in high-risk groups of people with diabetes.
2. The risks of oral hypoglycaemic therapy in patients with established coronary vascular disease and the cardiovascular effects of insulin-induced hypoglycaemia.
3. The effects of cardiovascular drugs (beta-blockers and ACE inhibitors) on metabolic control in diabetes.
4. The indication for the use of aspirin in diabetes.
5. The indication for hormone replacement therapy in women with diabetes.
6. The observational data that describes the unmet need of cardio-vascular protection and actual use of cardiovascular drugs in diabetes.

The pharmacological treatment of established coronary vascular disease and risk reduction in high-risk groups of people with diabetes

The use of antihypertensive agents and cholesterol-lowering agents in the primary and secondary prevention of vascular disease in diabetes is described in Chapters 5 and 6 respectively. The therapeutic approach to acute intervention following an acute myocardial infarction or unstable angina pectoris is described in Chapter 4. We therefore discuss (i) the management of stable angina pectoris in people with diabetes, (ii) the secondary prevention of coronary vascular disease with beta blockers and ACE inhibitors and (iii) randomized controlled trials of cardiovascular drugs that have attempted to improve long-term outcome in high-risk individuals with diabetes and established cardiovascular disease.

Symptomatic management of stable angina pectoris in diabetes

In the management of stable angina pectoris, the aim of treatment is to relieve symptoms by reducing myocardial ischaemia and thus the morbidity and mortality associated with the condition. This may be somewhat of a challenge in some patients with diabetes as there may be a lack of classical symptoms due to autonomic dysfunction, resulting in silent ischaemia (see Chapter 3).

The symptomatic treatment of stable angina pectoris involves the use of agents for short-term relief and for longer-term management. For rapid symptom relief, all patients with angina should be prescribed a sublingual nitrate and be instructed how to use it appropriately, including prophylactic use in anticipation of exercise. Long-term anti-anginal management involves use of one or more of the following drug classes: oral nitrates, beta-blockers, calcium channel blockers and the potassium channel opening agent, nicorandil.[6] Calcium channel blockers, long-acting nitrates and nicorandil are all effective as first line anti-anginal agents compared with placebo,[7–10] although there is no convincing evidence that they improve outcome beyond providing symptomatic relief. The use of beta blockers results in more significant symptom relief than the use of other agents as monotherapy and thus they should be used for first line symptomatic treatment, unless otherwise contraindicated.[11,12] All beta blockers are equally effective in preventing angina and ischaemia during exercise. The dose of an indivual drug should be adjusted to reduce the resting heart rate to 55–60 beats/min.[6] In addition, beta-blockade in high-risk patients reduces cardiovascular morbidity and mortality.[13]

There are no convincing data to suggest that management of stable angina pectoris in individuals with diabetes should deviate from this strategy. However, a theoretical argument exists which suggests that the efficacy of nitrate drugs may be compromised in patients with diabetes. This has been postulated to occur due to depletion of intracellular sulphydryl groups, which are essential for the biotransformation of exogenous nitrates within arterial smooth muscle[14] and may give rise to the phenomenon of nitrate tolerance. However, this has not been explored in any clinical trial setting.

The use of agents to modify coronary risk factors has been addressed elsewhere in Chapters 5 and 6, and later in this section in the discussion on the Heart Outcomes Prevention Evaluation (HOPE) and Losartan Intervention for Endpoint Reduction in hypertension (LIFE) studies. Later in the chapter we will also discuss the role of antiplatelet therapy in cardiovascular disease.

Secondary prevention of CHD: role of beta-blockers

Data from several prospective studies indicate that the use of beta-blockers at the time of myocardial infarction reduces mortality in diabetic and non-diabetic individuals (Chapter 4). Thus the ISIS 1 study of intravenous atenolol[15] and the MIAMI study of intravenous metoprolol[16,17] followed by oral therapy for 15 days showed a clear trend towards benefit that was greatest in the diabetic subgroups. Longer term use of beta-blockade is also protective (Fig. 7.1). In a randomized trial of propranolol in 3837 patients (465 with diabetes), started 5–21 days following myocardial infarction, a 28% reduction in mortality was observed in the treatment group, which resulted in the termination of the study after 24 months.[18] There is also evidence that the benefits of beta-blockade may be greater amongst diabetic and other high-risk groups. Kjekshus et al[19] conducted an observational cohort study of 2024 patients, including 340 with diabetes. Mortality at 1 year was significantly less in the non-diabetic compared with the diabetic patients (10% versus 17%), although mortality in diabetic individuals who received beta-blockers was 10% against 23% if these were not used. Beta-blockade was an indepen-

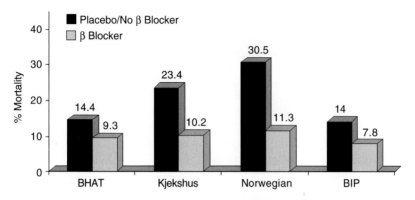

Figure 7.1   The effect of beta-blocker (chronic treatment) in diabetic patients following myocardial infarction.

dent predictor in multivariate analysis of 1-year survival following discharge.

A meta-analysis of nine major long-term secondary prevention trials involving almost 14 000 patients[13] examined whether there are subsets who benefit to a greater or lesser extent from long-term beta-blockade, up to 24 months post myocardial infarction. Overall mortality was 24% lower in those patients who received beta-blockers. The greatest absolute benefit was observed in subgroups with the highest baseline risk, but lower-risk patients also derived benefit.

The Norwegian Timolol Multicentre Study was a double-blind placebo-controlled study designed to evaluate whether long-term treatment with timolol 10 mg BD would reduce mortality and re-infarction in survivors of acute MI.[20] The study recruited 1884 patients, 99 (5.3%) of whom had a diagnosis of diabetes before the onset of myocardial infarction. Treatment with timolol was initiated 7–28 days post MI and was associated with a 39% reduction in total mortality and a 28% reduction in re-infarction after 33 months. A retrospective evaluation of the diabetes subgroup revealed a reduction of 66.6% in cardiac deaths, 56.6% in sudden deaths and 82.7% in re-infarctions, all of which were significant. Mortality in the placebo group was almost 50% greater in the diabetic patients and mortality in timolol group was similar in both diabetic and non-diabetic

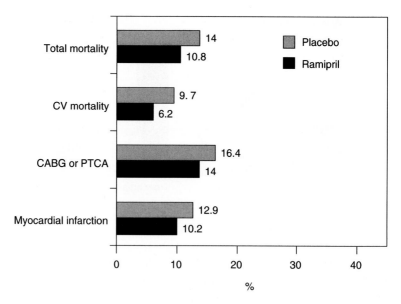

Figure 7.2   The effect of Ramipril and secondary outcomes in patients with diabetes (Micro-Hope study).

patients. Jonas et al[21] performed a retrospective study of the long-term effects of beta-blockade over a 3-year period in a cohort with diabetes and coronary artery disease. In this analysis, data were obtained from diabetic patients screened for the Bezafibrate Infarction Prevention (BIP) study, consisting of 2723 patients with type 2 diabetes, 19% of the original 14 417 screened for entry into the BIP study. Patients were divided into two categories, those receiving chronic beta-blocker therapy (911, 33%), of whom the majority received a cardioselective agent, and those who were not (1812, 67%). There was a significantly reduced mortality of 44% in the beta-blocker group and a reduction in cardiac mortality of 42%. Beta-blocker use was a significant independent predictor of survival over 3 years. Although these data are observational , they tend to support the findings of the Norwegian Timoldol study.

In conclusion, the majority of evidence for the beneficial effects of beta-blocker use in patients with diabetes is derived from analysis of subgroup data rather than dedicated randomized studies. Diabetes per se is not a contraindication to the use of beta-blockers and there is some evidence that diabetic individuals have more to gain from their use. In view of this, the introduction of beta-blocker therapy should be considered in all diabetic patients immediately following myocardial infarction as an effective secondary prevention strategy.

Secondary prevention of CHD: role of ACE inhibitors

Heart failure accounts for most of the excess mortality observed in diabetic individuals following myocardial infarction.[22,23] ACE inhibitors reduce left ventricular dysfunction and dilation and the progression to congestive cardiac failure during and following MI. There is strong evidence, both in the general population and in subgroup analyses in diabetic individuals, to support the use of ACE inhibitors in patients who have had myocardial infarction and who have left ventricular dysfunction. Several major studies have shown a reduction in overall mortality and in morbidity from further myocardial infarction and hospitalizations due to heart failure when ACE inhibitors are initiated during the immediate phase following myocardial infarction, in the first few days or weeks and when continued as long-term therapy. The acute use of ACE inhibitors following myocardial infarction is described in Chapter 4. Thus a meta-analysis of 15 trials involving over 100 000 patients who were treated with an ACE inhibitor within 36 hours of acute MI and continued for at least 4 weeks confirmed these beneficial effects.[24] Use of ACE inhibitors was associated with a reduction in mortality of around 6% and benefits were particularly evident in those patients who appeared to be at greatest risk of an event.

Several studies have evaluated the benefits of longer-term therapy with ACE inhibition initiated beyond the acute phase of myocardial infarction and in individuals found to have impaired left ventricular systolic function. Initially published in 1991, Studies of Left Ventricular Dysfunction (SOLVD)[25] has been one of the largest trials of ACE inhibitor use and provides evidence that the drug reduces mortality in patients with all grades of heart failure. Over 2500 patients were recruited (1284 placebo, 1285 enalapril), the majority of whom had evidence of ischaemic heart disease and had suffered a previous MI.

After a mean follow-up of 41 months, therapy with enalapril resulted in a 16% reduction in mortality, although the greatest effects were observed within the first 3 months of therapy. More recently the findings of subgroup analyses have been published and confirm that enalapril reduced mortality in patients with diabetes to a similar degree as for non-diabetic individuals.[26] The absolute risk reduction for mortality in diabetic patients with chronic heart failure was 4.5% over a mean follow-up period of 4.5 years.

The Survival and Ventricular Enlargement (SAVE) study examined over a period of 42 months approximately 2200 patients with asymptomatic left ventricular dysfunction, who recorded a radionuclide ejection fraction of less than 40%.[27] Patients received either captopril (titrated to a dose of 50 mg TDS) or placebo, between 3 and 16 days following MI. Treatment with captopril resulted in a significant reduction in total mortality, cardiovascular mortality and progression to severe congestive heart failure of the order of 19%, 21% and 37%, respectively. Similar benefits were observed in the Acute Infarction Ramipril Efficacy (AIRE) study,[28] where subjects with clinical evidence of heart failure were randomized within 3 to 10 days of myocardial infarction, to receive ramipril or placebo for an average of 15 months. Almost 2000 patients were recruited (982 placebo, 1004 ramipril). Treatment with ramipril, in a final dose of 5 mg twice daily, resulted in a significant reduction in total mortality of 27% and of progression to severe congestive cardiac failure by 22%, compared with placebo. Finally, the Trandolapril Cardiac Evaluation (TRACE) study,[29] which recruited patients with ECHO evidence of left ventricular dysfunction (LVEF < 35%), showed similar benefits for ACE inhibition. In this study, 873 patients were randomized to receive placebo and 876 to trandolapril, which was started 3 days post myocardial infarction and titrated to a final dose of 4 mg daily. After follow-up for 24–50 months, treatment with trandolapril reduced total mortality by 22%, cardiovascular mortality by 25% and progression to severe heart failure by 29%. In each of these three studies, patients were selected on the basis of clinical evidence of left ventricular impairment and patients with diabetes were well represented: 22% of SAVE, 12% of

AIRE and 13% of TRACE cohorts, respectively, had diabetes. The impact of treatment within the diabetic subgroups was disclosed only in the latter study. However, it seems reasonable to apply the beneficial results to the diabetic population as a whole, especially when there is evidence of reduced systolic function or clinical evidence of heart failure following myocardial infarction.

Secondary prevention of CHD: role of beta-blockers and spironolactone in patients with heart failure

Conventional doses of beta-blockers can cause worsening of heart failure, which may be fatal. In recent years there has been increasing evidence to support the use of small doses of beta-blockers in patients with stable chronic heart failure to reduce its progression. Several trials involving therapy with carvedilol had to be terminated prematurely due to significant benefits on hospitalizations for worsening heart failure and a reduction in mortality of the order of 65%.[30] These beneficial effects are also seen with other beta-blockers, including bisoprolol[31] and metoprolol.[32] At present, however, only carvedilol and bisoprolol are licensed for the treatment of heart failure in the UK.

Further manipulation of the renin–angiotensin system beyond ACE inhibition, using spironolactone, a competitive inhibitor of aldosterone, is also beneficial in patients with heart failure. In the Randomized ALdactone Evaluation Study (RALES),[33] which recruited 1663 patients, treatment with spironolactone 25 mg daily produced a 30% reduction in mortality after a mean follow-up period of 2 years, which caused the trial to be terminated prematurely. Hospitalization from heart failure and symptom control were both also significantly reduced by active treatment. It has been estimated that the addition of spironolactone to conventional heart failure treatment prevented 72 premature deaths and 264 hospitalizations per 1000 patients over the study period. There has been no information in either of the above studies on any diabetes-specific data.

Therapies for reduction of cardiovascular risk in high-risk individuals

The large ACE inhibitor trials outlined above suggested that treatment with a variety of agents prevented or delayed serious cardiac events in both diabetic and non-diabetic individuals with established cardiac damage. However, the impact within individuals with normal left ventricular function who are at high risk of cardiovascular events was not clear and it was against this background that the Heart Outcomes Prevention Evaluation (HOPE) study was conducted.[34] The trial examined in excess of 9500 men and women in the age group 55 or over, without evidence of left ventricular systolic dysfunction and although all were at high risk of a future cardiac event, only half of those enrolled had a history of previous myocardial infarction. Subjects were randomized to receive either placebo or ramipril, titrated to 10 mg once daily. The results indicated that treatment with the ACE inhibitor significantly reduced acute coronary events (cardiovascular deaths by 26%, MI by 20%, heart failure by 23%) and progression of coronary atherosclerosis (revascularization procedures by 15%). The benefits of treatment were such that the study was terminated prematurely after a mean follow-up period of 4.5 years. The study recruited 3577 people with diabetes who were analysed separately as the Micro-HOPE sub-study (Fig. 7.2).[35] In these individuals, treatment with ramipril reduced the development of myocardial infarction by 22% (NNT = 9), stroke by 33%, cardiovascular death by 37% and total mortality by 24%. Although there were beneficial effects on blood pressure, the improvements in primary endpoints appeared to be independent of any antihypertensive effects.

More recently, the Losartan Intervention for Endpoint Reduction in hypertension (LIFE) study has been published.[36] This was designed as a multicentre double-blind randomized trial to find the most suitable antihypertensive drug for the reduction of cardiovascular disease in high-risk individual with hypertension. It compared treatment with an angiotensin II receptor antagonist, losartan, against beta-blocker using atenolol, to achieve a reduction of cardiovascular mortality and morbidity in patients aged 55–80 years with essential hypertension and ECG evidence of left ventricular hypertrophy. The study recruited over 9000 patients, including a subgroup of 1195 individuals with diabetes, one quarter of whom had established coronary vascular disease. Within the diabetes subgroup, treatment with losartan resulted in a

39% reduction in all-cause mortality compared with atenolol. Significant reductions in cardiovascular mortality (37%) and admissions for heart failure (41%) were also observed. These findings were more marked within a group who had not received antihypertensive therapy prior to entering the study. Although blood pressure fell significantly in all patients, as in the HOPE study, the benefits of treatment appeared to be independent of any antihypertensive effects.

Both the HOPE and LIFE studies demonstrated that significant benefits can be obtained from modification of the renin–angiotensin system in individuals at high risk of cardiovascular disease. As these data were being published, studies were already under design to look at the effect of combining both ACE inhibitors and angiotensin II antagonists. The Randomised Evaluation of Strategies for Left Ventricular Dysfunction (RESOLVD)[37] was a pilot study in patients with congestive cardiac failure which found that the combination of candesartan and enalapril was more beneficial in influencing left ventricular remodelling and improving ejection fraction than either agent alone. The ONgoing Telmisartan Alone and in combination with Ramipril Global Endpoint Trial (ONTARGET) is a large study due to take place involving over 23 000 patients, including patients with diabetes and evidence of end-organ damage. It will compare the effects of treatment with each of the agents alone and in combination, on cardiovascular death, myocardial infarction, stroke and hospitalization from cardiac failure and promises to provide new insights into the optimal preventative therapy for high-risk patients.

The risks of oral hypoglycaemic therapy in patients with established coronary vascular disease and the cardiovascular effects of insulin-induced hypoglycaemia

Metformin, a member of the biguanide group of oral hypoglycaemic drugs, is indicated for use in people with type 2 diabetes, especially in overweight and obese individuals, in whom dietary measures have failed. In a large randomized trials, treatment with metformin was associated with positive outcomes.[38] Biguanides act predominantly by inhibiting gluconeogenesis, thus lowering hepatic glucose production.[39] They may be associated with an associated risk of life-threatening lactic acidosis under clinical conditions that impair the oxidative removal of lactate, such as in the context of myocardial infarction, congestive cardiac failure or renal impairment. Thus biguanides are not recommended for use in these circumstances[40] and this is clearly documented in the data sheet.[41]

A recent population-based, observational study has been performed in Tayside, Scotland, to examine the incidence of contraindications to metformin in patients with type 2 diabetes receiving metformin over a 30-month time interval.[42] Data on 1847 subjects who redeemed prescriptions for metformin were studied. Of these, 3.5% were admitted with an acute myocardial infarction (71 episodes) and 4.2% were admitted with cardiac failure (114 episodes) during the period of study. The development of contraindications rarely resulted in discontinuation of metformin, for example only 17.5% stopped metformin after admission with acute myocardial infarction. In spite of this, however, there was only one episode of lactic acidosis recorded in 4600 patient years. This study rightly concluded that metformin, in spite of the potential for adverse events, appeared to be a safe oral hypoglycaemic agent and possibly therefore the perceived risk associated with its use has been overstated. A different view has been obtained from the United States, where metformin has only become available since the mid-1990s, although it is now used commonly. In a recently reported retrospective study in an outpatient pharmacy setting, almost one-quarter of patients who received a prescription for metformin had one or more absolute contraindications to its use,[43] including a history of heart failure. The incidence of lactic acidosis was not examined in this study, however within the first 14 months of availability of metformin in the US, 47 cases of metformin-induced lactic acidosis were reported and the majority of these had relative or absolute contraindications to its use.[44]

Interest in the cardiovascular effects of sulphonylurea drugs was generated in the 1970s by reports from the University Group Diabetes Program (UGDP) that tolbutamide, a first generation sulphonylurea, was associated with an increase in cardiac mortality.[45] Subsequently, there has been criticism about the design and statistical analysis within this trial. Sulphonylurea drugs stimulate insulin secretion from pancreatic beta cells by inhibiting potassium efflux. They are capable of antagonising the effect of drugs that operate by opening potassium channels,[46] although there are differences in the effects induced by first and second generation sulphonylurea drugs, respectively. Much of the evidence to suggest adverse effects has been extrapolated from in vitro experiments and it is not clear how relevant this is to the clinical situation in patients with type 2 diabetes who are taking these drugs, particularly as most patients at present will receive the newer agents. Furthermore, there did not appear to be any significant adverse cardiovascular outcomes amongst patients receiving sulphonylurea drugs within the UKPDS cohort.[47]

Sulphonylureas, especially the first generation agents, are capable of inducing hypoglycaemia which can be fatal.[48] Hypoglycaemia due to either sulphonylurea or insulin may induce adverse cardiac effects. Activation of counter-regulatory responses to hypoglycaemia will cause an increase in cardiac workload,[49] which in younger individuals with normal cardiac function may not be detrimental. However, in the elderly or in patients with underlying cardiac insufficiency, cardiac ischaemia may ensue, which can manifest as angina, arrhythmia or myocardial infarction, and can result in sudden death.[50,51]

The effects of cardiovascular drugs on metabolic control in diabetes

Beta-blockers

Historically there have been concerns that beta-blockers could exert detrimental effects in people with diabetes. Firstly, adverse effects on glucose metabolism have been suggested, although the selective beta$_1$-antagonists, which are more commonly advocated in the management of ischaemic heart disease, do not appear to be associated with these.[52,53] Secondly, in theory beta-blockade could alter the warning symptoms of hypoglycaemia by masking the beta-adrenergic-mediated symptoms of tachycardia and tremor. This is the case in some studies,[54,55] however there is also evidence that the glycaemic threshold for symptoms is higher in the context of beta-blockade and that certain symptoms such as sweating are in reality increased.[56] Finally, unselected beta-blockade may prolong the recovery from hypoglycaemia as stimulation of hepatic glycogenolysis and gluconeogenesis occurs via beta$_2$-receptors and this has been documented.[54,57] However, this problem does not appear to be associated with the cardioselective beta-blockers.[54,55] Furthermore, in the Norwegian Timolol Study[20] and BHAT study[18] described above, which were both randomized trials of beta-blockade in the post myocardial infarction setting, there was no reported increase in incidence of hypoglycaemia in those patients who received beta-blocker therapy. Finally, in two population-based case control studies, beta-blocker use was not associated with an increased risk of hospital admission for hypoglycaemia among patients who received either insulin or oral hypoglycaemic drugs.[58,59]

ACE inhibitors

In contrast to beta-blockers, ACE inhibitor therapy may be associated with an improvement in glycaemic control. Following incidental observations of improved blood glucose control after initiation of an ACE inhibitorion for treatment of hypertension,[60,61] a number of later studies have confirmed this tendency. Herings et al[58] performed a nested case-control study which examined hospital admissions for hypoglycaemia amongst patients with diabetes, who were treated with insulin or oral hypoglycaemic drugs. They found that current ACE inhibitor use was associated with a 2.4-fold increased frequency of admission for hypoglycaemia and as many as 14% of hospital admissions for hypoglycaemia might be attributable to therapy with an ACE inhibitor. These results were reproduced by a study with similar design from the Tayside region of Scotland.[59] ACE inhibitors in this study were associated with an increased frequency of hospital admissions for hypoglycaemia, with an odds ratio of 3.2. Separate analysis for insulin versus oral hypoglycaemic drugs revealed that use of the latter was associated with greater risk.

The role of aspirin in the prevention of cardiovascular disease in patients with diabetes

Aspirin for secondary prevention

The role of aspirin in the immediate management of acute myocardial infarction is discussed in Chapter 4. In patients with both acute unstable angina and stable angina pectoris, low dose aspirin (75 mg daily) is advisable to reduce the risk of subsequent vascular events[62] and should be continued for at least 4 years. There is considerable evidence that this is a cost-effective strategy for reducing the chance of developing both fatal and non-fatal vascular events, including myocardial infarction, in a secondary prevention population.[63] These guidelines also apply to patients with diabetes, although there may be an argument in favour of using a higher dose of aspirin in these patients (see below).

In patients with stable angina pectoris, several studies have shown that aspirin therapy significantly reduces the development of cardiovascular events. The US Physician's Health Study was a large double-blind trial of low dose aspirin for the primary prevention of cardiovascular disease.[64] The main study excluded individuals with previous vascular events such as MI, stroke and TIA, although a retrospective evaluation of a subgroup of 333 middle-aged males with chronic angina pectoris was performed.[65] There were 27 confirmed incident MIs during an average follow-up of 60.2 months. Treatment with aspirin 325 mg on alternate days conferred significant protection, since only seven of these MIs occurred in the aspirin arm (87%

risk reduction). Aspirin therapy was associated with a higher incidence of stroke (relative risk 5.4), but none of these events was fatal and less than one-third resulted in any long-term disability. The first prospective study of aspirin in patients with stable angina pectoris was performed in a Swedish population.[66] In this trial, 2035 patients who had stable angina pectoris for at least one month and who were all receiving a beta-blocker were randomized to receive aspirin 75 mg daily or placebo. Therapy with aspirin for 8485 patient years resulted in a significant reduction in the development of either myocardial infarction or sudden death by 34% and a reduction by 32% in vascular events. In this study a slight excess of haemorrhagic strokes and serious bleeds was recorded in the aspirin group, although neither of these events was statistically significant.

The most convincing evidence of the benefits of aspirin in secondary prevention was obtained from a large meta-analysis of 145 randomized trials, which collated data on treatment for 2 years of 20 000 people with a history of previous MI.[67] Aspirin therapy prevented the occurrence of 18 non-fatal recurrent MIs, 6 non-fatal strokes and 13 vascular deaths per 1000 people. Data on high-risk patients, including information on individuals with diabetes, demonstrated that antiplatelet treatment for a month or more significantly reduces the development of a vascular event, including non-fatal MI, non-fatal stroke and vascular death. Treatment with aspirin reduced the rate of myocardial infarction from 22% to 18% in diabetic patients and from 16% to 13% in non-diabetic subjects.

Aspirin for primary prevention

In contrast to the clear evidence of the benefits of aspirin for secondary prevention purposes, there is uncertainty about the role of aspirin as a primary prevention treatment for all people. A balance must therefore be struck between the perceived benefits and adverse effects of aspirin in the primary prevention setting. In all, four randomized trials have examined the benefits of aspirin in this context. In the US Physicians's Health Study[64] involving 22 071 individuals aged 40–84 years, aspirin was so effective in reducing the risk of first myocardial infarction compared with placebo (by 44%) that the study was terminated prematurely. Closer analysis of these data revealed that the major benefits were seen in those aged 50 and above. Subgroup analysis of this study revealed that aspirin reduced the incidence of MI in those with diabetes from 10.1% to 4%. In keeping with the secondary prevention studies, there was a higher incidence of stroke in the aspirin treated individuals, but this was not significant. The British Doctors' Trial of 5139 apparently healthy men reported around the same time.[68] In this, therapy with aspirin 500 mg daily was studied against placebo, however active treatment failed to show a significant impact on the occurrence of fatal or non-fatal MI, although the confidence intervals were very wide: 16% benefit versus 26% for adverse effects.

Around a decade later, two further primary prevention trials were published involving high-risk individuals. The first of these was based within a general practice setting in the UK.[69] Males with no prior history of vascular events, but who were estimated to fail within the top 20% at greatest risk of an event, were recruited after a search of primary care records. The study included a treatment arm with warfarin; 5085 individuals received active treatment with aspirin 75 mg daily, which resulted in a significant reduction in the risk of myocardial infarction of 20%. Treatment did not influence the development of fatal MI or total mortality. In the second, a large multi-centre trial involving patients with controlled hypertension,[70] low dose aspirin further reduced cardiovascular risk in 18 790 well-controlled hypertensive patients. Aspirin reduced the risk of major cardiac events by 15% and of MI by 36%, but there was no difference in the incidence of stroke. The study included 1501 patients and was the only study of the four that included women (47% of participants). The results for the diabetic subgroup reflected the overall study results. Non-fatal haemorrhage and minor bleeding episodes were more common with aspirin therapy (risk ratio 1.8), but fatal haemorrhage was no different between groups.

Data from both of these studies involving high-risk individuals support the findings amongst healthy individuals that treatment with aspirin is beneficial in reducing the risk of a first myocardial infarction. Whether aspirin could have a positive effect also on vascular deaths or the development of stroke was not clear as there were insufficient events recorded in any of the studies to detect this. It is useful to place these positive findings in context. Treatment of 10 000 persons with low dose aspirin would be successful in preventing 67 MIs in a primary prevention setting against 137 MIs in a secondary prevention setting, with no major difference in the occurrence of haemorrhagic stroke between the respective groups. However, a review of the data on adverse events in all four of the above studies[71] has yielded an approximate 1.7-fold increase in the risk of haemorrhage stroke associated with aspirin treatment.

Thus the balance of benefit against risks of aspirin must be considered before contemplating antiplatelet therapy in a primary prevention setting. This benefit over risk improves as the absolute risk of developing a myocardial infarction increases. Thus at one extreme, the benefits of aspirin in a secondary prevention setting vastly outweigh the adverse effects. However, this assessment in the primary prevention setting is not as clear. Assuming that 100 people are treated for 5 years with aspirin, at a coronary event risk of 1.5% per year, the NNT to prevent MI is 44, to prevent MI without causing cerebral or major haemorrhage is 53 and without causing minor haemorrhage is 77. In contrast, at a coronary event risk of 0.5% per year the corresponding NNTs are 133, 256 and 500 respectively.[72] In the light of these calculations, it is advisable that aspirin should only be prescribed for primary prevention purposes once efforts have been made to formally estimate future cardiac risk. This advice is in keeping with the strategy advocated by the Joint British societies, in their guidance for coronary heart disease prevention.[73]

Aspirin in patients with diabetes

Aspirin interferes with platelet function by suppressing the synthesis of thromboxane A_2 through its inhibitory action on the enzyme cyclo-oxygenase. Doses of 75–325 mg of aspirin were assessed in the Collaborative Study[67] and appeared to be equally effective across this dose range. According to a more recent meta-analysis, there is no evidence that medium doses of aspirin, i.e. more than 75 mg but less than 500 mg daily, are any more protective in patients with stable angina.[62] However, there is some in vitro evidence that aspirin is less effective as an antiplatelet agent in patients with diabetes when compared with the effects in non-diabetic subjects.[74] The production of thromboxane A_2 is increased in patients with diabetes,[75] probably as a result of accelerated platelet turnover.[76] Because of these data, some authors have advocated that the optimum dose of aspirin for chronic use in people with diabetes should be in the region of 300 mg daily.[77] Although increasing the dose of aspirin may influence other factors involved in platelet–endothelium interactions, it must be balanced against the potential adverse effects that can be associated with aspirin therapy, especially serious gastro-intestinal and intracerebral haemorrhage.[63] The largest study of aspirin in people with diabetes included patients with established retinopathy both with and without other vascular disease. The primary end-points in the trial were retinopathy and maculopathy, but cardiovascular events were recorded, thus it could be considered as a combined primary and secondary prevention trial.[78] The trial comprised 3711 patients, of whom 44% were female, and all received either aspirin 650 mg daily or placebo. Aspirin was associated with a reduction in fatal and non-fatal MI from 15% to 13%, which was not significant. A non-significant increase in fatal and non-fatal stroke from 4.2% to 5% was recorded. In spite of the higher doses of aspirin used in this study, the rate of major haemorrhage was also not significant and there were no adverse effects on retinal outcomes.

Alternative antiplatelet therapies

Clopidogrel seems to be as effective as aspirin in the prevention of cardiovascular events following MI. In a large randomized study involving over 19 000 patients with established vascular disease, clopidogrel 75 mg daily significantly reduced the risk of ischaemic stroke, myocardial infarction and vascular death when compared with aspirin 325 mg daily.[79] When clopidogrel is added to aspirin in patients with acute coronary syndromes, the risk of cardiovascular death, myocardial infarction or stroke is significantly reduced (by 19.1%) in comparison to treatment with aspirin alone.[80] It is not known whether this combination offers any advantage over aspirin alone in patients with myocardial infarction or stable angina. Dipridamole does not appear to offer any advantages for the prevention of coronary vascular disease.[67]

The use of hormone replacement therapy in women with diabetes

Observational studies show substantially lower rates of coronary heart disease in post menopausal women who have received oestrogen replacement therapy.[81–83] However, these positive effects of hormone replacement may represent selection bias on the basis of other factors. Women who choose to take hormone replacement therapy (HRT) are often healthier and may therefore have a lower risk of coronary artery disease. Furthermore, they are often from a higher socioeconomic standing and as such may have more access to healthcare information.[84]

Oestrogen exerts favourable effects on cardiovascular risk factors. However, the risk of endometrial cancer in the presence of an intact uterus is such that addition of a progestin is required under these circumstances. There have been previous concerns that adding a progestin could negate the positive effects of oestrogen, but these have been allayed by a large randomized controlled trial. In this, the effect of unopposed oestrogen was tested against placebo and combination therapy using three different progestins in 875 healthy post menopausal women over a 3-year period.[85] The results were encouraging as all types of hormone replacement exerted beneficial effects on cardiovascular risk factors, including a reduction in low-density lipoprotein cholesterol of around 20% and significant reductions in fibrinogen levels.

Disappointingly, in spite of the encouraging data from PEPI and the earlier observational studies, there is no convincing evidence that the use of HRT reduces the occurrence of major cardiovascular events in post menopausal women when tested prospectively. The Heart and Estrogen/progestin Replacement Study (HERS)[86] aimed to establish whether treatment with conjugated equine oestrogen 0.625 mg/day with medroxyprogesterone acetate 2.5 mg/day could be effective in preventing recurrent coronary events in high-risk menopausal women with established coronary disease. In this study, 2763 women aged 44–79 years, 23% of whom had diabetes, were randomized to receive therapy with either active hormone replacement or placebo. Follow-up over an average of 4.1 years was associated with significant improvements in high-density lipoprotein cholesterol levels of 10% and reductions in low-density lipoprotein cholesterol levels of 11% compared with placebo. In spite of these favourable effects, hormone replacement failed to influence the development of fatal or non-fatal myocardial infarction, all-cause mortality or occurrence of unstable angina or congestive cardiac failure and was not associated with any significant effects on the risk of stroke.[87]

In women with diabetes, the cardioprotective effects of oestrogen are lost and the risk of coronary vascular disease equates to men without diabetes.[88] There is evidence that HRT is prescribed less frequently in women with diabetes,[89] possibly due to a perception of adverse effects on cardiac risk factors and glycaemic control. However, recent data propose that these concerns are unfounded. Oral HRT appears to have no adverse effects on insulin sensitivity and there is a suggestion that unopposed oestrogen may even improve this.[90] Continuous combined HRT has been shown to exert beneficial effects on lipoprotein concentrations.[91] An observational study of glycaemic control amongst post menopausal women with type 2 diabetes found that users of HRT had lower glycosylated haemoglobulin values than non-users and there were no differences between women using unopposed oestrogen and combination preparations.[92]

In spite of the apparent benefits of HRT, the absence of good outcome data on cardiovascular events means that HRT should not at present be used routinely to influence cardiovascular outcomes, either in a primary or secondary prevention setting in women with or without diabetes. However, the reassuring evidence on the lack of adverse effects on metabolic parameters in women with diabetes suggests that there are no grounds to refrain from prescribing HRT for these women if it is indicated for other reasons such as relief of menopausal symptoms.

Uptake of secondary prevention therapies in clinical practice

The Action on Secondary Prevention through Intervention to Reduce Events (ASPIRE) study[93] has highlighted the need for effective implementation of secondary prevention measures following myocardial infarction. ASPIRE, which was set up by the Epidemiology and Prevention Committee of the British Cardiac Society, collected data from throughout the United Kingdom and revealed gross undermanagement of coronary heart disease risk factors in survivors of myocardial infarction, particularly of lipids and blood pressure. In patients who had survived 3 months following myocardial infarction, 78% of men and 86% of women had a cholesterol level of 5 mmol/l or more. Furthermore, only 38% were receiving a beta-blocker, 17% an ACE inhibitor, 10% a lipid lowering drug and 75% aspirin. In a similar European survey involving nine countries,[94] the records of 3569 patients with established coronary vascular disease, including 641 with diabetes, were examined to determine the uptake of secondary preventive measures. Disappointingly, 53% had raised blood pressure (systolic > 140 mmHg and/or diastolic > 90 mmHg) and 44% had a total cholesterol > 5 mmol/l. Of patients who were post MI, 81% were receiving antiplatelet therapy, 58% beta-blockers, 38% ACE inhibitors and 32% lipid-lowering drugs. A follow-up study performed in 1999–2000 was extended to involve 15 European countries, including the UK. This involved over 8000 patients, including 740 with previously diagnosed diabetes. Unfortunately no significant improvement was shown in the prevalence of modifiable risk factors or the use of pharmacological agents proven to be of benefit in the prophylaxis of recurrent cardiovascular events.[95]

Several UK studies provide evidence to suggest that patients with diabetes do not receive adequate secondary prevention measures following myocardial infarction. Review of 275 patients, including 86 with diabetes one year following first MI, showed that most were given beta-blockers and aspirin appropriately.[96] However, fewer patients with diabetes than without received ACE inhibitors, even in the presence of left ventricular dysfunction, and a lower percentage received lipid-lowering therapy (27.5 versus 37.9%). In another study which followed patients after a first myocardial infarction, only 23% of patients with diabetes against 52% of those without diabetes received a beta-blocker on discharge from hospital.[97] Although some of these individuals had contraindications to the use of a beta-blocker, 35% of the diabetic and 18% of non-diabetic patients did not receive a beta-blocker in spite of not having any contraindications to their use.

Similar data highlighting the underuse of secondary prevention measures have been obtained from two population-based studies in people with diabetes in the Tayside region of Scotland, using the DARTS database. In the first of these,[98] survivors of first acute myocardial infarction over an 18-month period were studied, 147 patients with type 2 diabetes and 256 comparators who were randomly identified. The percentages of patients with type 2 diabetes who suffered an acute myocardial infarction and who received acute treatment with aspirin, thrombolytic therapy and beta-blockers were 34%, 16% and 11%, respectively. These data were consistently poor across all age ranges. In another study within the same population,[99] over half of males and almost three-quarters of females with diabetes and established macrovascular disease had a total cholesterol measurement recorded of 5.0 mmol/l or more (Fig. 7.3). Although these data were collected between 1993–94 and 1996–98, respectively, both studies confirm that a clear opportunity exists to improve the implementation of pharmacological measures that are known to be effective in the management of coronary vascular disease in individuals with type 2 diabetes.

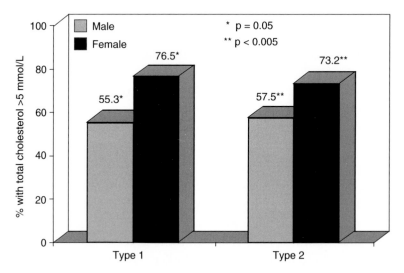

Figure 7.3   Poor targeting of secondary prevention measures in patients with diabetes and established macrovascular disease.

It is unclear why poor targeting of secondary prevention therapies should occur in high-risk individuals with diabetes, but perhaps concerns regarding possible adverse effects or perceived contraindications to certain treatments, especially beta-blockers, could play some part. Nevertheless, this is an important issue which needs to be addressed by all who are involved in the management of patients with diabetes to reduce mortality and morbidity from vascular events.

References

1. Gray RP, Yudkin JS. Cardiovascular disease in diabetes mellitus. In: Pickup J, Williams G, eds. Textbook of Diabetes. Blackwell Scientific: Oxford, 1997.
2. Evans JM, Wang J, Morris AD. Comparison of cardiovascular risk between patients with type 2 diabetes and those who had a myocardial infarction: cross sectional cohort studies. Brit Med J 2002: 324:939–42.
3. Haffner SM, Lehto S, Ronnemaa T et al. Mortality from coronary heart disease in subjects with type 2 diabetes and in nondiabetic subjects with

and without prior myocardial infarction. N Engl J Med 1998;339:229–34.

4. Garcia MJ, McNamara PM, Gordon T, Kannel WB. Morbidity and mortality in diabetics in the Framingham population. Sixteen-year follow-up study. Diabetes 1974;23:105–11.

5. World Health Organization (Europe) and International Diabetes Foundation (Europe). Diabetes care and research in Europe: the St. Vincent declaration. Diabet Med 1990;7:360.

6. Fihn SD, Williams SV, Daley J, Gibbons RJ. Guidelines for the management of patients with chronic stable angina: treatment. Ann Intern Med 2001;135:616–32.

7. Weiss RJ, Hicks D, Bittar N et al. A double-blind, placebo-controlled trial of sustained-release diltiazem in patients with angina. Sustained-Release Diltiazem Study Group. Clin Ther 1993;15:1069–75.

8. Ezekowitz MD, Hossack K, Mehta JL et al. Amlodipine in chronic stable angina: results of a multicenter double-blind crossover trial. Am Heart J 1995;129:527–35.

9. Chrysant SG, Glasser SP, Bittar N et al. Efficacy and safety of extended-release isosorbide mononitrate for stable effort angina pectoris. Am J Cardiol 1993;72:1249–56.

10. Kishida H, Murao S. Effect of a new coronary vasodilator, nicorandil, on variant angina pectoris. Clin Pharmacol Ther 1987;42:166–74.

11. Savonitti S, Ardissiono D, Egstrup K et al. Combination therapy with metoprolol and nifedipine versus monotherapy in patients with stable angina pectoris. Results of the International Multicenter Angina Exercise (IMAGE) Study. J Am Coll Cardiol 1996;27:311–16.

12. Rees-Jones DI, Oliver IM. A comparison of the anti-anginal efficacy of nifedipine alone and the fixed combination of atenolol and nifedipine. Br J Clin Practice 1994;48:174–7.

13. The Beta-Blocker Pooling Project Research Group. The Beta-Blocker Pooling Project (BBPP): subgroup findings from randomised trials in post infarction patients. Eur Heart J 1988;9:8–16.

14. McVeigh G, Brennan G, Hayes R, Johnston G. Primary nitrate tolerance in diabetes mellitus. Diabetologia 1994;37:115–17.

15. ISIS-1 (First International Study of Infarct Survival) Collaborative Group. Randomised trial of intravenous atenolol among 16,027 cases of suspected acute myocardial infarction. Lancet 1986;ii:57–66.

16. The MIAMI Trial Research Group. Metoprolol in Acute Myocardial Infarction (MIAMI): a randomised placebo-controlled international trial. Eur Heart J 1985;6:199–226.

17. Malmberg K, Herlitz J, Hjalmarson A, Ryden L. Effects of metoprolol on mortality and late infarction in diabetics with suspected acute myocardial infarction. Retrospective data from two large studies. Eur Heart J 1989;10:423–8.

18. Beta-blocker Heart Attack Trial research Group. A randomised trial of

propranolol in patients with acute myocardial infarction. 1. Mortality results. J Am Med Assoc 1982;247:1707–14.

19. Kjekshus J, Gilpin E, Cali G et al. Diabetic patients and beta-blockers after acute myocardial infarction. Eur Heart J 1990;11:43–50.

20. Gundersen T, Kjekshus J. Timolol treatment after myocardial infarction in diabetic patients. Diabet Care 1983;6:285–90.

21. Jonas M, Reicher-Reiss H, Boyko V et al. for the Bezafibrate Infarction Prevention (BIP) study group. Usefulness of beta-blocker therapy in patients with non-insulin dependent diabetes mellitus and coronary artery disease. Am J Cardiol 1996;77:1273–7.

22. Stone PH, Muller JE, Hartwell T et al. The effect of diabetes mellitus on prognosis and serial left ventricular function after acute myocardial infarction: contribution of both coronary disease and diastolic left ventricular dysfunction to the adverse prognosis. The MILIS Study Group. J Am Coll Cardiol 1989;14:49–57.

23. Lehto S, Pyorala K, Miettinen H et al. Myocardial infarct size and mortality in patients with non insulin dependent diabetes mellitus. J Intern Med 1994;236:291–7.

24. Garg R, Yusuf S. Overview of randomised trials of angiotension-converting enzyme inhibitors on mortality and morbidity in patients with heart failure. Collaborative Group on ACE Inhibitor Trials. J Am Med Assoc 1995;273:1450–6.

25. The SOLVD Investigators. Effect of enalapril on survival in patients with reduced left ventricular ejection fractions and congestive heart failure. N Engl J Med 1991;325:293–302.

26. Shindler DM, Kostis JB, Yusef S et al. Diabetes mellitus, a predictor of morbidity and mortality in the studies of left ventricular dysfunction (SOLVD) trials and registry. Am J Cardiol 1996;77:1017–20.

27. Pfeffer MA, Braunwald E, Moye LA et al. Effect of captopril on mortality and morbidity in patients with left ventricular dysfunction after myocardial infarction. N Engl J Med 1992;327:669–77.

28. The Acute Infarction Ramipril Efficacy (AIRE) Study Investigators. Effect of ramipril on mortality and morbidity of survivors of acute myocardial infarction with clinical evidence of heart failure. Lancet 1993;342:821–8.

29. Kober L, Torp-Pedersen C, Carlsen JE et al. A clinical trial of the angiotensin-converting-enzyme inhibitor trandolapril in patients with left ventricular dysfunction after myocardial infarction. N Engl J Med 1995;333:1670–6.

30. Packer M, Bristow MR, Cohn JN et al. The effect of carvedilol on morbidity and mortality in patients with chronic heart failure. US Carvedilol Heart Failure Study Group. N Engl J Med 1996;334:1349–55.

31. CIBIS-II investigators and committees. The cardiac insufficiency bisoprolol study (CIBIS-II): a randomised trial. Lancet 1999;353:9–13.

32. Hjalmarson A, Goldstein S, Fagerberg B et al. Effects of controlled-

release metoprolol on total mortality, hospitalisations and well-being in patients with heart failure: the Metoprolol CR/XL Randomised Intervention Trial in congestive heart failure (MERIT-HF). The MERIT-HF Study Group. J Am Med Assoc 2000;283:1295–302.

33. Pitt B, Zannad F, Remme WJ et al. The effect of spironolactone on morbidity and mortality in patients with severe heart failure. Randomised Aldactone Evaluation Study Investigators. N Engl J Med 1999;341:709–17.

34. The Heart Outcomes Prevention Evaluation (HOPE) investigators. Effects of an angiotensin-converting enzyme inhibitor, ramipril, on cardiovascular events in high-risk patients. N Engl J Med 2000;342:145–53.

35. The Heart Outcomes Prevention Evaluation (HOPE) investigators. Effects of ramipril on cardiovascular and microvascular outcomes in people with diabetes mellitus; results of the HOPE study and MICRO-HOPE substudy. Lancet 2000;355:253–9.

36. Lindholm LH, Ibsen H, Dahlof B et al for the LIFE study group. Cardiovascular morbidity and mortality in patients with diabetes in the Losartan Intervention for Endpoint reduction in hypertension study (LIFE): a randomised trial against atenolol. Lancet 2002;359:1004–10.

37. McKelvie RS, Yusuf S, Pericak D et al. Comparison of candesartan, enalapril and their combination in congestive heart failure: randomised evaluation of strategies for left ventricular dysfunction (RESOLVD) pilot study. Circulation 1999;100:1056–64.

38. UK Prospective Diabetes Study (UKPDS) group. Effect of intensive blood-glucose control with metformin on complications in overweight patients with type 2 diabetes (UKPDS 34). Lancet 1998;352:854–65.

39. Stumvoll M, Nurjhan N, Perriello G et al. Metabolic effects of metformin in non-insulin-dependent diabetes mellitus. N Engl J Med 1995;333:550–54.

40. Bailey CJ, Turner RC. Drug therapy—metformin. N Engl J Med 1996;334:574–9.

41. Lipha Pharmaceuticals: *Glucophage Pharmaceutical Data Sheet*, 1999.

42. Emslie-Smith AM, Boyle DI, Evans JM et al. Contraindications to metformin therapy in patients with type 2 diabetes: a population-based study of adherence to prescribing guidelines. Diabet Med 2001;18:483–8.

43. Horlen C, Malone R, Dennis B et al. Frequency of inappropriate metformin prescriptions. J Am Med Assoc 2002;287:2504–5.

44. Misbin RI, Green L, Stadel BV et al. Lactic acidosis in patients with diabetes treated with metformin. N Engl J Med 1998;338:265–6.

45. The University Group Diabetes Program. A study of the effects of hypoglycaemic agents on vascular complications in patients with adult onset diabetes. Diabetes 1970;19(Suppl 2):747–830.

46. Howes LG, Sundaresan P, Lykos D. Cardiovascular effects of oral hypoglycaemic drugs. Clin Exp Pharmacol Physiol 1996;23:201–206.

47. UK Prospective Diabetes Study (UKPDS) Group. Intensive blood-glucose control with sulphonylureas or insulin compared with conventional treat-

ment and risk of complications in patients with type 2 diabetes (UKPDS 33). Lancet 1998;352:837–53.

48. Ferner RE, Neil HAW. Sulphonylureas and hypoglycaemia. Br Med J 1988:296:949–50.

49. Fisher BM, Heller SR. Mortality, cardiovascular morbidity and possible effects of hypoglycaemia on diabetic complications. In: Frier BM, Fisher BM, eds. Hypoglycaemia in Clinical Diabetes, pp. 111–46. John Wiley: Chichester, 2000.

50. Duh E, Fenglos M. Hypoglycaemia-induced angina pectoris in a patient with diabetes mellitus. Ann Intern Med 1994;121:945–6.

51. Frier BM, Barr StCG, Walker JD. Fatal cardiac arrest following acute hypoglycaemia in a diabetic patient. Pract Diabetes Int 1995;12:284.

52. William-Olson T, Fellenius E, Bjorntrop P, Smith U. Differences in metabolic responses to beta-adrenergic stimulation after propranolol and metoprolol administration. Acta Med Scand 1979;205:201–209.

53. Ekberg G, Hansson BG. Glucose tolerance and insulin release in hypertensive patients treated with cardioselective beta-receptor blocking agent metoprolol. Acta Med Scand 1982;211:7–12.

54. Lager I, Smith U, Blome G. Effect of cardioselective and non-selective beta-blockade on the hypoglycaemic response in insulin-dependent diabetics. Lancet 1979;1:458–62.

55. Deacon SP, Karunanayke A, Barnett D. Acebutolol, atenolol and propranolol and metabolic response to acute hypoglycaemia in diabetes. Br Med J 1977: 2:1255–7.

56. Hirsch IB, Boyle PJ, Craft S, Cryer PE. Higher glycaemic thresholds for symptoms during beta-adrenergic blockade in IDDM. Diabetes 1991;40:1177–86.

57. Abramson E, Arky R, Woeber K. Effects of propranolol on hormonal and metabolic responses to hypoglycaemia. Lancet 1966;2:1386–90.

58. Herings RM, de Boer A, Stricker BH et al. Hypoglycaemia associated with use of inhibitors of angiotensin-converting enzyme. Lancet 1995;345:1195–8.

59. Morris A, Boyle DIR, McMahon AD et al for the DARTS/MEMO collaboration. ACE-inhibitor use is associated with hospitalisation for severe hypoglycaemia in patients with diabetes. Diabet Care 1997;20:1363–7.

60. Ferriere M, Bringer J, Richard J et al. Captopril and insulin sensitivity. Ann Intern Med 1985;102:134–5.

61. Rett K, Jaunch KW, Wicklmayr M. Hypoglycaemia in hypertensive diabetic patients treated with sulphonylureas, biguanides and captopril (letter). N Engl J Med 1988;319:1609.

62. Eccles M, Freemantle N, Mason J. North of England evidence based guideline development project: guideline on the use of aspirin as secondary prophylaxis for vascular disease in primary care. North of England Guideline Development Group. Br Med J 1998: 316:1303–9.

63. Patrono C. Aspirin as an anti-platelet drug. N Engl J Med 1994;330: 1287–94.

64. Steering Committee of the Physician's Health Study. Final report on the aspirin component of the ongoing Physician's Health Study. N Engl J Med 1989;321:129–35.

65. Ridker PM, Manson JE, Gaziano JM et al. Low-dose aspirin therapy for chronic stable angina. A randomised, placebo-controlled clinical trial. Ann Intern Med 1991;114:835–9.

66. Juul-Moller S, Edvardsson N, Jahnmatz B et al. for the Swedish Angina Pectoris Aspirin Trial (SAPAT) Group. Double-blind trial of aspirin in primary prevention of myocardial infarction in patients with stable chronic angina pectoris. Lancet 1992;340:1421–5.

67. Antiplatelet Trialists' Collaboration. Collaborative overview of randomised trials of antiplatelet – I: prevention of death, myocardial infarction and stroke by prolonged antiplatelet therapy in various categories of patient. Br Med J 1994:308:81–106.

68. Peto R, Gray R, Collins R et al. Randomised trial of prophylactic daily aspirin in British male doctors. Br Med J 1988:296:313–16.

69. The Medical Research Council's General Practice Research Framework. Thrombosis prevention trial: randomised trial of low-intensity oral anticoagulation with warfarin and low dose aspirin in the primary prevention of ischaemic heart disease in men at increased risk. Lancet 1998;351:233–41.

70. Hannson L, Zanchetti A, Carruthers SG et al. for the HOT study group. Effects of intensive blood-pressure lowering and low-dose aspirin in patients with hypertension: principal results of the Hypertension Optimal Treatment (HOT) randomised trial. Lancet 1998;351:1755–62.

71. Hebert PR, Hennekens CH. An overview of the 4 randomised trials of aspirin therapy in the primary prevention of vascular disease. Arch Intern Med 2000;160:3123–7.

72. Sanmuganathan PS, Ghahramani P, Jackson PR et al. Aspirin for primary prevention of coronary heart disease: safety and absolute benefit related to coronary risk derived from meta-analysis of randomised trials. Heart 2001;85:265–71.

73. Wood D, Durrington P, Poulter N et al. Joint British recommendations on prevention of coronary heart disease in clinical practice. Heart 1998;80(Suppl 2):S1–S29.

74. Mori T, Vandongen R, Douglas A et al. Differential effect of aspirin on platelet aggregation in IDDM. Diabetes 1992;41:261–6.

75. Davi G, Catalano I, Averna M et al. Thromboxane biosynthesis and platelet function in type 2 diabetes mellitus. N Engl J Med 1990;322:1769–74.

76. DiMinno G, Silver MJ, Cerbone AM, Murphy S. Trial of repeated low-dose aspirin in diabetic angiopathy. Blood 1986;68:886–91.

223

77. Colwell JA. Aspirin therapy in diabetes. Diabet Care 1997;20:1767–71.
78. EDTRS investigators. Aspirin effects on mortality and morbidity in patients with diabetes mellitus. J Am Med Assoc 1992;268:1292–300.
79. CAPRIE steering committee. A randomised, blinded trial of clopidogrel versus aspirin in patients at risk of ischaemic events. Lancet 1996;348:1329–39.
80. Mehta SR, Yusuf S. The clopidogrel in unstable angina to prevent recurrent events (CURE) trial programme; rationale, design and baseline characteristics including a meta-analysis of the effects of thienopyridines in vascular disease. Eur Heart J 2000;21:2033–41.
81. Sullivan JM, Van der Zwaag R, Hughes JP et al. Estrogen replacement and coronary artery disease. Effect on survival in post menopausal women. Arch Intern Med 1990;150:2557–62.
82. Sourander L, Rajala T, Raiha I et al. Cardiovascular and cancer morbidity and mortality and sudden cardiac death in post menopausal women on oestrogen replacement therapy. Lancet 1998;352:1965–9.
83. Stampfer MJ, Colditz GA, Willett WC et al. Post menopausal estrogen therapy and cardiovascular disease. Ten year follow-up from the nurses' health study. N Engl J Med 1991;325:756–62.
84. Barrett-Connor E. Post-menopausal estrogen and prevention bias. Ann Intern Med 1991;115:455–6.
85. The Writing Group for the PEPI Trial. Effects of estrogen or estrogen/progestin regimens on heart disease risk factors in post-menopausal women. J Am Med Assoc 1995;273:199–208.
86. Hulley S, Grady D, Bush T et al. Randomised trial of estrogen plus progestin for secondary prevention of coronary heart disease in post-menopausal women. Heart and Estrogen/progestin Replacement Study (HERS) Research Group. J Am Med Assoc 1998;280:605–13.
87. Simon JA, Hsia J, Cauley HA et al. Postmenopausal hormone therapy and risk of stroke. The Heart and Estrogen/progestin Replacement Study (HERS). Circulation 2001;103:638–42.
88. Gordon T, Castelli WP, Hjortland MC et al. Diabetes, blood lipids and the role of obesity in coronary heart disease risk for women. The Framingham Study. Ann Intern Med 1977;87:393–7.
89. Feher MD, Isaacs AJ. Is hormone replacement therapy prescribed for postmenopausal diabetic women? Br J Clin Practice 1996;50:431–2.
90. Sattar N, Jaap AJ, MacCuish AC. Hormone replacement therapy and cardiovascular risk in post-menopausal women with NIDDM. Diabet Med 1996;13:782–8.
91. Manning PJ, Allum A, Jones S et al. The effect of hormone replacement therapy on cardiovascular risk factors in type 2 diabetes: a randomised controlled trial. Arch Intern Med 2001;161:1772–6.
92. Ferrara A, Karter AJ, Ackerson LM et al. Hormone replacement therapy is associated with better glycaemic control in women with type 2

diabetes: The Northern California Kaiser Permanente Diabetes Registry. Diabet Care 2001;24:1144–50.

93. ASPIRE Steering Group. A British Cardiac Society Survey of the potential for the secondary prevention of coronary disease: ASPIRE (Action on Secondary prevention through Intervention to reduce Events) principal results. Heart 1996;75:334–42.

94. EUROASPIRE Study Group. EUROASPIRE. A European Society of Cardiology survey of secondary prevention of coronary heart disease; principal results. European Action on Secondary Prevention through Intervention to Reduce Events. Eur Heart J 1997;18:1569–82.

95. EUROASPIRE II Study Group. Lifestyle and risk factor management and use of drug therapies in coronary patients from 15 countries; principal results from EUROASPIRE II Euro Heart Survey Programme. Eur Heart J 2001;22:554–72.

96. Chowdhury TA, Lasker SS, Dyer PH. Comparison of secondary prevention measures after myocardial infarction in subjects with and without diabetes mellitus. J Intern Med 1999;245:565–70.

97. Younis N, Burnham P, Patwala A et al. Beta blocker prescribing differences in patients with and without diabetes following a first myocardial infarction. Diabet Med 2001;18:159–61.

98. Donnan PT, Boyle DIR, Broomhall J et al for the DARTS/MEMO collaboration. Prognosis following first acute myocardial infarction in type 2 diabetes: a comparative population study. Diabet Med 2002;19:448–55.

99. Brennan G, Devers M, Boyle D et al. Implications of cholesterol management guidelines for diabetes: a population-based study. Diabetologia 1999;42(Suppl 1):A6.

chapter 8

Coronary heart disease in patients with diabetes – non-pharmacological treatment

Klas Malmberg, Henrik Enhörning and Lars Rydén

Introduction

Coronary interventions in the form of coronary artery bypass grafting (CABG) and percutaneous coronary interventions (PCI) are routine procedures in the modern management of patients with coronary artery disease. It was noted at an early stage that subjects with diabetes mellitus had more complications and a decreased long-term survival following such procedures compared to non-diabetic patients.[1] A major challenge with PCI in patients with diabetes has been the high rate of restenosis.[2] Furthermore, the unexpected result of the Bypass Angioplasty Revascularisation Investigation (BARI) study[3] initiated a continuing debate about whether CABG should be the preferred intervention in the patient with diabetes.[4,5] This chapter describes the advantages and disadvantages of current invasive treatment strategies among people with diabetes.

Percutaneous coronary interventions

The high proportion of restenosis is still a major limiting factor for long-term success following all PCI techniques. Consistent reports demonstrate that diabetes is an independent predictor for restenosis.[6,7] Early reports documented a restenosis rate of 50–70% in patients with diabetes compared to 25–40% in the non-diabetic patient following balloon angioplasty. Other techniques, such as coronary atherectomy or Rotablator® (Boston Scientific Corporation Northwest Technology Center, Redmond WA, USA) have not decreased the rate of this complication to any important extent among patients with diabetes. The diabetic condition may influence several of the complex pathophysiological events causing restenosis:[8]

- The metabolic alterations that are linked to diabetes may accelerate smooth muscle cell proliferation induced by the PCI initiated intravascular injury.
- Besides endothelial dysfunction, a procoagulant state, with decreased fibrinolytic capacity and increased platelet stickiness, characterizes patients with diabetes mellitus.
- There is also evidence of overexpression of several growth stimulating factors that may promote processes ending with a restenosis.
- Advanced glycosylation end-products in the vessel wall induce inflammatory cell response, thereby promoting smooth muscle cell proliferation.
- As well as the procoagulant and hyperproliferative state, people with diabetes also have microvascular abnormalities that further potentiate the development of restenosis. Recent research shows that vasa vasorum at the site of an atherosclerotic plaque increases in proportion to plaque mass. The diabetic patient is prone to develop

microvascular proliferation at other locations and such events may further contribute to the excessive neointimal information, which is the hallmark histological finding in diabetic restenosis.

- All of these potential mechanisms are related to hyperglycaemia and some to hyperinsulinaemia as well.

In addition to a high restenosis rate, several studies report that patients with diabetes are more prone to develop in-hospital complications, such as increased periprocedural myocardial injury, compared to non-diabetic patients.[6] This is most apparent in insulin-treated patients and in women. The most consistent finding is the increased long-term mortality amounting to about 40% within 10 years.[9] Diabetes is an independent predictor of long-term mortality following PCI. Interestingly, it has been shown that diabetic patients undergoing PCI have a more rapid progress of their native coronary artery disease than diabetics not undergoing PCI and non-diabetic subjects.[10] Perhaps this relates to the fact that diabetic blood vessels are more sensitive to injury caused by the mechanical instrumentation.

Coronary stenting in the diabetic patient

In general, the introduction of coronary stenting caused a 25–30% reduction in the rate of restenosis. For the diabetic population, studies of the impact of stenting has been conflicting.[11] Stenting reduces the restenosis rate in the diabetic patient, but not to the same extent as in non-diabetic subjects, and the rate of in-stent restenosis in diabetic subjects compared to non-diabetic subjects seems to be higher. In a recent study, comprising 1474 patients out of whom 225 had diabetes, the rate of restenosis after 6 months of follow-up was 24% in non-diabetic subjects compared to 35% in non-insulin treated diabetics and 49% in patients on insulin. Several studies have shown a similar pattern with an increase both in event and restenosis rate in patients on insulin.[7] Most of these studies did not take into account that patients on insulin are often older with longer diabetes duration and more frequent micro- and macrovascular complications of their diabetes. Moreover, the patients are often less well controlled as regards their metabolic state than those not on insulin. In the study quoted there was an increased vessel lumen narrowing in patients with diabetes (regardless of antidiabetic treatment) compared to those without diabetes. It may be concluded that coronary stenting even in the diabetic patient contributes to a more favourable outcome after PCI as regards restenosis. However, diabetes is still a powerful predictor of unfavourable clinical events and mortality following PCI.

Adjunctive therapies
Antithrombotic therapy
Since people with diabetes have more vascular complications during and after a PCI, efforts have been directed towards platelet stabilization and anticoagulation with special reference to blockade of the glycoprotein GPIIb/GPIIIa receptor. In several large-scale randomized trials GPIIb/GPIIIa inhibitors improved the safety profile following PCI with or without stenting.[12,13] Subgroup analysis from these clearly indicates that patients with diabetes seem to benefit proportionately more than non-diabetic patients as regards target vessel revascularization, myocardial infarction and death.[14] A combined analysis of three studies using the GPIIb/GPIIIa inhibitor abciximab showed a one-year mortality reduction from 4.5% to 2.5% in patients with diabetes compared to 2.6% and 1.9% among the non-diabetic subjects.[15] Similar trends have also been observed with other GPIIb/GPIIIa inhibitors. Thus it has been suggested that the combination of glycoprotein inhibitors and stents should be preferred in patients with diabetes.[16] It must be acknowledged that this recommendation is based on retrospective subgroup analysis from relatively small patient populations that are rather poorly defined as regards their diabetes and its treatment.

Endothelial stabilization
Another potential target when attempting to improve the outcome following PCI is impaired endothelial function. Several reports suggest that intensive lipid lowering with statins improves endothelial function.[17,18] Although statins have not been successful in preventing restenosis after PCI in the general perspective a recent report

indicated favourable results in diabetic patients. Thus, statin therapy markedly improved clinical outcomes and reduced the proliferative response after coronary stenting when given to such patients. This effect was independent of the cholesterol lowering capacity, an interesting finding that needs to be verified in a prospective randomized trial. It underlines the importance of an aggressive secondary preventive treatment in patients with diabetes.

Brachytherapy

Excessive neointimal formation is a main feature of restenosis in patients with diabetes. Therapeutic actions targeted to inhibit this proliferative response should therefore be of particular interest. Intracoronary gamma radiation (brachytherapy) may be of special value. Preliminary data from a recent randomized trial showed a substantial reduction in in-stent and in-lesion restenosis rate following gamma radiation in diabetic patients. However, recent reports indicate that late stent thrombosis may be a major problem, but this has not been evaluated specifically in diabetic patients.

Metabolic control

Many of the metabolic perturbations that relate to restenosis and clinical events following PCI in patients with diabetes are linked to hyperglycaemia.[8] There are no randomized trials on the impact of meticulous blood glucose control on the restenosis rate. A recent cohort study indicated that patients with good metabolic control at the time of PCI had an increased event-free survival. In fact, HbA1c was an independent predictor of long-term prognosis. This indicates that metabolic control at the time of the procedure may be of crucial importance for development of restenosis and myocardial injury. Randomized trials are urgently needed and at least one such trial (Insulin Diabetes Angioplasty, IDA) is presently ongoing.

Sulphonylureas and preconditioning

The mechanism of action of traditionally used sulphonylureas, represented by glibenclamide, is to inhibit the opening of the ATP-

231

sensitive potassium channels, thereby stimulating insulin secretion (see Chapter 7). Glibenclamide is not specific to the pancreatic β-cell. ATP-dependent potassium channels in smooth muscle cells, myocytes, mitochondria and the vascular endothelium are also influenced. In most species the ATP-dependent potassium channels are important for ischaemic preconditioning, a phenomenon that is myocardiopro-tective in the setting of myocardial ischaemia followed by reperfu-sion.[19] Apart from inactivation of preconditioning, inhibition of ATP-dependent potassium channels may disturb coronary vasorelax-ation and preserve an untouched myocardial contractile strength. Normally these factors protect an energy-depleted myocyte.

The second generation of sulphonylureas represented by glimepiride may be less harmful compared with the first generation of these drugs. In particular the effects of these novel compounds are more specifically related to the pancreatic ATP-dependent potassium channels, while they are less active in myocardial and vascular tissue. This concept was recently tested in a PCI study randomizing patients to either glibenclamide or glimepiride. As a measure of ischaemia the amount of ST-segment shift and the time to onset of anginal chest pain was studied.[20] Following placebo and glimepiride the time to onset of pain was prolonged and the mean ST-segment shift reduced compared to glibenclamide. This suggests a compromised adaptation to ischaemia after glibenclamide treatment.

In a large retrospective cohort study comparing long-term outcome in patients with diabetes following coronary intervention with PCI or CABG, survival following PCI was lower than after CABG. Interest-ingly, this difference was only apparent among PCI patients on sulphonylureas.[21] This concept has further support from a registry study in diabetic patients undergoing direct PCI for acute myocardial infarction. Early mortality was significantly higher in patients on sulphonylureas compared to those on insulin or diet.[22] Early mortal-ity was primarily due to pump failure culminating in cardiogenic shock. A similar trend was seen in the GUSTO IIb trial.[23] All these observations have a substantial contributory value as background information to new prospective clinical trials recruiting patients from this increasing, and in many respects hitherto not well treated, population of type 2 diabetics.

Coronary artery bypass grafting

The proportion of diabetic patients among patients undergoing CABG has been reported as varying from 6 to 54%. Almost all studies report on an approximately two-fold increase in short- as well as long-term mortality in these patients. In a recent Swedish study, diabetic patients had a different preoperative risk factor pattern including more frequent three-vessel disease, hypertension, angina pectoris, intermittent claudication and obesity.[24] During surgery the period of aortic cross-clamping was longer and they also received more grafts. In this study the 30-day mortality was almost 7% among diabetic patients compared to 3% in those without diabetes, and that was persistent after 2 years of follow-up. The mortality did not differ in patients with different antidiabetic treatment. In a multivariate analysis, diabetes was an independent predictor of long-term mortality. Patients with diabetes tended to have more myocardial infarctions but the most striking finding was the almost three-fold increase in stroke during long-term follow-up. This confirms previous findings among diabetic subjects undergoing CABG. Despite this higher morbidity and mortality CABG improved the quality of life to a similar extent among non-diabetic and diabetic patients.

The mechanism behind the higher mortality in diabetic patients is poorly understood. Patients with diabetes often suffer from more extensive coronary artery disease and as a group they often have more compromised left ventricular function. However, even if such factors are included in multivariate statistical analysis, diabetes remains an independent predictor of increased morbidity and mortality. In a recent study, comprising more than 2000 consecutive diabetic patients undergoing CABG, there was an almost linear relationship between hospital mortality and mean peri-operative blood glucose value.[25] In fact, the average blood glucose during two preoperative days was an independent predictor of postoperative mortality in addition to well-known factors as congestive heart failure, renal failure and emergency surgery. Strategies for effective control of peri-operative hyperglycaemia have not been tested in randomized trials looking into morbidity and mortality following CABG in patients with diabetes. Such studies seem to be urgently needed.

In summary, available evidence indicates the patients with diabetes undergoing CAGB carry an increased risk of peri-operative complications and decreased long-term survival compared to non-diabetic patients. Symptomatically they benefit to the same extent as non-diabetic patients and should have the same opportunity for invasive evaluation and treatment as non-diabetic patients. This is further supported by recent data from the FRISC II trial. In this trial patients with unstable angina or non-Q-wave myocardial infarction were randomized to either acute invasive evaluation and treatment or to a more conservative arm.[26] The overall results showed that the invasive strategy was superior in preventing death and new myocardial infarction during the first year of follow-up. In the diabetic subgroup the overall event rate was more than doubled, although these subjects experienced the same relative benefit from the invasive approach as non-diabetic subjects. This once more underlines that the diabetic population should be considered for an invasive approach on the same indications and for the same contraindications as non-diabetic patients.

Bypass surgery versus percutaneous coronary interventions in multi-vessel disease

The optimal revascularization modality in people with diabetes and multi-vessel coronary artery disease is under extensive debate. This controversy started with the Bypass Angioplasty Revascularization Investigation (BARI).[3] A total of 1829 patients with multi-vessel disease

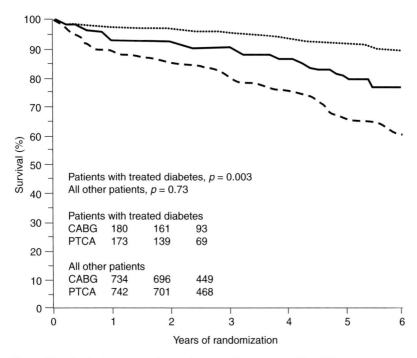

Figure 8.1 Survival among patients who were being treated for diabetes at baseline (heavy lines) and all other patients (light lines). Patients assigned to CABG are indicated by solid lines, and those assigned to PTCA by dashed lines. (From reference 3.)

were randomized to CABG or multi-vessel PCI. There was no overall difference in the 5-year survival rate between the two treatment group. In a subgroup analysis of the diabetic patients (subjects treated with insulin or oral hypoglycaemic agents) there was a distinct survival advantage in the CABG groups. The survival curves started to separate after 6 months and the difference increased during the complete 5-year period of follow-up (Figure 8.1). The 5-year all-cause mortality rate was 34% in diabetic patients randomized to PCI, compared to 19% in patients in the CABG group. Among diabetic subjects who were eligible but not randomized, who tended to have less advanced coronary artery disease, there was no survival difference but a clear trend in the same direction. The BARI finding has recently been extended to 7 years of follow-up.[27] The 7-year mortality rate was 44% in those treated with PCI compared to 24% in those treated with CABG.

Some retrospective cohort studies have not confirmed the BARI results. As outlined, eligible patients in the BARI study who were not randomized had a more similar mortality regardless of treatment modality compared to those within the study. However, the outcome in this registry is not inconsistent with the main findings. Thus, most available data indicate that CABG should be the preferred intervention in diabetic patients with multi-vessel disease.[28] Further analysis of the BARI trial indicates that the use of the left internal mammary artery (LIMA) is crucial for the result among people with diabetes.[29] The LIMA graft is more resistant to arteriosclerosis and has a long-term patency that is by far superior to that for a vein graft. One hypothesis is that the survival advantage noted by CABG with the LIMA grafts relates to prolonged myocardial protection within the extensive left anterior descending coronary artery territory. This may be especially important in the diabetic patient with a high risk for restenosis and frequent silent ischaemia following PCI. Another finding from the recent BARI analysis is that patients allocated to CABG had a much more favourable outcome following a new myocardial infarct compared to those randomized to PCI.[30] This is of particular importance for the diabetic patient who is more prone to develop new coronary events. It highlights the advantages of complete revascularization in this particular group of patients.[21] It is reasonable to suppose that the prognosis will improve with complete revascularization in the case of a new event.

The BARI results were derived before the introduction of coronary stenting, GPIIb/IIIa receptor blockers and brachytherapy. It is well known that the use of stents will decrease the complication rate following PCI. Some results from the Arterial Revascularization Therapy Study (ARTS) comparing multi-vessel coronary stenting with CABG have recently been released.[31] This still ongoing study revealed one-year interim results covering more than 200 patients with diabetes. These indicate that patients with diabetes still do better with CABG. One-year mortality was 6.3% in the PCI group compared to 3.1% in the CABG group. The rate of myocardial infarction was more than double in those randomized to PCI and stenting. Cerebrovascular events were, however, more prevalent after CABG. It was concluded CABG is preferable to stenting in diabetic patients with multi-vessel disease, but that it carries a significant excessive risk of stroke.

Diabetes and heart transplantation

Diabetes mellitus has been considered as a contraindication or at least a relative contraindication to heart transplantation, mainly because of the predicted increase risk of complications such as infection and worsening metabolic control due to corticosteroid immunosuppression. The introduction of cyclosporin has, however, allowed a substantial reduction in the steroid dosage. There are now several (relatively small) reports indicating that heart transplantation can be safely performed in the diabetic patients with the same short- and mid-term results as in non-diabetic patients.[32–37] One report concludes that diabetic patients with end-organ damage such as impaired renal function or typical symptoms of peripheral or autonomic polyneuropathy have the same complication rate and prognosis as patients without such complications and also non-diabetic patients during 2 years of follow-up.[38] Most studies indicate that metabolic control is more difficult to achieve after transplantation. It is also well-known that heart transplantation could induce diabetes in non-diabetic patients and that this may be predicted by a family history of diabetes.[39] This is probably due to the use of corticoid steroids, but it should also be kept in mind that heat failure per se is an insulin-resistant condition.

In summary, it seems that heart transplantation in this fast growing patient population can be performed with an acceptable complication rate and that diabetes no longer should be a contraindication for heart transplantation in carefully selected cases.

Conclusions

Non-pharmacological treatments have an important role to play in the management of coronary heart disease in people with diabetes. Coronary artery bypass grafting, incorporating a left internal mammary graft, is the treatment of choice for diabetic patients with multi-vessel disease. Percutaneous coronary interventions are of benefit in patients with more limited disease. As developments are made in adjunctive therapy, and newer methods become available to reduce the rates of restenosis, the role of PCI in patients with diabetes may become clearer. For patients with severe congestive cardiac failure, heart transplantation should be considered in selected patients.

References

1. Salomon NW, Page S, Okies JE et al. Diabetes mellitus and coronary artery bypass. Short-term risk and long-term prognosis. J Thorac Cardiovasc Surg 1983;85:264–71.
2. Ellis SG, Narins CR. Problem of angioplasty in diabetics. Circulation 1997;96:1707–10.
3. The Bypass Angioplasty Revascularization Investigation (BARI) investigators. Comparison of coronary bypass surgery with angioplasty in patients with multivessel disease. N Engl J Med 1996;335:217–25.
4. Simoons ML. Myocardical revascularization—bypass surgery or angioplasty? N Engl J Med 1996;335:275–7.
5. Kurbaan AS. Revascularization in diabetics: time to change practice? Br J Cardiol 2001;8:686–7.
6. Stein B, Weintraub WS, Gebhart SSP et al. Influence of diabetes mellitus on early and late outcome after percutaneous transluminal coronary angioplasty. Circulation 1995;91:979–89.
7. Kastrati A, Schomig A, Elezi S et al. Predictive factors of restenosis after coronary stent placement. J Am Coll Cardiol 1977;30:1428–36.
8. Aronson D, Bloomgarden Z, Rayfield EJ. Potential mechanisms promoting restenosis in diabetic patients. J Am Coll Cardiol 1996;27:528–35.
9. Kip KE, Faxon DP, Detre KM et al. Coronary angioplasty in diabetic patients. The National Heart, Lung and Blood Institute Percutaneous Transluminal Coronary Angioplasty Registry. Circulation 1996;94:1818–25.
10. Rozenman Y, Sapoznikov D, Mosseri M et al. Long-term angiographic follow-up of coronary balloon angioplasty in patients with diabetes

mellitus. A clue to the explanation of the results of the BARI study. J Am Coll Cardiol 1997;30:1420–5.

11. Lincoff AM. Does stenting prevent diabetic arterial shrinkage after percutaneous coronary revascularization? Circulation 1997;96:1374–7.

12. Lincoff AM, Califf RM, Moliterno DJ. Complementary clinical benefits of coronary artery stenting and blockade of platelet glycoprotein IIb/IIIa receptors. N Engl J Med 1999;341:319–27.

13. Topol EJ, Ferguson JJ, Weisman HF et al for the EPIC investigator group. Long-term protection from myocardial ischemic events in a randomized trial of brief integrin B3 bloackade with percutaneous coronary intervention. J Am Med Assoc 1997;278:479–84.

14. Marso SP, Lincoff M, Ellis SG et al for the EPISTENT investigators. Optimizing the percutaneous interventional outcomes for patients with diabetes mellitus. Results of the EPISTENT (Evaluation of Platelet IIb/IIIa inhibitor for Stenting Trial) diabetic substudy. Circulation 1999;100:2477–84.

15. Bhatt DL, Marso SP, Lincoff et al. Abciximab reduced mortality in diabetics following percutaneous coronary intervention. J Am Coll Cardiol 2000;35:922–8.

16. Sabatine MS, Braunwald E. Will diabetes save the platelet blockers? Circulation 2001;104:2759–61.

17. Weis M, Pehlivanli S, Meiser BM, von Scheidt W. Simvastatin treatment is associated with improvement in coronary endothelial function and decreased cytokine activation after heart transplantation. J Am Coll Cardiol 2001;38:814–18.

18. Penny WF, Ben-Yehuda O, Kuroe K et al. Improvement of coronary artery endothelial dysfunction with lipid lowering therapy: heterogeneity of segmental response and correlation with plasma-oxidized low density lipoprotein. J Am Coll Cardiol 2001;37:766–74.

19. Yellon DM, Dana A. The preconditioning phenomenon: a tool for the scientist or a clinical reality? Circ Res 2000;87:543–50.

20. Klepzig H, Kober G, Matter C et al. Sulfonylureas and ischaemic preconditioning: a double-blind, placebo-controlled evaluation of glimepiride and glibenclamide. Eur Heart J 1999;20:439–46.

21. O'Keefe JH, Blackstone EH, Sergeant P, McCallister BD. The optimal mode of coronary revascularization for diabetics. A risk-adjusted long-term study comparing coronary angioplasty and coronary bypass surgery. Eur Heart J 1998;191:696–703.

22. Garratt KN, Brady PA, Hassinger NL et al. Sulfonylurea drugs increase early mortality in patients with diabetes mellitus after direct angioplasty for acute myocardial infarction. J Am Coll Cardiol 1999;33:119–24.

23. McGuire DK, Emanuelsson H, Granger CB et al for the GUSATO IIb investigators. Influence of diabetes mellitus on clinical outcomes across the spectrum of acute coronary syndromes. Findings from the GUSTO-IIb study. Eur Heart J 2000;21:1750–8.

24. Herlitz J, Wognsen GB, Emanuelsson H et al. Mortality and mobidity in diabetic and nondiabetic patients during a 2-year period after coronary artery bypass grafting. Diabetes Care 1996;19:698–703.
25. 2000 CABGs
26. Wallentin L, Lagerqvist B, Husted S et al for the FRISC II investigators. Outcome at 1 year after an invasive compared with a non-invasive strategy in unstable coronary-artery disease: the FRISC II invasive randomised trial. Lancet 2000;356:9–16.
27. The Bypass Angioplasty Revascularization Investigation (BARI) investigators. Seven-year outcome in the Bypass Angioplasty Revascularisation (BARI) by treatment and diabetic status. J Am Coll Cardiol 2000;35:1122–9.
28. Weintraub WS, Stein B, Kosinski A et al. Outcome of coronary bypass surgery versus coronary angioplasty in diabetic patients with multivessel coronary artery disease. J Am Coll Cardiol 1998;31:20–2.
29. The Bypass Angioplasty Revascularization Investigation (BARI) investigators. Influence of diabetes on 5-year mortality and morbidity in a randomized trial comparing CABG and PTCA in patients with multivessel disease: the Bypass Angioplasty Revascularization Investigation (BARI). Circulation 1997;96:1707–10.
30. Detre KM, Lombardero MS, Brooks MM et al. The effect of previous coronary artery bypass surgery on the prognosis of patients with diabetes who have acute myocardial infarction. Bypass Angioplasty Investigation Investigators. N Engl J Med 2000;342:1040–2.
31. Serruys PW, Unger F, Sousa JE et al for the Arterial Revascularization Therapies Study Group. Comparison of coronary-artery bypass surgery and stenting for the treatment of multivessel disease. N Engl J Med 2001;344:1117–24.
32. Rhenman MJ, Rhenman B, Icenogle T et al. Diabetes and heart transplantation. J Heart Transplant 1988;7:356–8.
33. Badellino MM, Cavarocchi NC, Narins B et al. Cardiac transplantation in diabetic patients. Transplant Proc 1990;22:2384–8.
34. Faglia E, Favales F, Mazzola E et al. Heart transplantation in mildly diabetic patients. Diabetes 1990;39:740–2.
35. Ladowski JS, Kormos RL, Uretsky BF et al. Heart transplantation in diabetic recipients. Transplantation 1990;49:303–5.
36. Munoz E, Longuist JL, Radovancevic B et al. Long-term results in diabetic patients undergoing heart transplantation. J Heart Lung Transplant 1992;11:943–9.
37. Tenderich G, Schulte-Eistrup S, Petzoldt R, Koerfer R. Cardiac transplantation in patients with insulin-treated diabetes mellitus. Exp Clin Endocrinol Diabetes 2000;108:249–52.
38. Aleksic I, Czer LS, Freimark D et al. Heart transplantation in patients with diabetic end-organ damage before transplantation. Thorac Cardiovasc Surg 1996;44:282–8.

39. Depczynski B, Daly B, Campbell LV et al. Predicting the occurrence of diabetes mellitus in recipients of heart transplants. Diabet Med 2000;17:15–19.

chapter 9

Physical activity and exercise in type 2 diabetes

Alison F Kirk and Paul D MacIntyre

Introduction

Physical activity is an important component of good diabetes management. However, there is relatively little guidance for the promotion of physical activity in this group of people. This chapter reviews current literature on the potential benefits that people with type 2 diabetes can achieve by participating in physical activity, and provides important information for the promotion of physical activity in this population.

Physical activity, exercise and physical fitness

The terms physical activity, exercise and physical fitness are often used interchangeably when describing their relationship with health and disease. Standardization of this terminology is important in order to understand fully the true relationship.

Physical activity has been defined as 'any bodily movement produced by skeletal muscle that results in energy expenditure and includes a broad range of occupational, leisure and routine daily activities'.[1] Everybody therefore performs physical activity, although the amount and kind of physical activity performed varies from person to person.

Exercise is a component of physical activity and describes physical activity, which is planned and structured and done to improve and/or maintain physical fitness.

Physical fitness has been defined as 'a set of attributes that people have or achieve that relate to the ability to perform physical activity'.[2] Physical fitness is determined by a combination of regular physical activity and inherited genetic ability and can be related to athletic ability or health.

Current physical activity and exercise guidelines from the American College of Sports Medicine and Centers for Disease Control make important distinctions between physical activity and exercise. Traditional guidelines focus on the quantity and quality of exercise to develop and maintain cardiorespiratory fitness. Recent guidelines highlight the importance of accumulating physical activity, recommending activities which may not affect cardiorespiratory fitness, but which are beneficial for health.

Prevention of type 2 diabetes

There is now increasing evidence that many aspects of type 2 diabetes can be improved and possibly prevented by regular, frequent physical activity. The recent Finnish Diabetes Prevention Study[3] provides strong evidence that lifestyle changes in people with impaired glucose tolerance can prevent or delay the onset of type 2 diabetes. This study randomly assigned 522 men and women with impaired glucose tolerance to an intervention group, all of whom received an individualized diet and physical activity programme compared to a control group, who received standard care. Participants were followed for an average of 3.2 years. At 1-year follow-up the intervention group recorded significantly greater self-reported improvements in both diet and exercise. The intervention group also recorded significantly greater improvements at 1 year in the following clinical and metabolic variables:

- body weight
- waist circumference
- fasting plasma glucose concentration
- plasma glucose and serum insulin concentration 2 hours after oral glucose tolerance test
- HDL-C
- triglycerides
- blood pressure.

These changes, with the exception of HDL-C, were maintained at 2-year follow-up. Analysis of progression to type 2 diabetes showed that the cumulative incidence of diabetes was 58% lower in the intervention group compared to the control group.

The results of the National Institute of Health's Diabetes Prevention Study in the United States,[4] which compared the effectiveness of metformin with an intensive lifestyle intervention to delay or prevent type 2 diabetes, confirmed the results of the Finnish study, only with greater power. Both these studies highlight the importance of changes in lifestyle in people with impaired glucose tolerance to prevent or delay type 2 diabetes.

Management of type 2 diabetes

Physical activity has important physiological and psychological benefits for all people, but particularly for people with established type 2 diabetes. For this reason, physical activity and exercise are important components of good diabetes management.

Acute effects of exercise

Glucose levels

The increased metabolic demands that accompany exercise require an increase in fuel mobilization from storage sites and an increase in fuel oxidation in the working muscle. Fuel mobilization and utilization during exercise is controlled by a precise endocrine response. Generally, in normal healthy individuals, arterial insulin levels decrease and levels of glucogon, cortisol, epinephrine and norepinephrine levels increase during exercise. This precise endocrine response ensures arterial glucose levels change very little during exercise up to a moderate intensity.

Few studies have evaluated the acute metabolic response to exercise in people with type 2 diabetes. During mild to moderate exercise most people with type 2 diabetes exhibit decreases in blood glucose levels.[5-7] This response often persists into the post exercise period. Minuk et al[5] investigated the metabolic responses to exercise in seven obese people with type 2 diabetes, maintained on diet or sulphonylurea therapy, compared to seven obese non-diabetic controls. Exercise consisted of 45 minutes on a cycle ergometer at 60% of maximal aerobic power. In people with diabetes blood glucose levels fell by approximately 2.5 mmol/l during the 45-minute exercise session, while in control subjects blood glucose levels did not change. In people with diabetes this lower level of glycaemia was maintained into the post-exercise period.

The reason why blood glucose levels decrease during mild to moderate exercise remains controversial. Earlier studies attributed the decrease to an inadequate exercise associated increase in hepatic glucose production coupled to a normal increase in muscle glucose utilization.[5] The reduced rise in glucose production is suggested to be due to the failure of insulin to fall during exercise, as it does in control subjects and/or to the hepatic effects of hyperglycaemia present in people with type 2 diabetes.[5] In more recent studies a greater increase in glucose utilization and a decrease in plasma insulin levels has been described.[6]

In contrast to moderate intensity exercise, short-term high intensity exercise has been shown to increase blood glucose levels during and for up to one hour after exercise. This rise in blood glucose has been associated with an exaggerated counterregulatory hormone response. Kjaer et al[8] studied the effects of maximal exercise on glucoregulation in seven people with type 2 diabetes and seven healthy controls. The exercise protocol involved cycling at 60% of maximum aerobic power for 7 minutes followed by 3 minutes at 100% of maximum aerobic power and a further 2 minutes at 110% of maximum aerobic power. In people with diabetes plasma glucose concentrations increased and remained elevated for one hour post-exercise. Plasma glucose concentrations in control subjects did not change significantly during exercise.

Insulin resistance

Insulin resistance is a major feature of type 2 diabetes (see Chapter 1). Several studies have demonstrated that acute exercise increases insulin sensitivity. Devlin et al[9] demonstrated that a single session of high-intensity exercise at 85% of maximum aerobic power significantly increased peripheral and splanchnic insulin sensitivity, persisting for 12 to 16 hours post-exercise in a group of men with type 2 diabetes.

There is no consensus regarding the optimal intensity and duration of exercise required to improve insulin sensitivity. Recently it has been shown that improvements in insulin sensitivity after walking at a high intensity (75% of maximum aerobic power) with a short duration and at a moderate intensity (50% of maximum aerobic power) with a longer duration were nearly identical and significantly higher than in sedentary controls.[10] The beneficial effects of light-intensity activity on insulin sensitivity have also been demonstrated. Usui et al[11] showed that an acute 30-minute session of light intensity (40 to 50% of maximal aerobic power) cycling in obese people with type 2 diabetes improved insulin sensitivity.

The effect of an acute bout of exercise on insulin action is lost within a few days. Heath et al[12] illustrated that trained individuals lose much of their enhanced sensitivity to insulin within a few days of exercise termination. However, a single bout of exercise restores insulin sensitivity to the same level as in the trained state.

Research suggests that frequent exercise performed at a low to moderate intensity is required to facilitate glucose reduction and improved insulin sensitivity in people with type 2 diabetes. However, most studies investigating the effects of acute exercise on glucose levels and insulin resistance in people with type 2 diabetes have used relatively small study groups, controlled by diet or oral hypoglycaemic therapy. Further research with larger and more diverse diabetic populations is required to understand fully the effects of acute exercise in people with type 2 diabetes.

Long-term effects of exercise

Metabolic control

Regular, frequent physical activity holds important benefits for people with type 2 diabetes. A summary of potential benefits is illustrated in Table 9.1. Several studies have reported favourable changes in glycosylated haemoglobin after physical activity training of variable type, duration and intensity.[13–16] The favourable effect of frequent exercise

---

Table 9.1 Potential benefits of physical activity in type 2 diabetes

- Improve glycaemic control
  - Blood glucose levels
  - Insulin resistance
- Improve cardiovascular risk profile
  - Lipid profile
  - Blood pressure
  - Cardiorespiratory fitness
  - Body composition
- Enhance quality of life

on the requirements for hypoglycaemic medication has also been documented.[17,18] Fujinuma et al[17] investigated the effect of 3 to 4 weeks of supervised exercise in 78 people with type 2 diabetes. Compared to a control group of non-exercisers, a significantly greater number of participants in the exercise group discontinued or reduced their insulin dose. Of the 56 people allocated to the exercise group, 10 participants discontinued insulin injections and 36 reduced the number of insulin injections per day.

The majority of research investigating the effect of exercise in the management of type 2 diabetes has incorporated structured, supervised exercise programmes. A study by Walker et al[14] demonstrated that with correct education and encouragement an unsupervised exercise programme could also be carried out successfully. Participants in this study were 11 women with type 2 diabetes and 20 non-diabetic controls. All participants were encouraged to walk for one hour on 5 days per week for 12 weeks. At 12-week follow-up significant improvements in body mass index, body fat, HbA1c, total cholesterol and LDL cholesterol were recorded. This study is limited, however, by a lack of randomization.

Favourable changes in glucose control usually deteriorate within 72 hours of the last exercise session in people with type 2 diabetes,[9] and improved glycaemic control with prolonged periods of frequent exercise participation is largely due to the cumulative effects of individual exercise bouts as opposed to the long-term adaptations to physical activity training.[9,12] As a result, people with type 2 diabetes should participate in frequent exercise to sustain the glucose-lowering effects of exercise.

Not all studies have reported improvements in glycaemic control in response to exercise. Skarfors et al[19] studied the long-term effects of exercise training in a group of men over 60 years with type 2 diabetes. Exercise training incorporated supervised exercise sessions, twice weekly at 75% of maximal aerobic power for 45 minutes. At 2-year follow-up significant improvements in maximal aerobic power were demonstrated, but no accompanying beneficial effects were shown in metabolic variables when compared to controls. Similar findings have been reported by Ligtenberg et al.[20] In a randomized, controlled trial the effects of exercise were investigated in a group of 92 obese, elderly (over 55 years) people with poorly controlled, advanced type 2 diabetes. The exercise intervention included individual, supervised exercise at an intensity of 60 to 80% of maximal aerobic power for 50 minutes, three times a week for 6 weeks. For a further 20 weeks participants exercised at home, with encouragement being given for 6 weeks after the end of supervised exercise. Significant between-group differences were recorded in self-reported physical activity levels and maximal aerobic power at 6-week and 6-month follow-up. No changes were recorded in glucose tolerance or insulin sensitivity throughout the study.

The results of these studies could suggest that exercise is more effective for improving glycaemic control during earlier stages of diabetes. Consistent with this suggestion, Barnard et al[21] demonstrated that the effect of exercise and diet on glycaemic control is related to treatment of diabetes, the effect of diet and exercise interventions being greatest in those participants receiving no medication or oral hypoglycaemic agents, compared with participants taking insulin. These results stress the need for an early emphasis on lifestyle modification in the management of people with type 2 diabetes.

Cardiovascular benefit

Exercise has also been associated with improvements in cardiovascular risk profile in people with type 2 diabetes. Research has shown that after exercise training they experience favourable changes in lipid profile, including total cholesterol,[14,16,20] triglycerides,[15,16,22,23] high-density lipoprotein (HDL)-cholesterol[23] and low-density lipoprotein (LDL)-cholesterol,[14,16] blood pressure,[23] cardiorespiratory fitness[20,24-26] and psychological well-being.[27]

Lehmann et al[23] investigated the effect of an individualized, moderate intensity aerobic exercise programme in people with type 2 diabetes. Exercise was performed under supervision once weekly and participants were encouraged through goal setting, self-monitoring and social support to include a further three exercise sessions a week.

At 3-month follow-up participants in the experimental group recorded significant improvements in physical activity levels, blood pressure, waist to hip ratio and plasma lipids compared to controls, with a 20% reduction in triglycerides and an increase in high-density lipoprotein subfractions. There were no changes in glycaemic control (HbA1C) in the experimental group, however the control group increased on average by 0.6%.

In recent years the effect of resistance training on cardiovascular risk has been demonstrated. Honkola et al[16] evaluated the effects of an individualized, progressive resistance training programme on blood pressure, lipid profile and glycaemic control in people with type 2 diabetes. A moderate-intensity, high-volume, low-resistance supervised resistance training programme was carried out for 5 months, twice weekly. At 5-month follow-up the experimental group, in comparison to the control group, recorded significant improvements in total cholesterol, LDL-cholesterol and triglycerides. Body weight and glycaemic control did not change significantly in the experimental group, but increased in the control group. The difference between groups in the change in body weight and glycaemic control achieved statistical significance. No significant changes were recorded in blood pressure in either group. This study, however, could be criticised for a lack of randomization and as a result the majority of men participated in the experimental group and women in the control group. These studies illustrate the benefits of exercise on cardiovascular risk factors, but only incorporate a relatively short-term follow-up period. Further evidence is needed to confirm that the benefits observed can be maintained over a longer period.

Low levels of cardiorespiratory fitness have been directly associated with cardiovascular disease and all cause mortality in the general population.[28] In a recent prospective cohort study similar findings were reported in people with type 2 diabetes. In this study, 1263 men (50 ± 10 years of age) with type 2 diabetes were followed for mortality for an average of 12 years. After adjustment for age, baseline cardiovascular disease, fasting plasma glucose level, high cholesterol, overweight, smoking status, high blood pressure and family history of cardiovascular disease, men with low cardiorespiratory fitness had an adjusted relative risk for all-cause mortality of 2.1, compared with fit men.[29] Kohl et al[30] demonstrated a similar inverse relationship between cardiorespiratory fitness and mortality in people with variable levels of glycaemic control. Although risk of death increases with higher glycaemic status, the adverse impact of hyperglycaemia on mortality appears to be reduced with increased fitness.

Maximal aerobic power (VO_2 max) is the classic measure of overall cardiorespiratory fitness and describes the highest oxygen uptake obtainable by an individual for a given form of exercise despite increased effort and work rate. Several studies have demonstrated that people with type 2 diabetes have a reduced oxygen consumption at submaximal[31,32] and maximal exercise when compared with healthy age-matched controls.[32–34]

The causes of this impaired exercise capacity are unknown. Research has shown a strong inverse association between cardiorespiratory fitness and development of type 2 diabetes.[31] This raises the possibility that reduced cardiorespiratory fitness may contribute to the development of type 2 diabetes and could potentially serve as a marker for individuals at high risk. There is also evidence to suggest that both central (cardiac)[33,36] and peripheral factors[37,38] may relate to the impaired exercise capacity associated with type 2 diabetes.

Several studies have reported improvements in VO_2 max as a result of exercise training in people with type 2 diabetes.[20,24–26] Ligtenberg et al[20] found significant improvements in VO_2 max in elderly people with type 2 diabetes after 6 weeks of moderate-intensity supervised exercise. After 15 weeks of individualized exercise at 40 to 60% of VO_2 max, Khan et al[39] also reported significant improvements in VO_2 max.

Psychological benefit
While the psychological effects of exercise have been extensively studied in the general population, only a few studies have investigated the association between physical activity and psychological well-being in people with diabetes. Stewart et al,[40] in a 2-year observational study, illustrated higher levels of physical activity to be

associated with overall better psychological functioning and well-being in both people with type 1 and type 2 diabetes. Glasgow et al[41] investigated the association between quality of life and demographic, medical history and self-management characteristics of people with diabetes. Quality of life was assessed using the physical functioning, social functioning and mental health scales of the Medical Outcomes study SF-20 questionnaire. A total of 2800 people with type 1 and type 2 diabetes were sent surveys. A response rate of 73.4% was obtained. Findings from the study revealed physical activity participation to be the only significant self-management behaviour predictive of enhanced quality of life.

In a recent randomized controlled trial, Lightenberg et al[27] assessed the influence of an exercise training programme on psychological well-being in 51 elderly people with type 2 diabetes. After 6 weeks of supervised training three times a week for one hour at 60 to 80% of VO_2 max, significant improvements were found in both VO_2 max and all subscales of the well-being questionnaire, except depression. At the end of the supervised exercise period participants were advised to continue training at home without supervision. A follow-up was conducted 14 weeks after the supervised exercise period. At this follow-up, although VO_2 max remained significantly higher than the control group, well-being scores had returned to baseline level. These results could suggest that social support achieved during supervised group exercise is an important factor for the enhanced psychological well being apparent after exercise training. The development of social support through family or friends should therefore receive high priority when developing individualized unsupervised exercise programmes for people with type 2 diabetes.

Physical activity habits in type 2 diabetes

Physical activity participation

Despite the potential benefits of exercise, it has been reported that 60 to 80% of people with type 2 diabetes are currently inactive.[42–44]

While people with diabetes report exercise rates similar to those of the general population, people with diabetes reported a significantly greater frequency of exercise relapse.[42] Furthermore, the greatest number of people with diabetes report low adherence to exercise recommendations, compared to other diabetes self care behaviours.[44]

Variables associated with physical activity participation

Limited research has examined variables associated with physical activity participation in people with diabetes. Hays and Clark[43] reported higher education and younger age as significant correlates of physical activity participation in people with type 2 diabetes. Krug et al[42] also reported an association between physical activity participation and age, but in contrast to the former study, they reported that older people with type 2 diabetes were more likely to exercise than younger people. Swift et al[46] found older age and greater time since diagnosis were associated with how long subjects had maintained regular physical activity. These findings could be related to the health belief model.[47] This model proposes that adherence with a health behaviour depends on the perceived severity of illness threat, perceptions of vulnerability to illness if no action is taken and the belief that the effectiveness of the behaviour outweighs barriers to making the change. Increasing age and duration of diabetes with the onset of diabetes complications may influence perceived susceptibility and severity of diabetes and may explain why people with type 2 diabetes delay initiating an exercise programme until a later age.

Among the cognitive variables self-efficacy (a person's confidence in their ability to carry out a behaviour) has been identified as an important predictor of exercise participation in people with type 2 diabetes. Kingery et al[48] examined the relationship of self-efficacy in predicting diabetes self-care behaviours, including diet, exercise and glucose testing in people with type 2 diabetes. Exercise self-efficacy proved to be a moderately strong predictor of exercise participation. However, of the three self-care behaviours, participants rated themselves lowest on exercise self-efficacy. These findings are consistent with a study conducted by Padgett,[49] and highlight the importance of physical activity interventions designed to enhance self-efficacy for improving exercise adherence in people with type 2 diabetes.

Other cognitive variables which have been shown to be associated with exercise participation in people with type 2 diabetes include perceived benefits and barriers to physical activity participation,[50] performance and outcome expectations,[48] motivation and physical activity knowledge.[43]

Wilson et al[50] reported that people with type 2 diabetes believe in the effectiveness of medicational treatments of diabetes, but report the lowest amount of belief in the effectiveness of exercise. This highlights the need to explain the rationale behind the effectiveness of exercise in the management of type 2 diabetes. Perceived benefits of exercise for people with type 2 diabetes include improving diabetes control and managing weight.[46] Reported barriers include physical discomfort from exercise, fears of reactions from low blood sugar, being too overweight to exercise and lack of support.[46,50] Identification of perceived barriers to physical activity participation and education on how to overcome them, i.e. monitoring of blood glucose, could significantly reduce reported barriers and therefore enhance adherence to physical activity.

Low motivation to participate in physical activity is a major factor associated with poor physical activity participation and drop-out in healthy individuals.[51] Hays and Clark[43] reported motivation for physical activity to be significantly associated with physical activity participation in people with type 2 diabetes. These findings suggest that effective methods for enhancing motivation should be included in the promotion of physical activity in people with type 2 diabetes. Goal setting and self-monitoring of progress are important sources of self-motivation. Martin et al[52] found that flexible exercise goals set by the individual in comparison to instructor-set goals significantly improved adherence to an exercise programme and long-term maintenance of physical activity following completion of the programme.

Physical activity knowledge has been shown to correlate poorly with physical activity behaviour in the general population.[53] Similar findings have been reported in people with diabetes.[54] Guion et al[54] assessed knowledge of exercise in people with type 2 diabetes. Questionnaire results revealed only 38% of respondents knew the recommended amounts of exercise. Consistent with previous research, a weak relationship was present between knowledge of recommended exercise amounts and actual reported physical activity participation. Similar findings have been reported for other health behaviours, suggesting that awareness of desired health practices is not sufficient for bringing about the adoption of health behaviour change.

Social support has been consistently correlated with physical activity participation in the general population.[55] People with type 2 diabetes report the least amount of social support for exercise, compared to other self-care behaviours.[50] Lack of social support is one of the most frequently cited barriers to exercise participation among people with type 2 diabetes.[46] These findings are highlighted by data reporting that although 76% of people with type 2 diabetes are advised to exercise regularly, only 21% receive instructions about the most beneficial type and amount. In comparison, 76% of people with type 2 diabetes receive dietary instructions.[56] A study by Marsden[57] reported that people with type 1 diabetes perceived a poor service for exercise from health professionals, indicating that they did not receive adequate exercise education, support or encouragement.

Physical activity prescription

Physical activity prescription in the general population

Traditional guidelines for exercise prescription, summarized in Table 9.2 from the American College of Sports Medicine (ACSM), result from research about the quality and quantity of exercise required to develop and maintain cardiorespiratory fitness. These guidelines recommend 20 to 60 minutes of moderate- to high-intensity endurance exercise (60 to 90% of maximum heart rate or 50 to 85% of maximum aerobic power) performed 3 to 5 days a week.[58]

Table 9.2 American College of Sports Medicine (ACSM) guidelines

ACSM recommendations to develop and maintain cardiorespiratory fitness:
■ A minimum of three, 20-minute, moderate to vigorous intensity exercise sessions a week

ACSM and CDC recommendations for health promotion and disease prevention:
■ Accumulate 30 minutes or more of moderate intensity physical activity on most, preferably all, days of the week

Changes in health do not necessarily parallel improvements in cardiorespiratory fitness. A review of physiological, epidemiological and clinical evidence outlined that participation in moderate intensity physical activity, which did not exert an effect on cardiorespiratory fitness, had the potential to improve health. In view of this new research the American College of Sports Medicine and Centers of Disease Control and Prevention (ACSM/CDC) developed additional exercise guidelines, described in Table 9.2, focusing on improving health. These guidelines recommend accumulating 30 minutes of moderate intensity physical activity (60 to 79% of maximum heart rate or 50 to 74% of maximum aerobic power) most days of the week.[59] These guidelines appear more acceptable to the whole population. A recent study assessing participation in these two guidelines in an obese population noted that the newer exercise guidelines were met by twice as many of the obese participants (34%) as the traditional recommendations (17%).[60]

Physical activity prescription in people with type 2 diabetes
The ACSM recently published a position statement outlining exercise prescription for people with type 2 diabetes.[61] These guidelines

257

recommend that people with type 2 diabetes who have no significant complications or limitations should achieve a minimum cumulative total of 1000 kcal per week in aerobic activity to facilitate weight management and achieve health-related benefits. The addition of a well-balanced resistance training programme will further help to improve and maintain muscular strength and body composition.

In view of research demonstrating that favourable changes in glucose tolerance and insulin sensitivity deteriorate within 72 hours of physical activity participation, frequent physical activity participation is important for people with type 2 diabetes. The guidelines encourage participation in physical activity on at least three non-consecutive days. Furthermore, a low to moderate intensity of physical activity (40 to 70% of maximum aerobic power) is recommended to achieve these metabolic improvements. The intensity of activity should be a comfortable level of exertion to minimize risk and maximize health benefit and, most importantly, to enhance the likelihood of adherence to the physical activity programme. It should be noted that the ACSM/CDC[59] recommend that to achieve health-related benefits, such as improvements in weight, blood pressure and lipid profile, physical activity should be performed at a minimum intensity of 50% of maximum aerobic power on most, if not every, days of the week.

If no contraindications to exercise exist, the type of exercise a person with diabetes performs is a matter of personal preference. Most of the research documenting the benefits of exercise for people with diabetes involves aerobic activity such as walking,[14] cycling,[13] rowing[24] or swimming.[21] Recent research with circuit type resistance training exercise has shown it improves glucose utilization and the plasma lipid profile associated with increasing muscle mass.[16] Physical activity should be performed for a cumulative duration of 30 minutes. When weight loss is the primary goal the duration should to be incrementally increased to one hour.[62] For previously sedentary people with no formal history of exercise an initial low intensity of exercise should be recommended, with a gradual progressive increase in workload. To prevent musculoskeletal injuries, a proper warm-up and cool-down period should be included.

Most people, including those with diabetes, can undertake exercise with a high level of safety. Exercise is not without risk and the recommendation that people with diabetes participate in an exercise programme is on the basis that the benefits outweigh the risks. To minimize possible risks when developing an exercise prescription, particular attention should be paid to appropriate screening, programme design, monitoring and patient education. The American Diabetes Association (ADA), in collaboration with the ACSM, recently published a position statement to further current understanding about the role of exercise in people with type 1 and 2 diabetes.[63]

Pre-exercise evaluation

Clinical assessment

Prior to participation in an exercise programme the ADA and ACSM recommend that people with diabetes have a medical evaluation to screen for the presence of micro- and macrovascular complications that could potentially deteriorate as a result of participation in exercise. Identification of existing complications will assist in the development of an individualized exercise prescription with minimal risk to the patient.

Exercise test

The ADA and ACSM also recommend an exercise tolerance test prior to participation in moderate- to high-intensity exercise if a person with diabetes is at a high risk for underlying cardiovascular disease based on one of the following criteria:

- age > 35 years
- type 2 diabetes of > 10 years' duration
- type 1 diabetes of > 15 years' duration
- presence of any additional risk factor for coronary artery disease
- presence of microvascular disease (retinopathy or nephropathy, including microalbuminuria)
- peripheral vascular disease
- autonomic neuropathy.

This recommendation has been developed in view of the higher prevalence of sudden death[64] and silent ischaemia[65] in people with type 2 diabetes. It is important to note that the recommendation of preparticipation exercise screening in people with diabetes is not routinely followed in the UK. If resources are available this test can provide valuable information. The exercise test should be performed to evaluate for ischaemia, arrhythmia, abnormal hypertensive response to exercise or abnormal orthostatic responses during or after exercise. The stress test also provides information regarding initial aerobic capacity, specific precautions that may need to be taken and heart rate or perceived exertion that could be used to prescribe activities.

Exercise prescription for people with diabetic complications
An area of ongoing concern is the possible adverse effect of physical activity on existing complications of diabetes. People with diabetes complications are often told to refrain from exercise for fear of deterioration of the condition and development of further complications. This leads to further compromise of physical and cardiovascular conditioning. It is important to develop exercise prescriptions for individuals with diabetes complications that will result in improved participation in normal activities and psychosocial well-being, while minimizing risk of further deterioration. A summary of diabetic complications and physical activity recommendations is displayed in Table 9.3.

Retinopathy
In theory, physical activity and exercise could have a potential detrimental effect on diabetic retinopathy by raising systolic blood pressure. At present there is no evidence of an association between physical activity participation and development or progression of diabetic retinopathy. In the Wisconsin epidemiological study of diabetic retinopathy[66] higher levels of physical activity in women were associated with a reduced risk of having proliferative diabetic retinopathy and no association was found in men. The possibility that people with multiple diabetic complications could be less likely to

Table 9.3　Diabetic complications and physical activity recommendations

Diabetic complication	Physical activity recommendation
Retinopathy	Walking, swimming, cycling. Avoid strenuous, Valsalva-type or jarring exercise
Peripheral artery disease	Interval training (3-minute walk, 1 minute rest), swimming, stationary cycling, chair exercises
Peripheral neuropathy	Non-weight-bearing exercise (cycling, rowing, swimming). Avoid heavy weight bearing exercise (running, prolonged walking, step exercise). Emphasize foot care
Autonomic neuropathy	Water exercise, semi-recumbent cycling. Avoid exercise causing rapid body position, heart rate or blood pressure changes
Neuropathy	Light to moderate exercise

participate in exercise should not be overlooked. Bernbaun et al[67] assessed the effects of a 12-week moderate-intensity exercise programme in subjects with multiple diabetes complications including retinopathy. No deterioration of retinopathy was reported and significant improvements were recorded in exercise tolerance, glycaemic control and insulin requirements.

Activities such as walking, swimming, low-impact aerobics and cycling are encouraged for people with retinopathy. Strenuous anaerobic exercise, exercise involving Valsalva-type manoeuvres or jarring movements and activities that lower the head below the waist may be contraindicated.[68]

Peripheral artery disease

Research evaluating the effects of physical activity on peripheral artery disease in people with diabetes is limited. A number of studies evaluating the effects of physical activity for non-diabetic people with peripheral artery disease have reported improvements in symptoms. Hiatt et al[69] demonstrated, in a randomized controlled trial, that 12 weeks of exercise training for people with peripheral artery disease improved peak exercise performance, delayed the onset and progression of claudication pain during exercise and improved walking ability.

Interval training (e.g. 3-minute walk, 1-minute rest), swimming, stationary cycling and chair exercises are recommended activities for people with peripheral artery disease.[68]

Peripheral neuropathy

Limited research has evaluated the effects of physical activity for people with peripheral neuropathy. Complications of peripheral neuropathy, with the development of the insensate foot, and foot abnormalities indicate weight-bearing exercise, particularly prolonged walking, running or step exercise, should be undertaken with care or avoided. The repetitive stress and pressure from these types of exercise can lead to ulceration and fractures.

To minimize the risk of injury, non-weight-bearing exercise such as cycling, rowing, swimming and chair exercises should be encouraged. For people with neuropathy performing weight-bearing exercise, emphasis on foot care and decreasing foot pressure by proper footwear is essential.[68]

Autonomic neuropathy

Autonomic neuropathy is associated with a reduced aerobic capacity[70] and an increase in the risk of an adverse cardiovascular event or sudden death during exercise.[71] Hilstead et al[70] demonstrated a reduced maximal oxygen uptake accompanied by a impaired heart rate response to exercise in people with autonomic neuropathy in comparison to those with no autonomic neuropathy. Impaired heart rate response makes the use of heart rate to measure exercise intensity inappropriate for people with autonomic neuropathy. Instead, subjective perceptions of intensity using, for example, the rate of perceived exertion (RPE) scale should be used.[72] An illustration and description of this scale is shown in Table 9.4.

Table 9.4   The rate of perceived exertion scale

6	No exertion at all	13	Somewhat hard
7	Extremely light	14	
8		15	Hard (heavy)
9	Very light	16	
10		17	Very hard
11	Light	18	
12		19	Extremely hard
		20	Maximal exertion

Description of scale[38]
The scale requires a rating of perceived exertion during exercise, i.e. how strenuous the exercise feels. The perception depends mainly on muscle strain and fatigue and feelings of breathlessness. The scale goes from 6, 'no exertion at all', to 20, 'maximal exertion'. Instructions for the scale give additional anchor points: 9 corresponds to 'very light' exercise similar to walking slowly for some minutes, 13 is 'somewhat hard' exercise but still feels OK to continue. 17, 'very hard', is very strenuous, still able to continue but feeling very tired and having to push yourself. Finally 19 is 'extremely hard'. For most people this is the most strenuous exercise they have ever experienced.

In people with autonomic neuropathy the blood pressure response during exercise and to changes in posture may be abnormal, and ventilatory reflexes can be impaired. Tantucci et al[73] found that people with diabetic autonomic neuropathy had an increased respiratory rate and alveolar ventilation in response to submaximal incremental exercise, in comparison to both people with diabetes and no autonomic neuropathy and healthy controls.

Activities that cause rapid changes in body position, heart rate or blood pressure should be avoided. Water exercises and semi-recumbent cycling are recommended for those with orthostatic hypotension since the semi-recumbent posture and the pressure of water surrounding the body will help to maintain blood pressure.[74] The ability to recognize symptoms of hypoglycaemia are often reduced or absent in people with autonomic neuropathy. Awareness of hypoglycaemia and blood glucose monitoring before, often during and after exercise can help to protect against episodes of hypoglycaemia. In addition, thermoregulation may also be impaired. Loss of sweating may cause dry, brittle skin and contribute to ulcer formation. Proper foot care and adequate hydration should be encouraged and exercise in extreme temperatures should be avoided.[74]

Nephropathy

During and immediately after acute exercise the albuminuria excretion rate increases. This effect has been associated with the rise in systolic blood pressure during exercise.[75] No evidence is available to suggest this acute effect leads to renal impairment in the long term. With a cohort of 372 people with type 2 diabetes, Calle-Pascual et al[76] evaluated the effect of regular physical activity on the appearance of microalbuminuria. Results revealed the presence of normoalbuminuria is related to level of physical activity when corrected for blood pressure, duration of diabetes and glycaemic control. The higher the activity level, the higher the prevalence of normoalbuminuria.

At present it is generally recommended that people with nephropathy should avoid high-intensity strenuous physical activity,[77] but light- to moderate-intensity activity is safe and should be encouraged in this patient group.

Physical activity promotion

Despite substantial evidence showing potential health benefits of frequent physical activity for people with type 2 diabetes, physical activity is rarely included as part of diabetes management. Ary et al[56] reported that although 75% of people with type 2 diabetes are advised to exercise regularly, only 20% receive instructions about the most beneficial type and amount of exercise. In comparison, 73% of people with type 2 diabetes receive dietary instructions. A recent survey of diabetes health care professionals showed that they spend little time educating patients about physical activity and advice given is grossly inadequate and unstructured.[78]

The question of how to promote physical activity in people with type 2 diabetes has received little attention. The majority of research examining the effects of physical activity on diabetes management has used structured exercise programmes in which one exercise mode applies to all participants. Patient compliance in these studies is often disappointing and little assessment of the effectiveness of these interventions in the long term has been made.

The recent position statement on exercise and type 2 diabetes published by the ACSM provides some information on ways to promote adoption and maintenance of physical activity in people with type 2 diabetes.[61] The position stand highlights the use of the transtheoretical model of behaviour change[79] as a helpful framework for describing and predicting behaviour change. This model, illustrated in Fig. 9.1, was adapted to exercise by Marcus[80] in 1992 and, in recent years, has encouraged the use of physical activity interventions tailored to the specific needs of the individual. The stage of change model proposes that individuals move through five stages of change when adopting a new behaviour. These stages have been labelled: precontemplation (do not intend to change), contemplation (intend to change), preparation (have made some changes), action (actively engaging in a new behaviour) and maintenance (sustaining change over time). Progression from one stage to another is not always linear; at any point individuals can relapse to a previous stage.

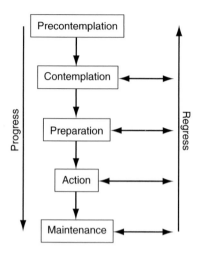

Figure 9.1 *Stage of exercise behaviour change*

Table 9.5 Appropriate strategies during each stage of exercise behaviour change

Stage of exercise behaviour change	Appropriate strategy
Precontemplation	Increase awareness of benefits of activity and risks of inactivity
Contemplation	Evaluation of expected or experienced benefits and costs of behaviour change
Preparation	Finding appropriate activities, realistic goal setting and developing social support
Action	Rewarding achievements, overcoming barriers
Maintenance	Varying activities, planning ahead to stay active

The stage of change model can be used to assess an individual's motivational readiness to become more active, and as a means of selecting appropriate cognitive behaviour strategies for the promotion of physical activity. Table 9.5 describes appropriate strategies to promote physical activity during each stage of exercise behaviour change.

This model has been applied successfully in the promotion of physical activity in the general population. In a randomized controlled trial, Marcus et al[81] compared the effectiveness of a self-help manual tailored to the individual's stage of exercise behaviour change with a standard self-help manual. Participants were 1559 employees from 11 manufacturing worksites. At one-month follow-up participants receiving the stage of behaviour change tailored intervention were significantly more likely to progress in stage of exercise behaviour change and in self reported physical activity levels. Movement within the stage of exercise behaviour change was significantly associated with changes in minutes of self-reported exercise per week.

In recent years, interventions to promote physical activity, based on the transtheoretical model, have been developed and implemented. One such intervention is motivational interviewing.[82] This intervention is described as a directive, client centred counselling style for helping clients examine and resolve ambivalence about behaviour change.[82] Motivational interviewing was originally developed to change problematic behaviours. Motivational interviewing explores conflicting feelings concerning a particular behaviour. Using reflective listening and open-ended questions an individual is encouraged to express self-motivational statements, problem solve their own barriers to change and formulate personal goals. Motivational interviewing is generally aimed at people in precontemplation and contemplation stages of change, where ambivalence to change is at its greatest.

Research on motivational interviewing has been focused mainly among addictive behaviours. In recent years reports of successful applications have emerged from studies of behavioural weight control programmes for people with type 2 diabetes and physical activity promotion interventions

A recent randomized pilot study examined the effectiveness of adding motivational interviewing strategies to a behavioural weight control programme for women with type 2 diabetes.[83] Participants who received motivational interviewing strategies had significantly better attendance, submitted more self-monitoring diaries, monitored their blood glucose more often and achieved better glucose control following treatment. Self-reported frequency of exercise and recording of caloric intake also improved, although not significantly. Harland et al[84] investigated the effectiveness of brief or intensive motivational interviewing, with or without financial incentive to promote physical activity. The proportion of participants reporting increased physical activity at 12 weeks was significantly greater in all intervention groups compared with controls. The proportion of participants increasing their activity did not differ between groups receiving brief or intensive motivational interviewing. However, a greater proportion of participants who received a combination of financial incentives and intensive interviewing increased their physical activity compared to other intervention groups.

Reported short-term increases in physical activity at 12 weeks were not maintained at one year, regardless of the intensity of intervention. The author concluded that brief interventions to promote physical activity are of questionable effectiveness. These conclusions should be interpreted with caution. Recently, Dunn et al recommended that a shift of 20 to 30% of sedentary people meeting minimum activity guidelines would be a major public health achievement.[85] In this study, 26% of the intervention group had increased physical activity at one year, although it is unclear whether they were meeting the current 1995 exercise guidelines recommended by the ACSM/CDC.[59] Furthermore, individuals in the control group received feedback of objective results (blood pressure, BMI, activity level, aerobic capacity, smoking and alcohol consumption), which is a motivational interviewing strategy and resulted in 23% of control increasing their physical activity at one year. This may have diluted the effect of motivational interviewing in the intervention group. Several additional limitations are inherent in this study and it is clear that further research is required to accurately assess the effectiveness of motivational interviewing on the promotion and maintenance of physical activity.

Exercise consultation is a relatively new cognitive behaviour intervention developed by Loughlan and Mutrie.[86] Similar to motivational interviewing, exercise consultation is an individualized counselling intervention which incorporates reflective listening, reviewing current physical activity behaviour, decisional balancing, social support and the development of realistic physical activity goals. Table 9.6 illustrates potential areas covered during an exercise consultation.

There are several important differences between the two interventions. Motivational interviewing is aimed primarily at individuals in precontemplation or contemplation stages of behaviour change. Miller states that motivational interviewing is most effective to 'start the process of change' and additional strategies are required to 'make the change'.[82] In comparison, exercise consultation is aimed at individuals in contemplation and preparation stages of behaviour change: individuals who are ready to change exercise behaviour. During exercise consultation the counsellor gives advice to the client, whereas during motivational interviewing the counsellor plays a passive role and encourages the participant to present their own arguments and strategies for change. Finally, exercise consultation does not focus on developing a long-term relationship; exercise consultations tend to be delivered in a single session lasting 20 to 30 minutes. Motivational interviewing involves a series of sessions and focuses on developing the participant's communication skills.

A number of well-conducted, randomized controlled trials have investigated the effectiveness of an exercise consultation process in middle- and older-aged adults in the general population.[87–89] Consistent findings from these studies provide strong evidence for the development of cognitive behavioural skills and the use of an exercise consultation process in physical activity promotion.

Research comparing the effectiveness of fitness assessment, exercise consultation and physical activity information alone demonstrated that at one year post-intervention only those participants receiving an

Table 9.6 Example of an exercise consultation

Decision balance table

Gains	Losses
1. Improve diabetes control	1. Time
2. Lose weight	2. Money
3. Feel fitter	

- Go through benefits of physical activity. Attempt to overcome perceived losses (time management, low cost activities)

Barriers to physical activity

Barriers	Strategies to overcome barriers
1. Physical discomfort from exercise	1. Individual exercise prescription avoids exercise which causes discomfort
2. Frightened of having hypos	2. Education on how to avoid hypos

Table 9.6 continued

3. Too overweight to exercise

4. Lack of support

3. Prescribe non-weight-bearing exercise. Possible initial home-based exercise programme to enhance confidence

4. Seek out social support (family and friends)

- Assess current/past physical activity status
- Go through current ACSM and ACSM/CDC exercise guidelines
- Look at potential activities

Goal setting

1 month	**3 months**	**6 months**
1. Walk back from work (5–10 minutes) at least 3 days/week	1. Increase walking to accumulate at least 30 minutes/day, 5 days/week	1. Complete sponsored 3 km walk

- Address issues of relapse prevention (indoor activities for wet days, ways to get back to exercise after holidays)
- Exercise and diabetes (avoiding hypos, foot care)

exercise consultation reported significantly more physical activity than at baseline. In addition, the exercise consultation was the preferred intervention among sedentary members of the general public.[87]

Calfas et al[88] investigated the effect of brief physician-led exercise counselling, compared to standard information on promoting physical activity. Consistent findings were recorded, with five out of the six physical activity measures recording significantly higher physical activity levels from baseline to 4 weeks follow-up in the experimental group compared to controls. In a similar large randomized controlled trial, Steptoe et al[89] evaluated the effectiveness of including brief, nurse-led behavioural counselling on healthy behaviour and cardiovascular risk factors in people with one or more modifiable cardiovascular risk factors. The intervention was stage of change tailored, incorporating the development of cognitive behavioural skills and targeting three health behaviours (smoking, diet and physical activity). Participants receiving behavioural counselling recorded favourable improvements in diet, physical activity and smoking habits at 4 and 12 months from baseline assessment, compared to controls. No significant difference, however, was found in cardiovascular risk factors.

Current research provides modest support for the use of exercise consultation for physical activity promotion in diabetic populations. A study of 34 people with type 1 diabetes showed significant improvements in physical activity levels at 30 days using exercise consultation.[90] A recent randomized, controlled trial of 26 people with type 2 diabetes assessed the effectiveness of exercise consultation compared to standard exercise information in promoting physical activity levels at 30 days. Self-report and electronic monitoring were used to assess physical activity levels. The study also assessed resultant quality of life. Participation in sport and exercise increased by 55% in the experimental group and decreased by 6% in control participants. Total physical activity counts per week increased by 3% in the experimental group and decreased by 9% in controls. A significantly greater number of patients receiving a consultation increased their stage of exercise behaviour change compared to controls. A positive trend in the experimental group compared to controls was apparent in most subscales of both quality of life questionnaires.[91] Both studies reported similar results, however they incorporated small patient numbers and short follow-up periods. Prospective research with significant numbers is required to assess the effectiveness of developing cognitive behavioural skills for the promotion of physical activity in diabetic populations.

Summary and conclusions

A substantial amount of evidence supports the hypothesis that regular, frequent physical activity and exercise have the potential to provide important health benefits for people with type 2 diabetes. What is unclear is how we promote physical activity in this population. In view of the complexity of type 2 diabetes, its complications and their effect on exercise capacity, an individualized physical activity prescription is undoubtedly required. An individualized physical activity prescription taking into account existing medical complications will help to maximize the benefits of physical activity and minimize the risks. This will in turn enhance adherence.

It is critical that physical activity behaviour changes are maintained. Although structured exercise programmes have been shown to be effective in the short term at increasing physical activity levels and providing important health benefits, these programmes are often time-consuming, reach a limited number of people and are relatively ineffective in the long term. Interventions that help people with type 2 diabetes to become more physically active and maintain this behaviour change in the long term are required.

Cognitive behavioural interventions such as motivational interviewing and exercise consultation have increasingly been shown to be effective at promoting and maintaining physical activity behaviour in the general population. These interventions have potential to be effective in a diabetes population. They allow for an individualized exercise prescription taking into account the individual's disease and motivational state. Cognitive behavioural strategies can be developed to help maintain physical activity behaviour change and education can be given to avoid adverse effects of exercise in diabetes. Finally, these interventions are relatively inexpensive and have the potential to reach a large number of people. With minimal training, cognitive behavioural interventions could be conducted by an existing member of the diabetes team or by an exercise physiologist. Further research is required to assess the effectiveness and acceptability of this intervention in routine diabetes management.

References

1. US Department of Health & Human Services; Public Health Service; Centers for Disease Control & Prevention; National Center for Chronic Disease Prevention & Health Promotion, Division of Nutrition & Physical Activity. Promoting Physical Activity: A Guide for Community Action. Human Kinetics, Champaign, IL, 1999.
2. Casperson CJ, Powell KE, Christenson GM. Physical activity, exercise and physical fitness: definitions and distinctions for health related research. Public Health Reports 1985;100:126–31.
3. Tuomilehto J, Lindstrom J, Eriksson J et al. Prevention of Type 2 diabetes mellitus by changes in lifestyle among subjects with impaired glucose tolerance. N Engl J Med 2001;344:1343–50.
4. Diabetes Prevention Program Research Group. Reduction in the incidence of Type 2 diabetes with lifestyle of metformin. N Engl J Med 2002;346:393–403.
5. Minuk H, Vranic M, Marliss E et al. Glucoregulatory and metabolic response to exercise in obese non insulin diabetes. Am J Physiol 1981;240:E458–64.
6. Glacca A, Groenewoud Y, Tsui E et al. Glucose production, utilisation, and cycling in response to moderate exercise in obese subjects with Type 2 diabetes and mild hyperglycaemia. Diabetes 1998;47:1763–70.
7. Larsen J, Dela F, Kjaer M, Galbo H. The effect of moderate exercise on postprandial glucose homeostasis in NIDDM patients. Diabetologia 1997;40:453.
8. Kjaer M, Hollenbeck C, Frey-Hewitt B et al. Glucoregulation and hormonal responses to maximal exercise in non-insulin-dependent diabetes. J Appl Physiol 1990;68:2067–74.
9. Devlin J, Hirshman M, Horton E, Horton E. Enhanced peripheral and splanchnic insulin sensitivity in NIDDM men after single bout of exercise. Diabetes 1987;36:434–9.

10. Braun B, Zimmermann M, Kretchmer N. Effects of exercise intensity on insulin sensitivity in women with non-insulin-dependent diabetes mellitus. J Appl Physiol 1995;78:300–306.

11. Usui K, Yamanouchi K, Asai K et al. The effect of low intensity bicycle exercise on the insulin-induced glucose uptake in obese patients with Type 2 diabetes. Diabetes Res Clin Pract 1998;41:57–61.

12. Heath G, Gavin J, Hinderliter J et al. Effects of exercise and lack of exercise on glucose tolerance and insulin sensitivity. J Appl Physiol 1983;55:512–7.

13. Trovati M, Carta Q, Cavalot F et al. Influence of physical training on blood glucose control, glucose tolerance, insulin secretion, and insulin action in non-insulin dependent diabetic patients. Diabetes Care 1984;7:416–20.

14. Walker K, Piers L, Putt R et al. Effects of regular walking on cardiovascular risk factors and body composition in normoglycemic women and women with type 2 diabetes. Diabetes Care 1999;22:555–61.

15. Raz I, Hauser E, Bursztyn M. Moderate exercise improves glucose metabolism in uncontrolled elderly patients with non-insulin-dependent diabetes mellitus. Israel J Med Sci 1994;30:766–70.

16. Honkola A, Forsen T, Eriksson J. Resistance training improves the metabolic profile in individuals with type 2 diabetes. Acta Diabetol 1997;34:245–8.

17. Fujinuma H, Abe R, Yamazaki T et al. Effect of exercise training on doses of oral agents and insulin. Diabetes Care 1999;22:1754–5.

18. Kevorkian G. Effects of exercise on the insulin levels in diabetics. J Vis Impair Blind 1986;80:954–5.

19. Skarfors E, Wegener T, Selinus I. Physical training as treatment for Type 2 (non-insulin-dependent) diabetes in elderly men. A feasibility study over 2 years. Diabetologia 1987;30:930–3.

20. Ligtenberg P, Hoekstra J, Bol E et al. Effects of physical training on metabolic control in elderly type 2 diabetes mellitus patients. Clin Sci 1997;93:127–35.

21. Barnard J, Jung T, Inkeles S. Diet and exercise in the treatment of NIDDM. Diabetes Care 1994;17:1469–72.

22. Taniguchi A, Fukushima M, Sakai M et al. Effect of physical training on insulin sensitivity in Japanese Type 2 diabetic patients. Diabetes Care 2000;23:857–60.

23. Lehmann R, Vokac A, Niedermann K et al. Loss of abdominal fat and improvement of the cardiovascular risk profile by regular moderate exercise training in patients with NIDDM. Diabetologia 1995;38:1313–19.

24. Brandenburg S, Reush J, Bauer T et al. Effect of exercise training on oxygen uptake kinetic responses in women with Type 2 diabetes. Diabetes Care 1999;22:1640–6.

25. Aliev T, Abdullaev N, Mirza-Zade V, Knyazev Y. Role of exercise in rehabilitation of coronary heart disease in cases combined with non insulin-dependent diabetes mellitus. Sports Med Train Rehabil 1993;4:53–5.
26. Mourier A, Gautier J, Kerviler E et al. Mobilisation of visceral adipose tissue related to the improvement in insulin sensitivity in response to physical training in NIDDM. Diabetes Care 1997;20:385–91.
27. Lightenberg PC, Godaert GLR, Hillenaar F, Hoekstra JBL. Influence of a physical training program on psychological well-being in elderly Type 2 diabetes patients. Diabetes Care 1998; 21:2196–7.
28. Blair SN, Kampert J, Kohl H et al. Influences of cardiorespiratory fitness and other precursors on cardiovascular disease and all-cause mortality in men and women. JAMA 1996;276:205–10.
29. Ming W, Gibbons L, Kampert J et al. Low cardiorespiratory fitness and physical inactivity as predictors of mortality in men with Type 2 diabetes. Ann Intern Med 2000;132:605–11.
30. Kohl H, Gordon N, Villegas J, Blair SN. Cardiorespiratory fitness, glycemic status, and mortality risk in men. Diabetes Care 1992;15:184–91.
31. Vanninen E, Uusitupa M, Remes J et al. Relationship between hyperglycaemia and aerobic power in men with newly diagnosed type 2 (non insulin-dependent) diabetes. Clin Physiol 1992;12:667–77.
32. Katoh J, Hara Y, Kurusu M et al. Cardiorespiratory function as assessed by exercise testing in patients with non-insulin-dependent diabetes mellitus. J Int Med Res 1996;24:209–13.
33. Regensteiner J, Bauer T, Reush J et al. Abnormal oxygen uptake kinetic response in women with type II diabetes mellitus. J Appl Physiol 1998;85:310–7.
34. Regensteiner J, Sippel J, McFarling E et al. Effects of non-insulin-dependent diabetes on oxygen consumption during treadmill exercise. Med Sci Sports Exercise 1994;27:875–81.
35. Wei M, Gibbons L, Mitchell T et al. The association between cardiorespiratory fitness and impaired fasting glucose and Type 2 diabetes mellitus in men. Ann Intern Med 1999;130:89–96.
36. Roy T, Peterson H, Snider H et al. Autonomic influence on cardiovascular performance in diabetic subjects. Am J Med 1989;87:382–8.
37. Liang P, Hughes V, Fukagawa V, Naomi F. Increased prevalence of mitochondrial DNA deletions in skeletal muscle of older individuals with impaired glucose tolerance: possible marker of glycaemic stress. Diabetes 1997;46:920–3.
38. Simoneau J, Kelley D. Altered glycolytic and oxidative capacities of skeletal muscle contribute to insulin resistance in NIDDM. J Appl Physiol 1997;83:166–71.
39. Khan S, Rupp J. The effect of exercise conditioning, diet, and drug therapy on glycosylated hemoglobin levels in type 2 (NIDDM) diabetics. J Sports Med Phys Fitness 1995;35:281–8.

40. Stewart A, Hays R, Wells K et al. Long-term functioning and well-being outcomes associated with physical activity and exercise in patients with chronic conditions in the medical outcomes study. J Clin Epidemiol 1994;47:719–30.

41. Glasgow R, Ruggiero L, Eakin E et al. Quality of life and associated characteristics in a large national sample of adults with diabetes. Diabetes Care 1997;20:562–7.

42. Krug L, Haire-Joshu D, Heady S. Exercise habits and exercise relapse in persons with non-insulin-dependent diabetes mellitus. Diabetes Educ 1991;17:185–8.

43. Hays L, Clark D. Correlates of physical activity in a sample of older adults with Type 2 diabetes. Diabetes Care 1999;22:706–12.

44. Ford E, Herman W. Leisure-time physical activity patterns in the US diabetic population: findings from the 1990 National Health Interview Survey. Diabetes Care 1995;18:27–33.

45. Anderson R, Fitzgerald J, Oh M. The relationship between diabetes-related attitudes and patients' self-reported adherence. Diabetes Educ 1993;19:287–92.

46. Swift C, Armstrong J, Beerman K et al. Attitudes and beliefs about exercise among persons with non-insulin-dependent diabetes. Diabetes Educ 1995;21:533–40.

47. Rosenstock IM. Historical origins of the health belief model. Health Educ Monogr 1974;2:1–9.

48. Kingery P, Glasgow R. Self-efficacy and outcomes expectations in the self-regulation of non-insulin dependent diabetes mellitus. Health Educ 1989;20:13–19.

49. Padgett D. Correlates of self-efficacy beliefs among patients with non-insulin dependent diabetes mellitus in Zagreb, Yugoslavia. Patient Educ Couns 1991;18:139–47.

50. Wilson W, Ary D, Bigard A et al. Psychosocial predictors of self-care behaviours (compliance) and glycemic control in non-insulin-dependent diabetes mellitus. Diabetes Care 1986;9:614–22.

51. Dishman RK, Ickes W. Self-motivation and adherence to therapeutic exercise. J Behav Med 1981;4:421–38.

52. Martin JE, Dubbert PM, Katell AD et al. Behavioural control of exercise in sedentary adults. J Consult Clin Psychol 1984;52:795–811.

53. King AC, Blair SN, Bild DE et al. Determinants of physical activity and interventions in adults. Med Sci Sports Exercise 1992;24:S221.

54. Guion WK, Carter CA, Corwin SJ. Knowledge of exercise in patients with diabetes mellitus. Med Sci Sports Exercise 2000;31:S361.

55. Wankel LM. Decision-making and social-support strategies for increasing exercise involvement. J Card Rehab 1984;4:124–35.

56. Ary D, Toobert D, Wilson W, Glasgow R. Patient perspective on factors contributing to non-adherence to diabetes regimens. Diabetes Care 1986;9:168–72.

277

57. Marsden E. The role of exercise in the well-being of people with insulin dependent diabetes mellitus: perceptions of patients and health professionals. 1996. Thesis/dissertation, University of Glasgow, Glasgow.

58. American College of Sports Medicine. Position stand on the recommended quality and quantity of exercise for developing and maintaining cardiorespiratory and muscular fitness in healthy adults. Med Sci Sports Exercise 1990;22:265–74.

59. Pate R, Pratt M, Blair S et al. Physical activity and public health: a recommendation from the Centers for Disease Control and prevention and the American College of Sports Medicine. JAMA 1995;273:402–407.

60. Weyer C, Linkeschowa R, Heise T et al. Implications of the traditional and the new ACSM Physical Activity Recommendations on weight reduction in dietary treated obese subjects. Int J Obes 1998;22:1071–8.

61. American College of Sports Medicine. Exercise and type 2 diabetes. Med Sci Sports Exercise 2000;32:1345–60.

62. Wallace J. Obesity. In: American College of Sports Medicine, ed. Exercise Management for Persons with Chronic Diseases and Disabilities. Human Kinetics, Leeds, 1997:106–11.

63. American Diabetes Association. Diabetes mellitus and exercise. Diabetes Care 2001;24:S51.

64. Balkau B, Jouven X, Ducimetiere P, Eschwege E. Diabetes as a risk factor for sudden death. Lancet 1999;354:1968–9.

65. Janand-Delenne B, Savin B, Habib G et al. Silent myocardial ischemia in patients with diabetes. Diabetes Care 1999;22:1396–400.

66. Cruickshanks K, Moss S, Klein R, Klein B. Physical activity and proliferative retinopathy in people diagnosed with diabetes before age 30 yrs. Diabetes Care 1992;15:1267–72.

67. Bernbaum M, Albert S, Cohen J, Drimmer A. Cardiovascular conditioning in individuals with diabetic retinopathy. Diabetes Care 1989;12:740–2.

68. Graham C, McCarthey P. Exercise options for persons with diabetic complications. Diabetes Educ 1990;16:212–20.

69. Hiatt W, Regensteiner J, Hargarten M et al. Benefit of exercise conditioning for patients with peripheral arterial disease. Circulation 1989;81:602-609.

70. Hilstead J, Galbo H, Christensen N. Impaired cardiovascular responses to graded exercise in diabetic autonomic neuropathy. Diabetes 1979;28:313–19.

71. Kahn J, Sisson J, Vinik A. QT interval prolongation and sudden cardiac death in diabetic autonomic neuropathy. J Clin Endocrinol Metab 1986;64:751–4.

72. Borg GAV. Psychophysical bases of perceived exertion. Med Sci Sports Exercise 1982;14:377–81.

73. Tantucci C, Bottini P, Dottorini L et al. Ventilatory response to exercise in diabetic subjects with autonomic neuropathy. J Appl Physiol 1996;81:1978–86.

74. Albright A. Exercise precautions and recommendations for patients with autonomic neuropathy. Diabetes Spectr 1998;11:231–7.

75. Dahlquist G, Aperia A, Carlsson L et al. Effect of metabolic control and duration on exercise induced albuminuria in diabetic teenagers. Acta Paediatr Scand 1983;72:895–902.

76. Calle-Pascual A, Martin-Alvarez P, Reyes C, Calle J. Regular physical activity and reduced occurrence of microalbuminuria in Type 2 diabetic patients. Diabetes Metab 2001;19:304–309.

77. Mogensen C. Nephropathy: early. In: Ruderman N, Devlin J, eds. The Health Professionals Guide to Diabetes and Exercise. American Diabetes Association, Alexandria, 1995:164–74.

78. Berlanga F, Eltringham-Cox A, Burr W, Nagi D. Physical activity in Type 2 diabetes. Its role and the current care pattern: a survey of diabetes health care professionals in the UK. Pract Diabetes Int 2000;17:60–1.

79. Proshaska J, Diclemente C. Stages and processes of self-change in smoking: towards an integrative model of change. J Consult Clin Psychol 1983;51:390–5.

80. Marcus B, Rossi J, Selby V et al. The stages and processes of exercise adoption and maintenance in a worksite sample. Health Psychol 1992;11:386–95.

81. Marcus BH, Emmons KM, Simkin-Silverman LR et al. Evaluation of motivationally tailored vs. standard self-help physical activity interventions at the workplace. Am J Health Prom 1998;12:246–53.

82. Miller W, Rollnick S. Motivational Interviewing: Preparing People to Change Addictive Behaviour. The Guilford Press, New York, 2001.

83. Smith D, Heckemeyer C, Kratt P, Manson D. Motivational interviewing to improve adherence to a behavioural weight-control program for older obese women with NIDDM. Diabetes Care 1997;20:52–4.

84. Harland J, White M, Drinkwater C et al. The Newcastle exercise project: a randomised controlled trial of methods to promote physical activity in primary care. BMJ 1999;319:828–32.

85. Dunn AL, Marcus BH, Kampert JB et al. Comparison of lifestyle and structured interventions to increase physical activity and cardiorespiratory fitness. JAMA 1999;281:327–34.

86. Loughlan C, Mutrie N. Conducting an exercise consultation: guidelines for health professionals. J Inst Health Educ 1995;33:78–82.

87. Loughlan C, Mutrie N. An evaluation of the effectiveness of the three interventions in promoting physical activity in a sedentary population. Health Educ J 1997;65:154–65.

88. Calfas K, Sallis J, Olderburg B, French M. Mediators of change in physical activity following an intervention in primary care: PACE. Prevent Med 1997;26:297–304.

89. Steptoe A, Doherty S, Rink E et al. Behavioural counselling in general practice for the promotion of healthy behaviour amoung adults at

increased risk of coronary heart disease: a randomised trial. BMJ 1999;319:943–8.

90. Hasler T, Fisher BM, MacIntyre P, Mutrie N. Exercise consultation and physical activity in patients with Type 1 diabetes. Pract Diabetes Int 2000;17:44–8.

91. Kirk AF, Higgins LA, Hughes A et al. A randomised controlled trial to study the effect of exercise consultation on the promotion of physical activity in people with Type 2 diabetes: a pilot study. Diabet Med 2001;18:877–83.

chapter 10

Managing heart disease and diabetes in primary care: applying the evidence in practice

Alastair Emslie-Smith, Jon Dowell and Frank Sullivan

Introduction

The evidence laid out in the preceding chapters of this book presents a formidable challenge for all health professionals working in primary care as they seek to provide effective care to their patients with diabetes. We will discuss some theoretical aspects of diabetic care from a primary medical care perspective then describe regional, local and consultation-based approaches to meeting those challenges.

At least 2% of the patients on a practice list have diabetes (Table 10.1). The prevalence of diabetes is steadily rising, as is the complexity of the health-care interventions that we are required to provide for this group of patients as our understanding of the cardiovascular risk associated with diabetes deepens. For many chronic conditions in primary care, the 'rule of halves' obtains: half of all affected patients

Table 10.1 Implications of diabetes

- Diabetes is common—2% of the population overall, 4% of those aged over 35, 10–20% of those over 65.
- The prevalence of type 2 diabetes may double in the next 10 years due to an ageing and increasingly obese population[1]
- Up to 50% of patients already have vascular complications by the time of diagnosis, early detection of the disease is therefore crucial, yet 50% of those with diabetes are still undiagnosed[2]
- Type 2 diabetes costs the UK NHS £1.83 billion/year (4.2% of its total budget); 41% of this is spent on the inpatient care of late complications and only 11% in primary care[3]
- Increasing evidence shows that tight glycaemic and blood pressure control prevents vascular complications, but that multiple drug regimes will often be needed to achieve this[4-6]
- New approaches to treatment and pharmaceutical developments (e.g. use of ramipril for primary cardiovascular prevention[7,8] and new drugs to combat obesity and smoking) add further opportunities, challenges and dilemmas to our practice
- Patients with both type1[9] and type 2[10] diabetes are very poor at adhering to drug regimes
- Diabetes care is prominent in the current emphasis on quality and clinical governance within primary care
- There is an increasing shift in emphasis towards primary care and community provision of diabetes services

are unknown to the practice, of those who are known, only half are being treated (25%) and of the treated patients only half are effectively controlled (12.5%)[11](Fig. 10.1).

With recent changes in the criteria for diagnosis of diabetes,[12] and ever more rigorous standards of control proposed,[13] the situation in diabetes is uncertain, but unlikely to be better than that described by

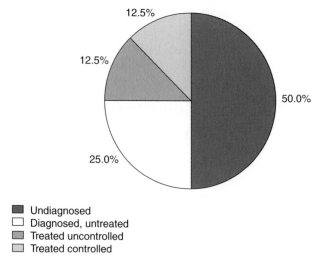

Fig. 10.1 *The rule of halves*

this axiom. Recent studies in Tayside, UK have shown that less than 20% of diabetic patients obtain sufficient blood glucose monitoring strips to test themselves daily[14] and that less than a third of patients redeem sufficient prescriptions for oral hypoglycaemic agents to take their medication as directed.[10]

Diabetes also accounts for an increasing amount of doctor and nurse consultations in primary care because of the health problems experienced by this group compared to the unaffected population and the shift from hospital to primary care for many patients. A study in Trent, UK demonstrated a doubling of service provision in primary care between 1990 and 1995.[15]

To minimize the development of cardiovascular complications in our practice diabetic populations, efforts in primary care must be concentrated in three main areas:

■ Early and accurate diagnosis of diabetes.
■ Structured and organized assessment, monitoring and management of all patients with diabetes, both at practice level and in an

integrated way with all other health professionals caring for people with diabetes in the locality.

■ The development of techniques to maximize adherence to advice and treatment recommendations in patients with diabetes.

Early and accurate diagnosis of diabetes in primary care

The WHO criteria for the diagnosis of diabetes[12] have recently been adopted in the UK, and for most primary care clinicians the diagnosis in acute presentations is fairly clear-cut, guided by their local laboratory colleagues[16] (Table 10.2).

Table 10.2 Algorithm for the diagnosis of diabetes

1. Classical symptoms (e.g. polyuria, polydipsia, unexplained weight loss) plus one of the following:

■ random venous plasma glucose concentration ≥ 11.1 mmol/l
   or

■ fasting venous plasma glucose concentration ≥ 7.0 mmol/l
   or

■ venous plasma glucose concentration ≥ 11.1 mmol/l (2 hour sample in oral glucose tolerance test)

2. No symptoms, i.e. incidental finding of glycosuria or hyperglycaemia

■ Diagnosis should not be based on a single venous plasma glucose measurement

■ Additional testing on another day with a value in the diabetic range is essential (using either fasting or random values, or samples taken 2 hours following glucose load)

■ If fasting or random values are not diagnostic, the 2-hour value should be used

> **Table 10.3 Presentations of diabetes in primary care**
>
> **Classical symptoms:**
> thirst, polyuria, polydipsia, nocturia, tiredness, weight loss, pruritis, skin infection
>
> **Investigation of related conditions:**
> vascular occlusion, renal impairment, visual impairment, erectile dysfunction, paraesthesia, cranial nerve palsy

The diagnosis may be considered in symptomatic patients without classical symptoms, during investigation of related conditions or as an unexpected finding of glycosuria or hyperglycaemia (Table 10.3). The sensitivity and specificity of the different tests will be influenced by the prior probability of disease, which varies according to the patient's clinical state, age, sex, ethnic group and other therapies.

Screening for diabetes

Up to 50% of people with diabetes already have complications by the time they are diagnosed.[17] Early detection of diabetes is most important. It therefore might be concluded that the widespread screening for diabetes in the adult population should be a worthwhile exercise. Conversely, Goyder and Irwig have argued that in the absence of good trials demonstrating benefit, there should be 'a move from screening for the disease itself to screening for risk factors'.[18] The periodic, opportunistic, screening of high-risk patients, preferably by measurement of fasting plasma glucose, including those who are obese, of Asian or Afro-Caribbean origin, or who have a family history of diabetes or a past history of gestational diabetes, is good practice. Recent WHO guidelines on the diagnostic criteria for diabetes recommend subsequent annual fasting plasma glucose measurements for people shown by oral glucose tolerance testing to have impaired glucose tolerance (IGT = fasting plasma glucose < 7.0 mmol/l; 2 hour (post-glucose) ≥ 7.8 and < 11.1 mmol/l) or impaired fasting glucose (IFG = fasting plasma glucose 6.1–6.9 mmol/l; 2 hour (post-glucose) ≤ 7.8 mmol/l).

Test performance characteristics in different patient groups are also important when considering screening for diabetes.[19] The purpose of screening is to enable us to prevent ill-health in those with occult disease.[20] Hyperglycaemia doubles the 5-year risk of a cardiovascular event.[21] The high levels of cardiovascular and other complications in diabetic patients have prompted many to propose a variety of blood and urine screening tests for populations arguing that earlier diagnosis and hence earlier treatment might reduce the complications.[22–24] There is evidence that microvascular complications are reduced by early diagnosis, but for the macrovascular disease the control of other risk factors, e.g. hypertension, may be most important.

Structured/organized care

At practice level
Greenhalgh's 1994 thesis[25] that the features of well structured care were the three Rs of:

1. Registration
2. Recall
3. Regular review

has recently been vindicated by a systematic review conducted by Griffin[26] on five trials which randomised 38%[27] to 88%[28] of clinic attendees to continuing hospital care or shared care. This review concluded that

'Unstructured care in the community is associated with poorer follow up, greater mortality and worse glycaemic control than hospital care. Computerised central recall, with prompting for patients and their family doctors, can achieve standards of care as good or better than hospital outpatient care, at least in the short term. The evidence supports provision of regular prompted recall and review of people with diabetes by willing general practitioners and demonstrates that this can be achieved, if suitable organisation is in place.'

A systematic approach to the provision of diabetic care in the practice provides benefits for patients and staff alike:

- A team approach is vital, involving GPs, nurses and support staff who are interested, motivated and committed to providing a high standard of care.
- Agreed practice protocols must be developed and regularly reviewed, clearly identifying the roles and responsibilities of the different members of the practice team in recall, monitoring, treatment and education.
- Protected time, as in dedicated mini-clinics, allows appropriate time and attention to be given to the monitoring, care, education and support of patients with diabetes. Relationships and trust built up by medical and nursing staff with patients and their families encourage attendance and compliance.
- A comprehensive register and an effective recall and follow-up system must be maintained, either manually or on computer, with capacity to identify clinic defaulters and irregular attendees. The development of central district registers can greatly assist practices in this, providing systems exist to regularly compare and update data held centrally with practice held information.
- A clear system of record keeping, using dedicated diabetes record inserts in the medical records or within the practice's computer system, is beneficial, allowing process and outcome measures to be compared over time.
- Standard patient information leaflets and educational materials should be adopted by the practice, ensuring the availability of consistent and high-quality information to patients.
- Involvement of community or practice-based podiatrists, dieticians and clinical psychologists in the practice diabetes team brings significant advantages.

Near patient testing

New technology allowing analysis of serum lipid levels and microal-buminuria in primary care gives the GP instant access to helpful clinical information during the consultation. Rigorous quality control and regular calibration with local laboratory standards is vital if such tools are to be used. Regular maintenance and calibration of glucose meters, including those owned by patients, is important. Unfortunately the cost of much useful equipment, e.g. HbA1c meters, is beyond the financial scope of most practices. The new NHS has yet to develop the infrastructure necessary to provide the quality control necessary for effective near patient testing.

Cardiovascular disease and the annual complications review

- A detailed history should be taken to elicit any symptoms of angina.
- The presence of left ventricular hypertrophy is a powerful predictor of the risk of a cardiovascular event—screening for LVH by electrocardiography would seem worthwhile, but is rarely carried out as part of routine reviews in practice.
- Structured medication review should maximize the pharmacological aspects of primary and secondary cardiovascular risk prevention (aspirin, ACE inhibitors, statins, beta-blockers, etc.) (see Chapter 7).
- Lifestyle advice, in relation to smoking, diet and aerobic exercise, is a key component (see Chapter 9).

Cardiovascular risk factor intervention

Over 70% of people with diabetes die from macrovascular disease and type 2 diabetes is compounded by the metabolic syndrome of hypertension, dyslipidaemia, insulin resistance and obesity. The importance of tight blood pressure, lipid and glycaemic control has been well demonstrated in recent large-scale clinical trials. The UKPDS demonstrated the clear benefit of obtaining a blood pressure of 144/82 mm Hg or less and that the use of angiotensin-converting enzyme inhibitors or beta-blockers was equally effective.[29] Up to 30% of diabetic patients with hypertension will require three or four different classes of antihypertensive in combination[30] (see Chapter 5). Such evidence as this places a responsibility on practitioners to develop methods of implementing and auditing evidence-based guidelines in this important area. For example, although people with diabetes benefit significantly from aspirin, beta-blockers, statins and angiotensin-converting enzyme inhibitors after myocardial infarction, a recent study has shown that these drugs are less likely to be commenced than in patients without diabetes.[31] Evidence from the HOPE (Heart Outcomes Prevention Evaluation) study demonstrated the major impact in lowering cardiovascular death (37% risk reduction) if patients with diabetes were treated with ramipril.[7] The introduction of practice pharmacist support and the availability of more sophisticated prescribing data makes this task easier. Negotiation by primary care groups for extra prescribing funds for specific quality areas such as hyperlipidaemia may also facilitate improvement, as will a structured approach by all members of the practice team to the problems of drug concordance.

Intensive and sustained advice on appropriate lifestyle, particularly in the areas of dietary change, aerobic exercise and smoking is crucial. Smoking has been shown to be an even more significant a risk factor for cardiovascular disease in those with diabetes than in the non-diabetic population.[32-35] Guidelines from the Health Education Authority (HEA)[36] recommend that:

- GPs continue to advise smokers opportunistically to stop smoking at least once a year, give advice on and/or prescribe effective medicines (NRT or bupropion (amfebutamone)) and refer patients to specialist cessation services where extra support is considered necessary. They should also record the response to that advice and arrange follow-up where appropriate.
- Primary health care teams and hospitals should create and maintain accessible records on the current smoking status of patients.
- The provision of NHS smokers' clinics should reflect the level of demand (at least one or two clinics per HA and more if demand increases).
- Practice nurses should be prepared to encourage known smokers to stop and offer help where possible.

- GPs and practice nurses should receive training to enable them to encourage patients to give up smoking and should be able to provide accurate advice on NRT and bupropion. There should be national standards for training and service provision to ensure minimum standards of delivery.
- Other healthcare professionals should be encouraged to ask patients about smoking and advise smokers to quit.
- More should be done to encourage pregnant women to stop smoking.

Concordance with lifestyle and risk factor advice is more likely if the whole family, rather than just the individual patient, is encouraged to make behavioural changes. This is particularly challenging when working with ethnic groups in whom the prevalence of diabetes is higher than the overall population. Different cultural norms and traditions, particularly in dietary areas, must be understood and addressed with patients in whom communication barriers may exist.

Identification of patients at the highest risk of developing cardiovascular events allows efforts and resources to be channelled most effectively. Coronary risk prediction charts and computer programs such as that produced as part of the 'Joint British Recommendations on Prevention of Coronary Heart Disease in Clinical Practice'[37] are helpful in this. However, recent work has demonstrated that calculations based on the Framingham risk equation, such as the Joint British Recommendations and the New Zealand tables, considerably underestimate the number of patients with both type 2 and, in particular, type 1 diabetes who are at medium and high risk of developing cardiovascular disease and who would benefit from primary prevention strategies.[38] This work highlights the need for the development of a more accurate model for calculating cardiovascular risk in patients with diabetes.

Integrated care

Effective diabetes care depends on a structured, co-ordinated and integrated regional service, with a close working partnership between all professionals involved, and with their patients.

Since the early 1970s, individual practices and localities have described systems of structured care, often referred to as 'shared care' which were designed to complement hospital diabetic services for those who attended hospital.[39] Community-based services have also tried to make services universally available to those who were unable or unwilling to attend secondary care (40–60% of the total).[40,41]

Different patterns of shared care have been described:

- shifted, where patients are simply discharged to primary care[42,43]
- prompted, where a system for ensuring recall of patients is ensured[27,28]
- truly shared, where resources move with the patient and a great deal of support for practices occurs before, during and after the change.[25]

The development of multi-disciplinary Local Diabetes Service Advisory Groups (LDSAGs) to co-ordinate an integrated approach is an encouraging model. Effective communication channels are essential to make clinical information available to all professionals involved in patient care. The development of regional diabetes IT networks has the potential to enhance this process, overcoming the disadvantages of the patient-held 'shared-care card' approach.

Clear guidelines concerning referral criteria between primary care and their colleague diabetologists, podiatrists and dieticians is crucial, along with a flexible, sensitive and patient-centred approach to the sharing of care, including ease and speed of access to specialist help and advice. Diabetes specialist nurses have a central role in this (Fig. 10.2).

Education and training

Continuing professional development in diabetes care is an important responsibility for clinicians. A comprehensive programme of training appropriate to the needs of all professionals involved in diabetes care is an integral part of any local diabetes care system. The 'workshop' approach, where new developments are shared, clinical problems and issues are raised and local guidelines are discussed, is a particularly useful model.

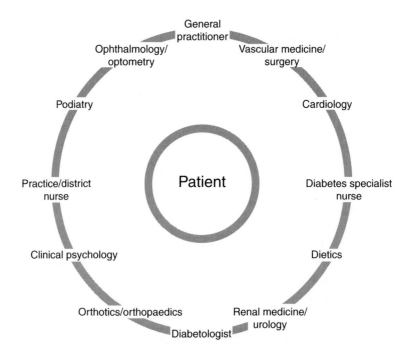

Fig. 10.2 *The ongoing care of patients with diabetes, in particular once they have developed vascular complications, involves a wide spectrum of health-care professionals*

Once within a structured care system, there is no shortage of evidence-based advice to primary care clinicians about how to treat the patients for whom they are responsible. Diabetes is a favourite condition for guideline developers. Of the first 40 guidelines produced by the Scottish Intercollegiate Guidelines Network (SIGN)[44] seven were on aspects of diabetes (Table 10.4), including guideline number 19 on the management of diabetic cardiovascular disease.[45] These have recently been superceded by an updated and expanded single National Guidelines for the Management of Diabetes (SIGN Guideline no. 55). It is essential that such national guidelines be adapted by local clinicians, perhaps within LDSAGs, to suit local needs. Guidelines produced and owned by local clinicians are more likely to be adopted and implemented to provide a common approach to the monitoring and treatment of diabetes and its complications.

Table 10.4 Scottish Intercollegiate Guidelines (SIGN) for diabetes care

SIGN 4: Prevention of visual impairment in diabetes and minimum dataset for collection in diabetes patients

SIGN 9: Management of diabetes in pregnancy

SIGN 10: Report on good practice in the care of children and young people with diabetes

SIGN 11: Management of diabetic renal disease

SIGN 12: Management of diabetic foot disease

SIGN 19: Management of diabetic cardiovascular disease

SIGN 25: Report on a recommended minimum dataset for collection in people with diabetes

SIGN 55: Management of Diabetes

Quality control and clinical governance

National Service Frameworks

The Department of Health in England and the Scottish Executive Health Department have both commissioned the development of Diabetes National Service Frameworks. The English Framework[46] seeks:

- To define practical, implementable and sustainable standards for the delivery of care, focused on the needs of people with diabetes, covering prevention, diagnosis, management and complications of type 1 and type 2 diabetes, and the management of diabetes in pregnancy.
- To ensure that top quality standards of care and treatment for diabetes are available in all primary care, local hospitals and specialist centres.
- To reduce unacceptable variations in care, while improving the overall quality of services.
- To pay particular heed to the needs of those who are disproportionately affected by diabetes, such as people from ethnic minority communities.

293

- To reduce the incidence of type 2 diabetes and improve the general health of all people with diabetes.
- To work jointly with partners on local delivery mechanisms, including health improvement programmes, long-term service agreements, clinical governance and local development plans.

Audit

The need to deliver high standards of diabetic care means that we must audit and monitor both process and outcome measures within our practice diabetic population. In local audit groups, professionals collaborate to share data and clinical information with one another, provide peer-group support and feedback to clinicians in a non-threatening, educative process, and to allow local targets and agreed standards to be developed. These help GPs to improve quality of care at practice level. Regional diabetes information technology networks and local audit facilitators can greatly assist this process. As an example, the SPICE PC (Scottish Programme for Improving Clinical Effectiveness in Primary Care) project[47] was recently developed by the Royal College of General Practitioners in Scotland (Table 10.5). This should allow general practitioners to audit and compare their quality of care with colleagues across the whole country, and will allow benchmarking of appropriate national quality standards to be developed. Other clinical governance and quality initiatives will serve a similar purpose.

Examples of innovative models of integrated diabetes care

The Tayside Regional Diabetes Network (Table 10.6)

There are approximately 11 000 people with diabetes (prevalence 2.5%) in the Tayside region of Scotland (population 391 000). The region is served by a major teaching hospital, two district general hospitals and 73 general practices. The DARTS (Diabetes Audit and Research in Tayside, Scotland) study began as a research project in 1996 whereby electronic linkage of a variety of data sources

Table 10.5 Scottish Programme for Improving Clinical Effectiveness in Primary Care (SPICE PC) audit criteria for type 2 diabetes

- Patients with type 2 diabetes under the age of 75 will have HbA1c measured annually
- Patients with type 2 diabetes will have an annual screening for eye problems according to locally agreed protocols
- Patients with type 2 diabetes will have an annual foot check according to locally agreed protocols
- Patients with type 2 diabetes will have an annual blood pressure check
- Where blood pressure is consistently greater than 140 systolic and/or 80 diastolic, attempts will be made to lower the blood pressure according to locally agreed protocols
- Patients with type 2 diabetes will have an annual check of serum creatinine and urinary protein
- Patients with type 2 diabetes will have an annual measurement of non-fasting total cholesterol
- Patients with type 2 diabetes will have an annual BMI measurement
- Patients with a BMI > 25 will have appropriate advice on diet and exercise
- All patients will be invited to attend a minimum of one educational session
- Smoking status will be recorded
- The practice will have an accurate computerized register that will include significant concomitant diseases, e.g. CHD, stroke, renal failure and long-term drugs for diabetes and chronic conditions

Table 10.6 Aims and objectives of the Tayside Regional Diabetes Network

- To provide comprehensive, patient-focused, integrated, seamless care for all people with diabetes, sensitive to local health needs, at the interface of the primary and secondary sectors, to achieve improved service and outcome for patients as well as efficient and effective use of resources
- To minimize premature morbidity and mortality in those with diabetes in Tayside
- To maximize quality of life by detecting and treating the disease and its complications at an early stage
- To provide equal access to high quality diabetes care for all the residents of Tayside
- To identify and register all those patients diagnosed with type 1 and type 2 diabetes in Tayside
- To foster close collaboration and communication among all health care professionals who care for people with diabetes in Tayside and to facilitate high quality diabetes care, research and audit
- To provide and assist with the analysis of data on various parameters at the individual, practice/clinic and regional level
- To provide education and evidence-based decision support mechanisms to patients, carers and health professionals involved in diabetes care in Tayside
- To develop and monitor professionally-led audit, evidence-based evaluation of practice and achievable quality standards for diabetes care in Tayside, within the context of the regional clinical governance framework

produced a comprehensive register of all patients with diabetes in the region.[48] The research project has subsequently developed into a major collaboration between primary and secondary care in

Tayside regional diabetes network

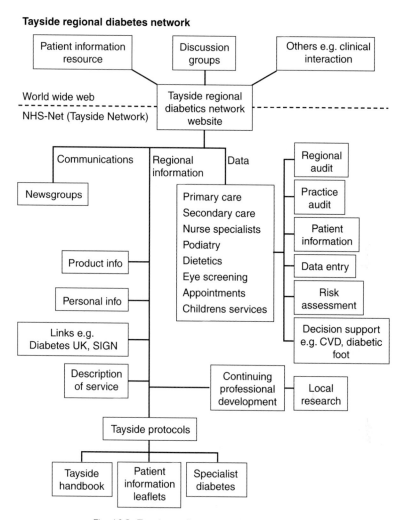

Fig. 10.3 *Topology of a managed clinical network*

Tayside to develop a powerful service tool. The register and information technology systems that have been developed to support it form the key part of a managed clinical network,[49] which facilitates comprehensive, integrated and seamless management of diabetes across the whole region (Fig. 10.3). The register receives information, electronically where possible, from primary and secondary care clinicians relating to their findings at diabetes monitoring and assessment appointments. It also has electronic links to the regional biochemistry database, the diabetic eye screening service, SMR data relating to hospital admissions and data relating to all encashed prescriptions within the region. A key component has been the work of nurse facilitators, who have visited each practice within the region to manually validate all primary care data.

In return, DARTS provides up-to-date feedback to clinicians in the region, showing aggregate practice or clinic-specific data for various process and outcome variables, comparing these with regional averages and, also, detailed patient-specific data highlighting process, outcome and reversible risk-factor analyses. Embedded within the system is a cardiovascular-risk calculator based on the Framingham risk equation. This high-quality audit and support system provides primary and secondary care clinicians with the information necessary to plan and target effective intervention to those patients at highest risk of developing vascular complications. In addition, the system acts as a prompt, to highlight patients who have not undergone monitoring and complication screening assessments within an agreed time-scale. Plans are in hand to develop a centralized recall system for primary care and an on-line appointment-booking system for hospital clinics.

In addition to this patient-specific information, which is encrypted, password protected and available only to clinicians via the NHS Intranet, a website[49] has been developed (Fig. 10.4). This provides a wide range of information for healthcare professionals in the form of an online diabetes handbook, developed in a collaborative exercise between primary and secondary care, containing locally adapted protocols and evidence-based guidelines for the management of all aspects of diabetes. For patients there is a wide variety of regularly updated patient information leaflets which guarantee the provision of accurate and consistent advice to patients with diabetes throughout the region.

The network is administered under the umbrella of the Tayside Diabetes Advisory Group (a local diabetes service advisory group),

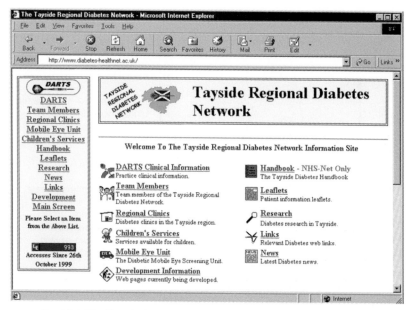

Fig. 10.4 *The Tayside Regional Diabetes Network website (www.diabetes-healthnet.ac.uk)*

which is made up of patients and healthcare professionals derived from all relevant disciplines. A subgroup composed of primary and secondary care clinicians takes responsibility for the ownership and appropriate use of the data within the register and for the development and self-regulation of audit and evidence-based quality standards for diabetes care across the region.

The Ladywood Community Diabetes Service (Fig. 10.5)

The Ladywood Primary Care Group is responsible for provision of primary care services in a highly deprived inner-city Birmingham constituency. The population of 126 000 includes 64% who are Asian or Afro-Caribbean. The prevalence of diabetes is over 4%, more than twice the national average. The population is served by a district general hospital, employing three diabetologists, and 38 general practices, mostly single-handed.

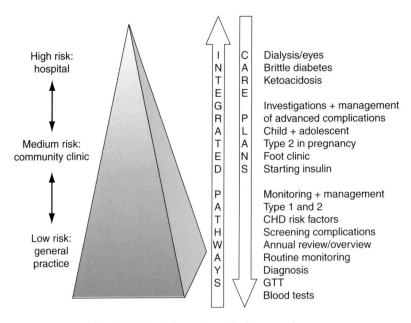

Fig. 10.5 *The Ladywood model of integrated care*

In 1998 the relatively small specialist hospital diabetes team were delivering many aspects of diabetes care to around 50% of the local diabetic population, overloading this service. Primary care provision for diabetes was unstructured in many cases. There was almost no dietetic or podiatry provision in the community. The level of diabetic care offered to the elderly, housebound and ethnic minorities was recognized as being poor, and there was wide variation in training and enthusiasm for diabetes care in general practice.

The service has been redesigned to provide systematic and integrated care for all people with diabetes in the locality. It aims to address these problems, recognizing the anticipated doubling in workload over the next 10 years and the need to improve the long-term health of patients with diabetes while also reducing the escalating costs of treating the complications of diabetes. The resulting model, The Ladywood Community Diabetes Service, has been cited as an example of good practice in *Testing Times*,[50], the Audit Commission's report on diabetes service provision in England and Wales.

The service utilizes integrated care pathways across primary and secondary care, supported by evidence-based clinical guidelines and served by a comprehensive computerized diabetes information system (the Westman Data Information System, developed in Salford) via the NHS NET. The diabetes information system (DIS) describes patients' access to services as they move between three levels of care, defined by clinical need. Clinical need is assessed according to the presence and degree of diabetes complications and cardiovascular risk. Those with low to moderate clinical need receive all diabetes care except for eye screening in general practice. Those with moderate to high need are in a shared-care arrangement between primary care and a consultant-led community clinic team based in a community diabetes clinic. This expert team advises and supports general practice colleagues with management guidance. The relatively small number of people with high to very high need receive a greater proportion of their diabetes care from hospital-based secondary and tertiary care services. The system is a fluid one, allowing people to move between these levels of care in a seamless way.

Each level offers activity appropriate to its degree of expertise and specialization, with the expert community team and hospital teams discharging to lower levels where clinically appropriate, with a management plan and guidelines for re-referral.

Each general practice wishing to provide diabetes services contracts with the primary care group to provide care to a contractual standard. The contract includes performance management targets for both the recording of information and the way in which it is used. Appropriate training, IT support and remuneration are provided to make that involvement possible. All general practices involved have had clinical staff trained to Certificate level on the University of Warwick Primary Diabetes Care Course. The course provides multidisciplinary training and reflects the issues surrounding the delivery of services in a multicultural context.

The Ladywood Community Diabetes Clinic is located in a large local health centre. It is staffed by an expert community team made up of a consultant diabetologist, diabetes specialist nurses, a dietitian with Asian language skills, a health care assistant and a senior podiatrist. As the service develops, GP diabetes intermediate specialists will be trained and appointed. The team has a key role in the continuing education, training and support of colleagues in primary care and people with diabetes and their carers.

The community clinic provides:

- A service that is patient centred, flexible, easily accessed and that provides a good level of continuity of care.
- Assessment and management advice for those:
  - □ with poor or deteriorating diabetes control
  - □ developing complications
  - □ with high cardiovascular risk
  - □ requiring complex changes in therapeutic regimes.
- A fast-track referral into the secondary or tertiary sectors.

Communication between general practice and the community team is paperless, with all examination findings, the results of investigations, an up-to-date list of co-existing medical problems and current medication entered on the DIS, as well as referral details and questions, advice and management plans.

New ideas on managing poor treatment use

Health care professionals may be tempted to believe that advocating management based upon evidence-based medicine is sufficient. Unfortunately, this is not so, and there is ample evidence that patients fail to follow medical advice and treatment adequately. Large, population-based studies in Tayside, Scotland, have demonstrated that poor compliance to insulin therapy in patients with type 1 diabetes[9] and to oral hypoglycaemic medication in patients with type 2 diabetes[10] is extremely common. In this respect, diabetes and cardiovascular disease are not atypical and there is a large literature on the topic of non-compliance or non-adherence. For overviews see Myers and

Midence,[51] Meichenbaum and Turk[52] or Sacket and Haynes.[53] This is a complex problem which remains poorly understood but is undoubtedly the major barrier to effective care. It is also one that may best be identified and managed in primary care where the majority of preventive care is supervised.

The notion that patients should passively accept and follow medical advice (comply) has been criticized on both ethical and practical grounds.[54] Put simply, professionals have no right to expect legally competent patients to accept advice uncritically. In addition, the long-term adjustments in dietary and medication taking behaviours required of people with diabetes are not easy to make or sustain. Patients have been found to fail to comply both deliberately and accidentally, which reflects the two essential underlying problems.[55] First, patients have to believe in the value of the treatment being suggested for them as an individual. They must be 'got on board'. Second, they must be motivated to continue with both prescribed therapy and dietary measures, or 'kept on board'.

Getting the patient on board

A major shift in thinking towards 'concordance', has been advocated to induce a more constructive attitude and avoid conflict in the clinical situation.[56] This is often misunderstood to be a new word for compliance, but the definition currently offered[57] indicates the radical nature of the concept:

'The clinical encounter is concerned with two sets of contrasted but equally cogent health beliefs – that of the patient and that of the prescriber. The task of the patient is to convey his or her health beliefs to the prescriber; and that of the prescriber, to enable this to happen. The task of the prescriber is to convey his or her (professionally informed) health beliefs to the patient and of the patient to entertain these. The intention is to assist the patient to make as informed a choice as possible about the diagnosis and treatment, about benefit and risk and to take full part in a therapeutic alliance. Although reciprocal, this is an alliance in which the most important determinations are agreed to be those that are made by the patient.'[57]

Previous attempts to improve treatment use have been, at best, only partially successful and the social science literature is beginning to explain why.[58,59] It appears that patients often struggle to come to terms with their illness, commonly without medical help, and may not come to fully believe in the rationale for treatment. This may be compounded by a clinical relationship and process that gives little attention to the patient's own priorities, a point perhaps illustrated by the relatively scant attention given to quality of life measures and patient preferences in publications based on the UKPDS.[60]

There are a number of psychological models to explain why patients fail to react rationally to health threats, why adjustment is difficult and why they may not consider it worthwhile.[55] The most all-encompassing model, Leventhal's self-regulatory model, is one of the few to explicitly include this emotional component, but it does not translate simply into a clinical approach (Fig. 10.6). This model

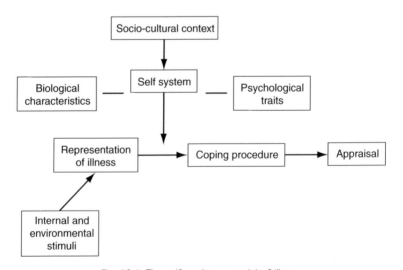

Fig. 10.6 *The self-regulatory model of illness*

conceptualizes the individual as an active problem solver whose behaviour reflects an attempt to close the gap between actual and ideal health status. Patients are considered to respond to illness in a dynamic way based upon their interpretation and evaluation of the illness and the perceived outcome of coping strategies. It contains three main stages:

1. The patient identifies the meaning of the health threat (representation) based upon concrete signs and symptoms as well as beliefs about the consequences and duration of the event.
2. The patient develops and implements an action plan or coping strategy.
3. The outcome of the action is appraised.

An important feature of this model is that these processes occur simultaneously at a cognitive and emotional level. In addition, there is a dynamic interaction between the three stages of meaning, coping and appraisal. Appraisal will be based upon the patient's understanding or 'representation' of the illness and coping or treatment strategies modified appropriately.[61] Likewise, their representation may change in the light of experience.

This model allows for the influence of personality, external context and experience over time (both past experience and progress with the current illness episode). It appears that there is increasing acceptance of and supporting evidence being accumulated for this model.[62]

All this suggests there is a problem with the conventional clinical relationship for at least some of these non-compliant patients.[63] This has been seen as an area of primary care expertise and there have been two trials that have attempted to introduce patient-centred approaches to address this.[64,65] Unfortunately, neither succeeded, probably because the practice nurses involved changed their approach very little.[66,67]

At present, the evidence is not clear about how poor medication use should be managed. It seems likely that convenient dosing is important and there is clear observational evidence that once or twice daily dosing is preferable to support this.[10,68] However, the research in this area remains generally problematic and there is little inconvertible evidence to help clinicians. One problem is that poor medication has been conceived as a single problem, whereas it increasingly seems a multi-factorial and highly individualized problem. The tailored responses that practitioners have been employing on an empirical basis for years are, however, extremely difficult to research.

The process of seeking concordance may be seen as a way of managing the legitimate differences in views between health care professionals and patients. At present there are a number of suggestions about how this may this be achieved, largely based on evidence regarding the effectiveness of communication in terms of clinical outcome or patient satisfaction.[58,69–72] There is currently no direct evidence that this approach improves treatment use, although some small studies have indicated that encouraging patients to be more active during consultations is effective.[73]

Consultation models will no doubt be developed and refined over the coming years to help define appropriate ways of managing patients for whom conventional care process is ineffective. The therapeutic alliance model (Fig. 10.7) was developed in the primary care setting for use with poorly controlled, non-compliant patients and reflects a complex consultation process.[74] Essentially, the task, when seeking concordance, is to explore patients' beliefs about their illness and treatment, partly in order to foster an empathic relationship. Information provision is then tailored to ensuring patients appreciate any necessary additional details, risks or options before discrepancies in the patient's situation are highlighted and they are helped to choose a response. Treatment goals are established for both parties before management is agreed and concordance has not been achieved if significant disparity exists between the two parties' views of the problem, treatment goals or solution. Where this occurs, the patient's view takes priority unless they are not competent to do so.

Unfortunately, there is also evidence that some patients may prefer and benefit from a directive consultation style.[75,76] This factor, along with the relatively brief training given to the practice nurses involved,

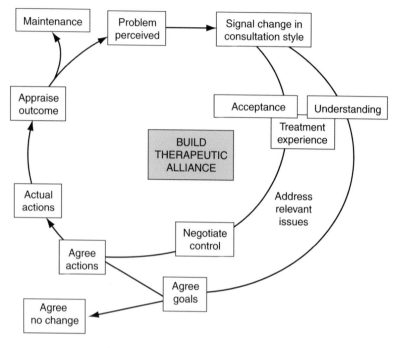

Fig. 10.7 *The therapeutic alliance model*

may account for the failure of existing trials of patient-centred diabetic care to produce significant improvements in care.[66] In contrast, the success of the intensive arm of the UKPDS and other pharmacy based interventions in the USA suggests there is merit in exploring the value of directive consultations, at least for selected patients.[77]

The skills required to develop a concordant approach are likely to need refining into a short consultation process that can match care to patients' needs more closely. If this is not done, the issue of non-compliance will remain, as patients will always be free to accept or reject advice as they wish.

Keeping patients on board

Assuming a diabetic arteriopathic patient does believe in the clinical goals they must still sustain rigorous attention to what they eat and

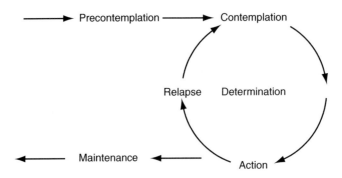

Fig. 10.8 *The transtheoretical model of change*

to what are frequently complex treatment regimes. A second major issue must also be considered—motivating patients to manage the necessary changes adequately. The difficulty lies in distinguishing which patients are in this category and which are simply reluctant to voice their loss of confidence in their care package. Poorly motivated patients may be managed by reducing barriers to compliance or increasing their motivation to overcome them. This is similar to any other behaviour change and may be considered in terms of the transtheoretical model (Fig. 10.8), which suggests there are six stages in the process of changing behaviour.[78]

It follows from this model that individuals require different support at different stages to promote change. Someone contemplating a change will need information and time to discuss their options, whereas someone who has recently changed their behaviour may need assistance with motivation to maintain that change. This mechanism forms the basis for therapeutic interventions such as motivational interviewing which attempt to highlight and reduce 'ambivalence' about change.[79,80] It is supported by evidence that an individual's stage in the model is strongly predictive of short term actions such as smoking cessation or exercise increase[81,82] (see Chapter 9).

Barriers such as practical difficulties managing treatment or ignorance of dietary matters can usually be rectified providing adequate motivation exists. When it does not, strategies for developing motivation, such as brief motivational interviewing, are likely to be more use than patient education.[83] This approach closely accords with the ethos of concordance and may become part of this process.

One concern is that consultations including such counselling require additional time. However, practitioners are used to organizing extended or repeated consultations when required for minor surgery or conditions such as depression. It is likely, therefore, that a proven strategy could be introduced into practice, but this should only be done once it has been shown it is an effective use of time.

Identifying barriers to care

Failure to achieve an optimal care package for an individual may be due to professional or patient factors. It may be helpful to break these down into the constituent aspects of performance—knowledge, attitude and skills (Table 10.7). All of these must be in place to achieve adequate performance. However, they obviously operate at different levels for professionals and patients. The process of defining and monitoring acceptable care is currently a sensitive professional issue. There are two main options: by process or by outcome. These serve different purposes and are probably both necessary to ensure that optimal care is sustained.

Conclusions

It is clear that optimal diabetic and vascular care cannot be achieved using the existing approach. Poor compliance remains a major reason for this, but more detailed understanding of patients' views and a new professional approach offer the potential to improve this. It is likely that significant refinements will be added to existing ideas about how non-compliant patients should be managed in the next few years. However, these have not yet been fully developed or evaluated.

Table 10.7 Barriers to care

	Professional	Patients
Knowledge	Needs to know enough of the evidence to give appropriate advice	Need to understand enough about their disease and its management to select and apply management plan
Attitude	Needs to care about maintaining skills and knowledge, must recognize patient's role and importance of organizing care systematically	Need to make a constructive adjustment to their condition and be willing to develop effective relationships with health care professionals
Skills	Must be able to listen to, inform and empower patients Requires adequate clinical diagnostic skills	Must be able to communicate with health care professionals Must be able to manage medicines and diet adequately
Performance	Good performance requires regular review of the process and outcome	Good performance requires daily commitment to treatment plan and a willingness to work openly with carers

Acknowledgements

The help and guidance of Dr Sue Penfold, from The Ladywood Primary Care Group, Birmingham, in the drafting of the section entitled The Ladywood Community Diabetes Service, is acknowledged with thanks.

References

1. Amos AF, McCarty DJ, Zimmet P. The rising global burden of diabetes and its complications: estimates and projections to the year 2010. Diabet Med 1997;14 (Suppl 5): S1–85.
2. Harris MI, Flegal KM, Cowie CC et al. Prevalence of diabetes, impaired fasting glucose and impaired glucose tolerance in US adults. The third national health and nutrition examination survey, 1988–1994. Diabetes Care 1998;21:518–25.
3. Bottomley J, Baxter H, Lawlar D et al. CODE-2 UK: the current costs of type 2 diabetes in the UK. Value Health 1999;5:396.
4. DCCT research group. The effect of intensive treatment of diabetes on the development and progression of long-term complications in insulin-dependent diabetes mellitus. N Engl J Med 1989;329:977–86.
5. UK Prospective Diabetes Study (UKPDS) group. Intensive blood glucose control with sulphonylureas or insulin compared with conventional treatment and the risk of complications in patients with type 2 diabetes (UKPDS 33). Lancet 1998;352:837–53.
6. UK Prospective Diabetes Study (UKPDS) group. Glycemic control with diet, sulphonylurea, metformin or insulin in patients with type 2 diabetes mellitus. Progressive requirement for multiple therapies (UKPDS 49). JAMA 1999;281:2005–12.
7. Heart Outcomes Prevention Evaluation (HOPE) study investigators. Effects of an angiotensin-converting-enzyme inhibitor, ramipril, on cardiovascular events in high risk patients. N Engl J Med 2000;342:145–53.
8. Heart Outcomes Prevention Evaluation (HOPE) study investigators. Effects of ramipril on cardiovascular and microvascular outcomes in people with diabetes mellitus: results of the HOPE study and MICRO-HOPE substudy. Lancet 2000;355:253–9.
9. Morris AD, Boyle DIR, McMahon AD et al. Adherence to insulin treatment, glycaemic control and ketoacidosis in insulin dependent diabetes mellitus. Lancet 1997;350:1505–10.

10. Dannan PT, MacDonald TM, Morris AD, for the DARTS/MEMO Collaberation. Adherence to prescribed oral hypoglycaemic medication in a population of patients with type 2 diabetes: a retrospective cohort study. Diabet Med 2002;19:279–84.

11. Hart JT. Rule of halves: implications of increasing diagnosis and reducing dropout for future workload and prescribing costs in primary care. Br J Gen Pract 1992;42:116–19.

12. Alberti KGMM, Zimmet PZ for the WHO consultation. Definition, diagnosis and classification of diabetes mellitus and its complications. Part 1: diagnosis and classification of diabetes mellitus. Provisional report of a WHO consultation. Diabet Med 1998;15:539–53.

13. UK Prospective Diabetes Study Group. Cost effectiveness analysis of improved blood pressure control in hypertensive patients with type 2 diabetes: UKPDS 40. BMJ 1998;317:720–6.

14. Evans JMM, Newton RW, Ruta DA et al. Frequency of blood glucose monitoring in relation to glycaemic control: observational study with diabetes database. BMJ 1999;319:83–6.

15. Goyder EC, McNally P, Drucquer M et al. Shifting of care for diabetes from secondary to primary care, 1990–5: review of general practices. BMJ 1998;316:1505–506.

16. Kinmonth A. Diabetic care in General Practice. BMJ 1993;306:599–600.

17. UK Prospective Diabetes Study Group: UKPDS VIII. Study design, progress and performance. Diabetologia 1991;34:877–90.

18. Goyder E, Irwig L. Screening for diabetes: what are we really doing? BMJ 1998;317:1644–6.

19. Worrall G. Screening healthy people for diabetes: is it worthwhile? J Fam Pract 1991;33:155–60.

20. New Zealand Society for the Study of Diabetes. Screening for diabetes in asymptomatic individuals. NZ Med J 1995;108:464–5.

21. Koskinen P, Manttari M, Manninen V et al. Coronary heart disease incidence in NIDDM patients in the Helsinki heart study. Diabetes Care 1992;15:820–5.

22. Davies M, Day J. Screening for non-insulin-dependent diabetes mellitus (NIDDM): how often should it be performed? J Med Screening 1994;1:78–81.

23. Davies M, Alban-Davies H, Cook C, Day J. Self testing for diabetes mellitus. BMJ 1991;303:696–8.

24. Harris MI. Undiagnosed NIDDM: clinical and public health issues. Diabetes Care 1993;16:642–52.

25. Greenhalgh PM. Shared care for diabetes: a systematic review. Occasional paper 67. Royal College of General Practitioners, London, 1994.

26. Griffin S. Diabetes care in general practice: meta-analysis of randomised control trials. BMJ 1998;317:390–5.

27. Hurwitz B, Goodman C, Yudkin J. Prompting the clinical care of non-insulin dependent (type II) diabetic patients in an inner city area: one model of community care. BMJ 1993;306:624–30.

28. Diabetes Integrated Care Evaluation Team. Integrated care for diabetes: clinical, psychosocial, and economic evaluation. BMJ 1994;308:1208–12.

29. UK Prospective Diabetes Study Group. Efficacy of atenolol and captopril in reducing risk of macrovascular and microvascular complications in type 2 diabetes: UKPDS 39. BMJ 1998;317:713–20.

30. UK Prospective Diabetes Study Group. Tight blood pressure control and risk of macrovascular and microvascular complications in type 2 diabetes: UKPDS 38. BMJ 1998;317:703–13.

31. Boyle DIR, McMahon AD, Newton RW et al. Missed opportunities for secondary prevention of coronary disease in diabetes. Diabet Med 1998;15(Suppl 1):S57.

32. Klein R, Moss SE, Klein BEK, DeMets DL. Relation of ocular and systemic factors to survival in diabetes. Arch Intern Med 1989;149:266–72.

33. Moy CS, LaPorte RE, Dorman JS et al. Insulin-dependent diabetes mellitus mortality. The risk of cigarette smoking. Circulation 1990;82:37–43.

34. Ford ES, DeStefano F. Risk factors for mortality from all causes and from coronary heart disease among persons with diabetes. Findings from the National Health and Nutrition Examination Survey 1. Epidemiological follow-up study. Am J Epidemiol 1991;133:1220–30.

35. Stamler J, Vaccaro O, Neaton JD, Wentworth D. Diabetes, other risk factors, and 12-yr cardiovascular mortality for men screened in the multiple risk factor intervention trial. Diabetes Care 1993;16:434–44.

36. West R, McNeill A, Raw M. Smoking cessation guidelines for health professionals: an update. Thorax 2000;55:987–99.

37. Wood D, Durrington P, Poulter N et al. Joint British recommendations on prevention of coronary heart disease in clinical practice. Heart 1998;80(Suppl):S1–29.

38. Brennan G, Devers M, Boyle DIR et al. Implications of cholesterol management guidelines for diabetes: a population based study. Diabetologia 1999;42:16.

39. Thorn PA, Russell RG. Diabetic clinics today and tomorrow: mini-clinics in general practice. BMJ 1973;2:534–6.

40. Wood J. A review of diabetes care initiatives in primary care settings. Health Trends 1990;22:39–43.

41. Sullivan FM, Stearn R, MacCuish A. The role of general practitioners in diabetic eye care in Lanarkshire. Diabet Med 1994;11:583–5.

42. Hayes TM, Harries J. Randomised controlled trial of routine hospital clinic care versus routine general practice care for type II diabetics. BMJ 1984;289:728–73.

43. Hoskins PL, Fowler PM, Constantino M et al. Sharing the care of diabetic patients between hospital and general practitioners: does it work? Diabet Med 1993;10:81–6.

44. Scottish Intercollegiate Guidelines Network (SIGN) website: http://*www.sign.ac.uk.*

45. Management of diabetic cardiovascular disease: SIGN 19. Scottish Intercollegiate Guidelines Network, 1997.
46. Department of Health website: http://*www.doh.gov.uk/nsf/diabetes.htm.*
47. Royal College of General Practitioners (Scotland). Scottish Programme for implementation of Clinical Effectiveness in Primary Care (SPICE pc), 1999.
48. Morris AD, Boyle DIR, MacAlpine R et al. The diabetes audit and research in Tayside Scotland (DARTS) study: electronic record linkage to create a diabetes register. BMJ 1997;315:524–8.
49. Tayside Regional Diabetes Network website: http://*www.diabetes-health-net.ac.uk.*
50. Testing Times – a review of diabetes services in England and Wales. The Audit Commission 2000.
51. Myers L, Midence K. Adherence to Treatment in Medical Conditions. Overseas Publishers Association, Amsterdam, 1998.
52. Meichenbaum D, Turk D. Facilitating Treatment Adherence. Plenum, New York, 1987.
53. Sackett D, Haynes RB. Compliance and Therapeutic Regimens. John Hopkins United Press, London, 1976.
54. General Medical Council. Seeking patients' consent: the ethical considerations. General Medical Council, 1998.
55. Myers L, Midence K. Concepts and issues in adherance. In: Myers L, Midence K, eds. Adherence to Treatment in Medical Conditions, Harwood, London, 1998.
56. Blenkinsopp A, Bond C, Britten N et al. From compliance to concordance: achieving shared goals in medicine taking. Royal Pharmaceutical Society of Great Britain 1997; Merck Sharp and Dohme.
57. The 'Medicines Partnership' website: http://*www.concordance.org.*
58. Stewart M, McWhinney I, Buck C. The doctor/patient relationship and its effect upon outcome. J R Coll Gen Pract 1979;29:77–82.
59. Haynes RB, McKibbon KA, Kanani R. Systematic review of randomised trials of interventions to assist patients to follow prescriptions for medications. Lancet 1996;348:383–6.
60. UK Prospective Diabetes Study Group. Quality of life in type 2 diabetic patients is affected by complications but not by intensive policies to improve blood glucose or blood pressure control: UKPDS 37. Diabetes Care 1999;22:1125–36.
61. Nerenz DR, Leventhal H. Self-regulation theory in chronic illness. In: Weibe D, ed. Coping with Chronic Disease. Academic Press, 1983:13–37.
62. McGavock H, Britten N. A Review of the Literature on Drug Adherence. Royal Pharmaceutical Society, 1996 .
63. Horne R, Weinman J. Illness cognitions: implications for the treatment of renal disease. In: McGee HM, Bradley C, eds. Quality of Life Following Renal Failure. Harwood Academic Publishers, 2000:113–32.

64. Kinmonth AL, Woodcock A, Griffith S et al. Randomised controlled trial of patient centred care of diabetes in general practice: impact on current well being and future disease risk. BMJ 1998;317:1202–208.

65. Pill R, Stott N, Rollnick S, Rees M. A randomised controlled trial of an intervention designed to improve the care given in general practice to Type II diabetic patients: patient outcomes and professional ability to change behaviour. Fam Pract 1998;15:229–35.

66. Pill R, Rees ME, Stott NC, Rollnick SR. Can nurses learn to let go? Issues arising from an intervention designed to improve patients' involvement in their own care. J Adv Nurs 1999;29:1492–9.

67. Stott NC, Rees M, Rollnick S et al. Professional responses to innovation in clinical method: diabetes care and negotiating skills. Patient Educ Couns 1996;29:67–73.

68. Greenberg RN. Overview of patient compliance with medication dosing: a literature review. Clin Ther 1984;6:592–9.

69. Williams S, Weinman J, Dale J. Doctor–patient communication and patient satisfaction: a review. Fam Pract 1998;15:480–92.

70. Stewart M, Roter D. Communicating with Medical Patients. Sage Publications, Thousand Oaks, 1989.

71. Stewart MA. Effective physician–patient communication and health outcomes: a review. Can Med Assoc J 1995;152:1423–33.

72. Stewart M, Belle Brown J, Weston WW et al. Patient-centred Medicine: Transforming the Clinical Method. Sage Publications, Thousand Oaks, 1995.

73. Greenfield S, Kaplan S, Ware J et al. Patients' participation in medical care: effects on blood sugar control and quality of life in diabetes. J Gen Intern Med 1988;3:448–57.

74. Dowell J, Jones A. Achieving concordance in practice (abstract). Drug Utilisation Research Group, Annual Scientific Meeting, 1998, London.

75. Thomas KB. General practice consultations: is there any point in being positive? BMJ 1987;294:1200–202.

76. Thomas KB. The consultation and the therapeutic illusion. BMJ 1978;1:1327–8.

77. Sclar DA, Skaer TL. Effect of medication utilization review on Medicaid health care expenditures: a case study of patients with non-insulin-dependent diabetes mellitus. J Res Pharmaceut Econ 1991;3:75–89.

78. Prochaska JO, DiClemente CC. Stages and process of self-change of smoking: toward an integrative model of change. J Consult Clin Psychol 1983;51:390–5.

79. Butler C, Rollnick S, Stott N. The practitioner, the patient and resistance to change: recent ideas on compliance. Can Med Assoc J 1998;154:1357–421.

80. Rollnick S, Miller WR. What is motivational interviewing? Behav Cognit Psychother 1995;23:325–34.

81. DiClemente CC, Prochaska JO, Fairhurst SK et al. The process of smoking cessation: an analysis of precontemplation, contemplation, and preparation stages of change. J Consult Clin Psychol 1991;59:295–304.
82. Cardinal BJ. The stages of exercise scale and stages of exercise behaviour in female adults. J Sports Med Phys Fitness 1995;35:87–92.
83. Rollnick S, Heather N, Bell A. Negotiating behaviour change in medical settings: the development of brief motivational interviewing. J Ment Health 1992;1:25–37.

Index

Note: References to figures are indicated by 'f' and references to tables are indicated by 't' when they fall on a page not covered by the text reference.

SAVE study (captopril) 202–203
Scottish Intercollegiate Guidelines
    Network (SIGN), guidelines for
    diabetes care 292, 293t
screening for diabetes 285–286
sensory innervation of heart, and silent
    myocardial ischaemia 74–75
SHEP study, antihypertensive treatment
    142, 143, 144
silent myocardial ischaemia (SMI)
    and autonomic neuropathy
        angina perceptual threshold 74–75,
        77–78
        circadian rhythms 80
        noradrenaline uptake measurement
        78–79
        peripheral neuropathy 72
        prevalence of SMI 73
        subclinical neuropathy 75–77
    and clinical practice 87–88
    community-based studies 70–72
    history 65–67
    hospital-based studies 67–70
    prognostic significance of 80–87
simvastatin
    coronary heart disease outcomes 112,
        177, 178t, 179
    prescribing 188
sinus arrhythmia, abnormalities in
    autonomic neuropathy 46
smoking, and cardiovascular disease
    risk 289–290
SOLVD trial (enalapril) 111,
    201–202
SPICE PC audit criteria, for type 2
    diabetes 294, 296
spironolactone, secondary prevention of
    CHD 203
ST segment depression, and silent
    myocardial ischaemia 65–67
statins
    adverse effects 190
    after percutaneous coronary
        interventions 230–231
    coronary heart disease outcomes 179
        primary prevention studies 176, 177t
        secondary prevention studies 112,
        177–178
    drug interactions 189
    mechanism of action 186–187
    prescribing 187–188
Steno study
    cardiovascular disease outcomes
        159–160

glycaemic control, and cardiovascular
    disease risk 128–129
stenting, and restenosis 229–230
Stockholm Diabetes Intervention study,
    glycaemic control, and
    cardiovascular disease risk 125
STOP-2 study, antihypertensive
    treatment 142, 145, 150
STOP study, antihypertensive treatment
    142, 143
structured care 286–290
sudden and unexpected death see
    unexplained death
sulphonylureas
    and cardiovascular disease risk
        126–127, 129–131
    and percutaneous coronary
        interventions 231–233
    treatment risks 207
sympathovagal balance, autonomic
    neuropathy assessment 47–52
syndrome X, insulin resistance in
    and cardiovascular disease risk 6–8
    characteristics of 2–3
    and dyslipidaemia 13–14
    evolutionary role 5, 6f
    and free fatty acid metabolism 15–17
    and hypertension 11–13
    measurement of 3–4
    and metabolic control mechanisms
        4–5
    and pathogenesis of type 2 diabetes
        8–11
    and sedentary lifestyle 14–15
Syst-Eur study, antihypertensive
    treatment 142, 149–150

TAMI study group, thrombolysis, and
    myocardial infarction 101
Tayside Regional Diabetes Network,
    integrated care model 294, 296–299
telmisartan, ONTARGET study 205
therapeutic alliance model, in primary
    care 306–307
thrombolytic therapy, for myocardial
    infarction 100–102
timolol, secondary prevention of
    myocardial infarction 109–110,
    199–200
tolbutamide
    and cardiovascular disease risk
        126–127
    treatment risks 207
TRACE study (trandolapril) 202–203

training and education in diabetes care
291–292, 293t
trandolapril, secondary prevention of
myocardial infarction 202–203
type 1 diabetes
antihypertensive treatment 155–156
cardiovascular disease risk
and glucose levels 124–125
and glycaemic control 125–126
and plasma lipid levels 174–175
hypertension in, epidemiology
132–133
type 2 diabetes
antihypertensive treatment 156–160
cardiovascular disease risk
and glucose levels 123–124
and glycaemic control 126–131
and insulin resistance 6–8
and plasma lipid levels 174, 175
coagulation/fibrinolysis abnormalities
23–24
hypertension in, epidemiology
133–135
insulin resistance *see* insulin
resistance
pathogenesis 8–11
and physical activity *see* physical
activity
platelet abnormalities 24–25
vascular endothelial dysfunction *see*
vascular endothelial dysfunction

unexplained death, and autonomic
neuropathy 38–39
QT interval prolongation 41–43

therapeutic interventions 54–55, 56t
United Kingdom Prospective Diabetes
Study (UKPDS)
antihypertensive treatment 158–159
cardiovascular disease risk
and glycaemic control 129–131
and hypertension 133–135
University Group Diabetes Program
(UGDP), glycaemic control, and
cardiovascular disease risk 126–127
unstable angina 113–114

VA-HIT study, coronary heart disease
outcomes 112, 178t, 179, 179–180
Valsalva manoeuvre, autonomic
neuropathy assessment 43–45
vascular endothelial dysfunction
and hyperglycaemia 21–23
and inflammatory processes 25
and insulin resistance 19–21
blood pressure changes 12–13
free fatty acid effects 16–17
role of nitric oxide 17–19
VLDL (very low density lipoproteins)
properties of 172t, 173
see also plasma lipids
von Willebrand factor, and insulin
resistance 23–24

Western lifestyle, and insulin resistance
14–15
WOSCOPS study (pravastatin) 176, 177t,
179

Zocor *see* simvastatin